"Joanna [...] guide lights the
way for p[...] [t]wenty years as a
pediatric [...] [s]te, Ms. Breyer
describes the many situations such a parent might face and considers the various ways a parent might respond to a child's illness. In so doing, she provides
comfort during a confusing, shocking, and despairing time. Joanna Breyer's
counsel for parents who have lost a child—that the death of a child is nearly
unbearable, but that they will survive and emerge stronger—is exactly on
point, as I know all too well. This is a handbook for life events we don't ever
want to consider. I am grateful that Joanna Breyer has considered them so
thoughtfully.""

— Nancy Goodman, founder and executive director, Kids v Cancer

"Based on her extensive experience helping children with cancer and serious
illnesses and their families, Dr. Breyer has written this comprehensive, innovative, and useful book. She describes, in detail, the trajectory of serious illness in children and the stressors that they and their families face. Using
examples from her own practice as well as from others' clinical and research
work, Dr. Breyer provides a wealth of practical and effective strategies to help
them cope during and after treatment and when treatment fails. Not a "one-
size-fits-all" approach, she emphasizes the role of individual differences,
experiences, styles, personalities, and preferences. In addition, there is a listing of various resources to help parents navigate treatment and living with
childhood cancer. When a child is diagnosed with a serious medical condition,
parents often tell us that there is no roadmap or guidebook to tell them what
to expect and how best to help their child—this is that book."

— Mary Jo Kupst, Ph.D., emerita professor of pediatrics, Medical
    College of Wisconsin

"Joanna Breyer balances profound compassion with pragmatism to provide an
extraordinarily valuable guide to the management and care of sick children.
By using real examples and clinical vignettes, Breyer pierces through some the
most difficult barriers in medicine, and helps us navigate through complex
and forbidding landscapes. Written in the spirit of Jimmie Holland, the pioneering psychiatrist who studied the minds of cancer patients, Breyer's book
focuses its attention on children with cancer and other illnesses. This book
should be compulsory reading for anyone facing these terrifying conundrums
and life-altering decisions."

— Siddhartha Mukherjee, author of *The Emperor of All Maladies: A
    Biography of Cancer,* winner of the 2011 Pulitzer Prize in general
    nonfiction, and *The Laws of Medicine,* assistant professor of medicine
    at Columbia University

"*When Your Child Is Sick* is a wonder. Though I've known and admired Dr. Breyer throughout her tenure at Dana-Farber/Boston Children's, I stand in awe at how comprehensive this book is in guiding parents through maintaining confidence and alleviating fear during what can be an extremely challenging experience. Breyer is a former senior member of a team of experts that has vast experience with helping families trapped in the crisis of profound childhood illness. A great clinician, she is above all an inspired teacher who provides a treasure trove of advice for those facing the greatest fear parents have—that of losing a child."
>   —David G. Nathan, president emeritus, Dana-Farber Cancer Institute,
>   physician-in-chief emeritus, Boston Children's Hospital, Robert A.
>   Stranahan Distinguished Professor of Pediatrics, Harvard Medical
>   School

"This is definitely the book to read if you have a sick child. The author helps families navigate the complex course of pediatric illness by describing evidence-based psychological interventions that alleviate suffering in the patient and his family. This book is also an excellent guide for pediatric medical staff, who will learn working tools that improve the quality of their work and the quality of their patients' lives. I recommend it without hesitation and wish I'd had it earlier in my professional career."
>   —Maria Die Trill, Ph.D., president, International Psycho-Oncology Society

When Your Child Is Sick

A GUIDE TO NAVIGATING

the Practical and Emotional Challenges

of Caring for a Child Who Is Very Ill

Joanna Breyer, PhD

A TarcherPerigee Book

tarcherperigee

An imprint of Penguin Random House LLC
375 Hudson Street
New York, New York 10014

Most TarcherPerigee books are available at special quantity discounts for bulk purchase for sales promotions, premiums, fund-raising, and educational needs. Special books or book excerpts also can be created to fit specific needs.
For details, write: SpecialMarkets@penguinrandomhouse.com.

LIBRARY OF CONGRESS CATALOGING-IN-PUBLICATION DATA

Names: Breyer, Joanna.
Title: When your child is sick : a guide to navigating the practical and emotional challenges of caring for a child who is very ill / Joanna Breyer, PhD.
Description: New York, New York : A Tarcher Perigee Book, [2018] | Identifiers: LCCN 2018013195 (print) | LCCN 2018013240 (ebook) | ISBN 9780698407008 (e-book) | ISBN 9780147517586 (paperback)
Subjects: LCSH: Sick children—Care. | Children—Diseases. | Parent and child—Psychological aspects. | BISAC: HEALTH & FITNESS / Diseases / Cancer. | HEALTH & FITNESS / Diseases / General.
Classification: LCC RJ61 (ebook) | LCC RJ61 .B818 2018 (print) | DDC 618.92—dc23
LC record available at https://lccn.loc.gov/2018013195

Printed in the United States of America
1 3 5 7 9 10 8 6 4 2

Book design by Sabrina Bowers

This book is dedicated to
the many extraordinary children and families
I have worked with over the years
who taught me more than I can say about
love, death, healing, and resilience.

Contents

· · · · · · · · ·

PART III
WHEN YOUR CHILD'S TREATMENT DOES NOT WORK

Introduction

This book is for parents of children who have medical conditions requiring hospitalization and lengthy treatments. You are facing an unexpected, enormously upsetting, and unwelcome challenge. Having a child in the hospital repeatedly or over time is emotionally draining and disruptive to family life, not to mention hard in many practical ways. How your children, ill and healthy, react to the hospitalization may also cause you stress and worry. My hope is that this book will offer advice to help you and your children through this difficult experience.

I had the privilege of working as a psychologist for twenty-five years at Children's Hospital Boston and in several outpatient clinics at the Dana-Farber Cancer Institute. I counseled children and adolescents who had cancer, as well as their families. Over the years, I got to know many children and families in the most trying circumstances. I often marveled at the parents' strength as their child's treatments progressed and at the children's resilience as they flourished, despite their illness. I learned how different children are and that what helps one child might not help another. I appreciated the younger children who sometimes protested loudest at what they were expected to endure, and I worked with their parents to discover which simple tools and interventions could transform their understandable outrage and opposition into cooperation, mastery, and pride. I came to admire the adolescents whose lives were so dramatically upset by their illness and treatments and wondered at the range of their responses. I also came to respect the strength and courage of parents. Although my experience was primarily in working with children with cancer and their families, I hope that much of what follows will be relevant to parents of children hospitalized for a variety of reasons, such as a sudden severe injury or chronic conditions like cystic fibrosis, sickle cell anemia, diabetes, or chronic cardiac conditions.

In the coming chapters, I will describe a range of reactions that children may have to their hospitalization and treatment and possible interventions that may be useful in your family depending on the age, character, and temperament of your child and your parental style. You, as the parent, are the expert on your child; you are with them, know them, and are best suited to communicate their emotional needs to the medical team working to help them. However, the hospital is a new world, and in this foreign context, particularly at first, you may not always feel you know what is best for your child or what he or she needs. You will likely feel tired, sad, and scared much of the time, and taking care of yourself may require a considerable effort. It may be hard to believe how such a place can quickly become familiar.

This book has three sections:

Part I makes the hospital world a little more familiar to you by describing the people you are likely to meet and what their roles are. I will outline some of the challenges you may encounter and offer some ideas that other parents have come up with for how to deal with them. I suggest ways to talk directly with your child about his condition. I describe children's and adolescents' varied reactions to the stress of hospitalization and invasive treatments and give examples of ways to help them cope with the new demands they are facing. I talk about responses your other children may have and about interventions to help them. I detail some of the challenges you, your child, and your child's siblings face if your child needs a stem cell transplant. Finally, I discuss some of the issues you and your family may face when your child returns home after a long hospitalization.

In Part II, I address issues of "survivorship" that you and your child may face after your child's treatment is completed. Because I worked for many years in a childhood cancer survivorship clinic, my emphasis in this section is on childhood cancer survivors, although much of what I discuss will be relevant to children who have lived with or are living with other serious medical conditions.

Part III is for parents whose children are not healed by their treatments whatever their initial condition—who despite everybody's best efforts, over time, quickly or slowly get worse and cannot be cured. This section acknowledges the many different styles and approaches of parents and children in this situation. I discuss ways to make direct conversations a little more bearable and ways that you can acknowledge the situation indirectly. This section encourages you to trust your instincts and find comfort in this heartbreaking situation in whatever ways you can. The final chapter describes different ways in which people grieve and ways parents have honored and remembered their child as time passes.

Other families' stories are interspersed in boxes throughout the book. Many families generously gave me permission to quote part of their stories, and some children and parents have written directly about their experiences and how they would advise other parents. In instances when I could not reach a family I have changed their stories in ways to preserve their privacy. Although your story will be different, my hope is that it will be some comfort to know ways in which others have navigated this path before you.

My expectation is that different parts of the book will be relevant at different times, and my hope is that you will use the index and detailed chapter headings to find the topic of immediate interest to you.

PART I

. . . .

On Treatment

CHAPTER 1

· · · · · · · · · · · ·

Entering the Medical World

I f your child has to go into the hospital for a serious illness or accident, do not be surprised if you feel overwhelmed. Even if you are an experienced and terrific parent and your child has entered an excellent facility, the world of the hospital is very different from your world at home, where you are in charge. The experience can take over your life. You are dealing with practical challenges and many intense emotions— not only your own but also those of your sick or injured child, your partner, other family members, and your other children. It is hardly a wonder if you feel scared and worried.

If you have other children at home, you have to figure out how they will be cared for while your time and attention is devoted to your child in the hospital. If you are working, you may need to make arrangements so you can be absent when your child needs you in the hospital or when your other children need you at home. Financial concerns may add to your worries. You will likely feel pulled in a hundred different directions. Add to that the challenge of learning about the new world you have unexpectedly entered, and it can feel absolutely crushing. Becoming familiar with this world is key.

In this chapter I will describe the roles of the different staff you will meet in the hospital and ways to communicate effectively with them. I suggest ways you can help your child and yourself get accustomed to the facility. I'll also discuss some of the practical challenges that most parents face and suggest first steps to take to handle them.

GETTING TO KNOW THE HOSPITAL STAFF

One of the first and best things you can do to understand your child's situation is to get to know the medical staff and make them your partners in helping your child.

You will be confronted by a daunting cast of characters. Following is a general description of the people you are likely to meet and their role in caring for your child:

■ The **doctors** are in charge of your child's overall medical care. You likely encountered several doctors during your child's hospital admission and diagnosis, particularly if the admission was through the emergency room. After you are admitted, each new doctor may continue to ask you very similar questions about your child's symptoms and his prior medical history. The doctors have the best intentions about clearly communicating with you, but they may be covering many patients or use medical language that can be difficult to understand. Most doctors will be happy to repeat what they said in a nonmedical way because they want you to know what is going on. Ask each doctor what his or her role is so you can understand his or her place in your child's care. In a teaching hospital, especially, the number of doctors and nurses who visit can be confusing and irritating. A teaching hospital has a hierarchy of doctors at different levels of training:

> ▶ Medical students in their early medical training
> ▶ Residents in their fourth or fifth year of training
> ▶ Fellows beginning their specialized medical training, having completed their residencies
> ▶ The attending doctor who is in charge
> ▶ Specialists who will be consulted briefly only about a particular problem

The doctors are usually on rotating schedules. Find out which doctor is your child's primary doctor, and what the possibilities of continuity of care are both during your child's hospitalization and after discharge. Tips on how to get the information you need from the doctors and nurses follow in the section "Communicating with Your Medical Team" on page 8.

■ In some hospitals a **nurse practitioner** (a nurse with several years of extra clinical training) may be the primary medical provider who oversees your child's treatment. If so, he or she will be supervised by a senior doctor.

■ **Nurses** are responsible for the ongoing care of your child. You will see much more of them than you will of the doctors. Your child's nurse will give your child his medications and do some of the more complicated regular medical care required like dressing changes or postsurgery care. Nurses can work eight-, ten-, or twelve-hour shifts depending on the hospital. Over several weeks you will meet many nurses.

Some hospitals assign primary and secondary nurses to a child's team, but many hospitals do not. Often your child (and maybe you) will have favorite nurses, and you might wish that a particular nurse could be assigned to your family each time she comes in. But that may be difficult to arrange because of conflicting considerations in assigning nurses, such as the need to balance clinical care requirements.

There may be one or two nurses you feel do not work well with your child. If your child regularly appears unhappy when that nurse comes in or if you have repeatedly found this nurse not responding to requests you have made about his or her treatment of your child, then bring up your concerns with the **nursing supervisor** or the **charge nurse,** who is the head nurse in each shift. They will try to help, probably first speaking to the nurse concerned and, if that makes no difference, seeing what flexibility in scheduling they have to ensure that nurse is not assigned to your child.

■ **Nursing assistants** may help nurses by taking temperatures and blood pressure and helping with other routine tasks like bathing.

■ **Psychosocial clinicians**, including a social worker, resource specialist, psychologist, and/or psychiatrist may be on your child's medical team or available for special consultation about the emotional aspects of your child's care. The role of each will vary somewhat from hospital to hospital, as will the extent of psychosocial support available. Services can include providing ongoing emotional support, giving valuable information on available resources, being a liaison with or member of the medical team, providing child therapy, developing a behavioral plan to gain your child's cooperation with treatment, and other specialized consultations on pressing emotional issues. In most hospitals, a psychosocial clinician, usually a **social worker**, sometimes a **psychologist**, will meet with you soon after you come to the hospital and will ask you about your family and who is available to help through this crisis. This clinician will likely ask about your and your child's most pressing needs and can give you useful information about the hospital and available resources. He or she is there to offer practical help and emotional support. You may find some of the questions repetitive, even intrusive, but the information you give him or her will allow the medical team to be more respectful and understanding of your wishes and concerns. You are likely to be asked about your religious affiliations, family values, and financial circumstances. If you let the clinician know anything in your child's history (or your own) that could make it particularly difficult for your child or you to be in the hospital, you may avoid considerable discomfort and misunderstandings with the medical team. See the box below.

IMPORTANT FAMILY HISTORIES TO SHARE WITH YOUR MEDICAL TEAM

Following are examples of information to share with your medical team so that they will have a more complete understanding of how to interact with your family:

- A parent or another close family member who has just gone through a medical trauma, so the medical team will understand your intense reaction.

- A hard family event that involved considerable conflict, such as a divorce, which could affect how family members deal with one another, so the medical team can arrange to give separate updates to different family members.

- A family member who has a particular medical or psychological problem that might affect his or her behavior in the hospital, such as depression, alcoholism, or drug use, so inpatient staff can develop a preventative plan that could save you and your child unnecessary stress. For example, security staff can be forewarned that they may be called to escort an inebriated family member off the floor.

- Siblings who have special needs of their own that may frequently require your presence, so the medical team will understand why you are not at the hospital at particular times.

The psychosocial clinician will let you know which emotional support services are available directly in the hospital and will help you find appropriate referrals for services outside of the hospital. The clinician may also have useful suggestions about how to help your other children, who are likely to have their own strong reactions to what is happening. **Remember that strong reactions are normal and that consulting a psychosocial clinician does not mean you or your child have mental health problems.** Chapter 6 outlines circumstances when meeting a psychosocial clinician makes sense.

If psychosocial staff are not part of the routine care offered at your hospital, you may need to request a consultation with a psychiatrist, a psychologist, or a social worker.

■ A **psychiatrist** is the consultant of choice when your child could be helped by antianxiety, antidepressant, or other special medications if, for example, your child is showing extreme mood swings while taking prednisone or has become completely withdrawn.

Some hospitals or outpatient clinics also have psychiatrists available to meet with parents. If you have become depressed, are acutely anxious, are having a very hard time sleeping, or are having other disturbing symptoms and might benefit from medications, ask if a psychiatrist is available. Many hospitals can provide you with an outside referral if they do not have a psychiatrist on staff.

■ A **chaplain** is available in many hospitals to visit you and your child. If the chaplain is not of your faith, often he or she will have lists of people of other religious traditions who could visit you in the hospital. Some parents appreciate a visit from the chaplain even if he is of a different faith. Many hospital chaplains are knowledgeable about different ecumenical traditions and also understand the stress that hospitalization can cause a family.

■ A **child life specialist** works in the playroom, planning and organizing age-appropriate activities for children and adolescents. He or she will often bring activities to patients in their rooms if they cannot go to the playroom. Some child life specialists will help prepare a child for a particular medical procedure or go with a child into the treatment room. Sometimes the child life specialist will also be in charge of a resource room where you can find helpful information.

■ **Cleaning staff** will clean your child's room each day, usually in the morning. They will be aware of the strict rules about hygiene that the hospital has to follow. They have been trained to be meticulous and careful. Members of a hospital's cleaning staff often work for many years in the same hospital, and many are interested in the progress of the patients whose rooms they cover.

COMMUNICATING WITH YOUR MEDICAL TEAM

Working out who to talk to about what is likely to be key to your peace of mind in the hospital. Since a doctor is in charge of your child's treatment plan, major treatment decisions will be discussed with him or her. Sometimes the initial plan will be described by the doctor with the whole medical team present. (In our hospital, this was called the "Day One Talk," with the doctor, the primary nurse, and the psychosocial clinician present.) Get a binder to organize written information you are given and to include your own notes. You may add a separate section later for home care. Don't expect to remember even half of what is discussed initially. If you write notes or record the meeting, you can go back over it later and ask your nurse or the doctor to explain something further if there are parts you do not understand.

You can include in this binder a section on key test results, including lab results. Some parents like to track the results each day, others do not—this choice will depend on your style.

In a teaching hospital, the doctors do medical rounds each day, often in the morning. The team will likely include a medical student, the resident, the fellow, the attending doctor, and either your child's current nurse or the charge nurse. The team might gather in the hallway or in your child's room but they will always wish to examine your child briefly. They will probably have questions for you about your child's condition. Make a list of questions ahead of time, because their visit may be a short one.

In a regular hospital, find out if your child's primary doctor has a particular schedule for visits and keep a record so you know when you can next expect to see him or her to ask any questions you might have.

If you find you are getting confusing or even contradictory messages about treatment plans or anything else, you have several options. You can ask for clarification at the daily rounds, you can ask your child's primary nurse, or you can ask for a team meeting to which all relevant caregivers can be invited. If your child's hospitalization is likely to last several months, requesting a weekly or bimonthly team meeting may help ensure you and all caregivers remain on the same page.

Your primary nurse and the other nurses are good sources of information—particularly about the ongoing daily medical care your child will need. Some questions you have for your nurse may be medical questions about the details of your child's treatment that the doctors went over too quickly to be grasped. Some may be more practical: What do you do when you have been ringing the call button for ten minutes and no one has arrived? What do you do when your child's infusion machine is beeping? What care can you give your child and what would the nurses like you to leave to them?

It pays to consider the timing of your questions. A nurse will have more or less time to talk with you depending on the number of patients he or she is covering, what is going on with the other patients, and where she is in her shift. The change of shift is generally not a good time to get answers to questions because the nurses are sharing information with one another to be sure there is a smooth transition of care. You can ask the nurse for a specific time to go over general questions about your child's care; evenings might well be when he or she has the most time. A nurse may also be able to communicate any concerns you have with your doctor, because she may see the doctors more frequently than you do. The nurse will also likely be the person who goes over the details you need to know about your child's care at home as your child approaches discharge.

Communication also benefits from being a two-way street. You may have a lot of questions for your doctors and nurses, but you will also have important information to give them. You, as the expert on your child, can tell them, for example, how much warning your child needs before an intrusive medical procedure or what works best to help your child calm down when upset.

IF ENGLISH IS NOT YOUR FIRST LANGUAGE

If English is not your first language, most hospitals provide access to interpreters. Depending on the language, interpreters may work for the hospital or for an outside agency. Some interpreters who deal with your family face-to-face over time can become quite involved with your family. Most hospitals will have some interpreters who belong to a separate agency and may be available on a conference call or Skype for a particular medical conference or medical update. These interpreters are less likely to get to know your family. Sometimes the interpreter will have a dialect that you find hard to understand, particularly given the complicated medical subject matter. You may then want to ask if there is another translator available whose dialect is more familiar to you. It is sometimes tempting to have a family member with some knowledge of English to act as the interpreter, but, particularly if the medical situation is complicated or uncertain, it may be preferable to have an outside professional do the translating both because you want to be sure you are clear about the medical situation and because it may be hard for the family member to deliver bad news directly.

If you have come from abroad, ask a psychosocial clinician to contact your consulate or embassy and see if there are local organizations with connections to your country that have people or resources to help you.

GETTING ACCUSTOMED TO THE HOSPITAL

A new environment is stressful in any circumstances, and far more so if you have or are a sick child. The more your child becomes familiar with different places in the hospital, the less afraid he or she will be. If your child feels too sick to walk around, you can often take her out of her room in a wheelchair or cart and show her the playroom, where she can meet other children or talk with staff. You can use the wheelchair to help her get to know the layout of the floor and to show her other places in the hospital. You can help even a very young child understand that some places in the hospital are fun, like the playroom, resource room, gift shop, or entertainment area; many places are safe, like the kitchen or cafeteria; and only a few places are scary, like the treatment room. Most children are anxious if they have to go to the treatment room. Slow breathing and other strategies discussed in chapter 8 can help your child stay calm going in to the treatment room.

A few hospitals might have single rooms for all patients, but many hospitals do not. In this case, you and your child may need to get used to one or more roommates. This can be a chance to share information and experiences with another family. It can also be challenging for everyone, depending on what is happening with the roommate or his family. A baby may cry a lot, a family may keep late hours or watch TV when you would like you and your child to be able to sleep. The other child may be seriously ill, causing you to worry about what your child is overhearing. There may be many visitors when you feel your child needs peace. Bring these concerns up with psychosocial or nursing staff and they will find a way to discuss the situation with the other family and see what compromises can be worked out. If you feel your child's health is being adversely affected and if attempts at compromise have failed, you can reasonably ask to transfer rooms. But understand that single rooms may be in short supply because they are usually assigned based on medical priorities such as infection control, immune system disorders, severity of illness, or new diagnosis.

....

PRACTICAL CHALLENGES

Practical challenges include organizing your family's lives at home and in the hospital, mobilizing helpful support, and navigating financial stressors. Your particular situation could make any one of these challenges harder.

At the Hospital

Mobilizing support

Your family, friends, and neighbors might really want to help, but do not always know how. You may have to guide them. One of the first things you can do is to create an immediate plan to cover your child in the hospital and your children at home. You likely know who in the family could come right away to offer you or your other children needed support. If grandparents live nearby, perhaps they can either stay at home with your other children or be with your sick child at the hospital so you can go home for a break. Assign someone the task of organizing and coordinating friends and neighbors to collect your other children from school or take them to after-school activities. Later, you can revise your original plan when you know better what your child will need after some days in the hospital. Neighbors and friends may offer to bring cooked meals to your home. You can also ask one or two people to organize deliveries and space them evenly; several websites have been specially designed to make this easy to do. (See the box that follows.)

If your hospital is far from your home, those still at home may need more practical help and you may need some local help at the hospital. Perhaps family or friends can look up and distribute information about useful services nearby. Your psychosocial clinician can tell you about resources available through the hospital.

How to let others know what is happening

Your family and friends are probably very concerned and want to know what is happening. Responding to many people's requests for updates creates additional stress, so outsource the job to a helpful friend or family member who can send out group emails or open a Facebook page on which regular updates are posted about your child's progress—though you may want to be careful about the privacy levels you allow. You can always review it before it is posted if you wish, but delegating these updates to a family member can take the burden off you.

WEBSITES TO ORGANIZE HELP AND TO KEEP FAMILY AND FRIENDS UPDATED

www.caringbridge.org
To start your own free, ad-free, and protected website

- To share updates on health and to keep friends and family informed

- To receive good wishes and encouragement

- To coordinate everyday help through a planner (meals, rides, etc.)

lotsahelpinghands.com
This site can be used to organize help from friends and family and for communication

- To set up a care calendar (to organize meal deliveries, rides, etc.)

- To receive good wishes

- To set up a message board on which people can communicate helpful ideas

Mealtrain.com
This is a free website that helps coordinate getting meals to a family

- Creates free meal sign-ups

- Offers sample meal plans

- Sends reminders to participants before their scheduled day

Takethemameal.com
Facilitates coordinating meals for a family

- Creates individual sign-up sheets

- Allows friends to find your schedule

- Provides suggestions on good meals to transport, and recipes

- Offers the option of buying meals to send (frozen) in almost half of the states in the United States

Managing visitors

Once friends and relatives know your child is in the hospital, you may need some help in managing how many visitors come and when. Assign someone to be the gatekeeper, who can limit the number of visitors at any one time and can tactfully keep away those whom you and your child would rather not see in this situation. That your child needs to rest, that doctors come in at unexpected times, and that the hospital room is small are among the reasons parents sometimes give for why it might not be the best time to visit. If you are far away from home, this will be less of a problem.

At Home

Your children at home

Having a brother or sister rushed to the hospital and what follows can be extremely upsetting to children of any age, but particularly to younger siblings. Initially, siblings experience major disruptions in the routine of family life. They pick up on your emotions and are probably unhappy that they are seeing less of you as you are spending time with your child at the hospital. They may worry. Try to maintain the siblings' regular routine as much as you can (e.g., keeping your children at their regular school or seeing if someone else can take them to extracurricular activities). Try to arrange for them to stay at home with your partner, a grandparent, or a close friend. If your children are young and the plan is for them to stay with a grandparent, relatives, or friends, be sure to speak regularly with them on the phone and reassure them that you will all be coming home as soon as possible. Your psychosocial clinician will tell you about resources like SuperSibs that are available for brothers and sisters. For a description of typical sibling reactions and suggestions on how to help siblings, see chapter 5.

PROGRAMS OFFERED THROUGH ALEX'S LEMONADE STAND FOUNDATION

www.alexslemonade.org/campaign/supersibs

SuperSibs Comfort and Care Program

- Free

- Provides six mailings per year of age-appropriate support materials for brothers and sisters of children who have cancer in the US, ages 4–18

- Provides tool kits and periodic mailings with parents' tips for siblings

Offers emotional support and fun activities for siblings to reassure them of their special role in what is happening in the family and gives practical advice to parents

Sib Spot

- Offers resources and activities for siblings of different ages

- Parental supervision suggested

Sibling Ambassador Program

- Offers opportunities to siblings to share their experiences and stories with others

- Can include visiting schools, speaking at events, or meeting families

Eligibility: A sibling diagnosed with cancer, being treated, or out of treatment.

Website: www.alexslemonade.org/campaign/supersibs to start a new referral

Telephone: (610) 649 3034

Fax: (610) 649 3038

Address: 111 Presidential Blvd., Suite 203, Bala Cynwyd, PA, 19004 USA

Your Children's Schools

It is important for your children's school to know what is happening right away. You can make the first call to the school principal or your hospitalized child's teacher to tell them about your child's diagnosis and initial treatment plan, but consider asking someone else to handle giving the follow-up information. While your child is in the hospital, if he feels up to it, many hospitals have a tutor available at no cost, for an hour a day three or four times a week. Sometimes your child's teachers can send materials that the hospital tutor can use. There are also many ways in which a teacher and classmates can stay in touch with your child, including sending emails or texts. Utilizing Skype can allow a child to follow what is going on in his classroom from the hospital.

Your other children's teachers also need to know what is happening. Ask your children if they want to be asked how their brother or sister is doing, then share their preferences with their teacher. Many brothers and sisters told us they felt uncomfortable and irritated at being repeatedly asked such questions, but some liked being asked. Ask teachers to contact you immediately, perhaps by email, if they have any concerns about how your other children are doing in school. Seeing changes in your other children's behavior or school performance is not unusual, but benefits from being attended to immediately if possible. Teachers' reactions can run the gamut from lowering expectations excessively to being rigid and unsympathetic. Ideally, teachers continue to have reasonable expectations with occasional modifications depending on the home situation. Designate a friend or family member to keep your other children's teachers updated.

Financial Hardship

Unfortunately, in addition to the enormous stress you are already under, having a sick child can be very expensive. Even if you have health insurance, your expenses are likely to rise and your income to fall—in many cases dramatically. There are many out-of-pocket expenses related to your child's care that are not covered by health insurance, including meals for caregivers during long hospital stays and frequent clinic visits, co-payments, and deductibles, as well as travel and child care expenses. At the same time, many families experience a loss of income when parents must reduce their work schedule, take an unpaid leave, or even give up their job due to their child's illness and the care required. A social worker or a resource specialist is a good person with whom to raise any initial financial concerns that you may have.

IF YOU DO NOT HAVE INSURANCE

Few hospitals provide free care for families with no insurance, although immediate emergency care will be given. St. Jude Children's Research Hospital in Memphis, Tennessee, is an exception. No child will be denied treatment there because of a family's inability to pay. Generally, hospitals throughout the country are tightening their rules and are reluctant to start an experimental course of treatment like some stem cell transplants until they know the family has or will be getting insurance to cover most of the expense. If your child does not have health insurance, work with the financial staff at your hospital to apply for insurance coverage as quickly as possible.

IF YOU DO HAVE INSURANCE

If you do have insurance, you should call your insurance company as soon as possible and let them know that your child is ill. When you call, ask to speak with member services and be sure to ask the following questions:

- Is [name of hospital where you are seeking treatment for your child] in my plan's network?

- Am I eligible to have a case manager?

- What is my coverage for inpatient care?

- Are referrals or authorizations required for outpatient services?

- What is my coverage for prescription medications?

- How much are my co-payments and deductibles?

- Am I eligible for home care benefits?

Many pediatric patients who are covered by a parent's private health insurance plan are eligible for supplementary coverage through Medicaid. The benefits of obtaining supplemental insurance through Medicaid can be significant. The supplemental coverage often covers co-payments and deductibles required by the patient's primary insurance. And in many states, through a program called Premium Assistance, the parent who carries the private health insurance is eligible to receive reimbursement for the private health insurance premiums he or she pays. Unfortunately, many eligible patient families fail to access support from these two important programs because they never find out about them. (Note: While eligibility for Medicaid and Premium Assistance varies by state, the majority of states do offer these programs; families should be sure to ask the social worker or resource specialist about them and explore their eligibility.)

What You Can Do

Over the years I spent working with families, many shared the financial strains and hardships caused directly or indirectly by having a sick child. But it is only recently that investigators have focused on the many ways in which this can occur. Now many studies have documented substantial work disruptions, income loss, and material hardships (food, energy, or housing challenges), and some associated negative psychological impacts in families with a child with cancer.[1]

Other recent studies have found an association between poverty and some health outcomes in children with leukemia.[2] Although not everyone is affected to the same degree, significant and unanticipated material financial hardship can occur in families at all income levels.

As these results have been coming in, medical caregivers have become increasingly concerned about the related adverse effects and have begun to try to assess whether financial or material hardships exist in the family of a patient and to ameliorate them where possible. The growing evidence has led some caregivers to propose that psychosocial standards of care in pediatric oncology should include a routine assessment of risk for financial hardship at your child's diagnosis and at various times during treatment. Risk factors for financial hardship include current low income or financial hardship, being a single parent, living a long way from your child's treatment center, anticipating a long or difficult course of treatment, or having a job that is insecure or inflexible. So if you are in or find yourself moving into any one of these categories or even if there is a remote likelihood that you could down the road, what can you do?

1. Ask to meet with a resource specialist or social worker at your child's hospital immediately. He or she should be able to help you access concrete resource support such as assistance with parking fees, utility bill payments, or grocery cards. Many families are eligible for assistance from federal or state programs and/or philanthropic foundations or societies. Some funds are available based on the child's particular conditions—for example, from the Pediatric Brain Tumor Foundation, the Jeffrey Modell Foundation (for immune deficiency disorders), or the Wiskott-Aldrich Foundation (for Wiskott-Aldrich syndrome). Others have somewhat broader eligibility criteria such as the National Children's Cancer Society, the Bone Marrow Foundation, or the Family Reach Foundation. Others are more need-based than condition-related, such as the Patient Advocate Foundation, the National Patient Travel Center, or Next Step, or government-funded programs such as Medicaid, Supplemental Security Income (SSI), and the Women, Infants, and Children program (WIC). Please note that the availability of funds at philanthropic foundations as well as their eligibility guidelines varies widely, so the guidance of a knowledgeable resource specialist or social worker can be a tremendous help. (See Appendices A and B.)

2. If you are a single parent, ask the hospital staff if they have funds available specifically for those without partners.

3. Your resource specialist/social worker may also have access to hospital donor funds that are specifically earmarked for resource assistance. Hospitals that do provide this assistance are not allowed to advertise it, because it could be seen as a way to attract patients, but you should not be afraid to ask. For example, each year the resource specialists in the Pediatric Resource Program at Dana-Farber are able to help on-treatment families access $850,000 in support; this includes $400,000 from a variety of philanthropic foundations along with $450,000 from hospital donor funds earmarked for resource support. In addition, the program helps families access significant amounts of additional resources from several external sources that are difficult to track. This includes SSI payments, Premium Assistance payments, and savings through supplementary Medicaid coverage.

4. Seek out other parents or join a parent group in the hospital. Other parents are happy to share information on accessing extra financial resources and how to cope with income loss.

5. You can search the Web to see if resources from local, state, federal, or private sources could be available to compensate for a serious income loss or to address a particular financial stressor like an overdue rent payment. Try not to wait too long, because some of the organizations or agencies that do have funds available may take some time to process your request.

6. Consider whether you can temporarily adjust your budget in ways that would economize but not cause your family significant hardships, such as postponing planned expenses or buying generic brands. If you are already struggling financially, any further economy may be a significant hardship.

7. Although it may be difficult to accept the generosity, try to be grateful, not reluctant, should family, friends, or neighbors want to organize a fund-raising event for your child, be it an auction, a raffle, a sports event, or a yard or bake sale. It will help you and they will be glad to have something useful to do

8. Similarly, try to be grateful, not reluctant, should colleagues offer you some of their vacation time to be sure you can have your time out of the office paid.

9. Advocate for some flexibility in your work schedule and be sure to explore your eligibility for time off via the Family Medical Leave Act. How your employer reacts to the situation has a big impact. Employers vary greatly in their responses, and some jobs allow more flexibility than others. We found some employers were enormously sympathetic and translated their concern into allowing modified work schedules, time off as needed, and a guaranteed return to the same job when circumstances allowed it. Others were more rigid and had strict rules about family and sick leave. In a two-parent family, parents sometimes decided who would work and who would not, based on the relative flexibility of each job and employer and who carried the family health insurance. Single parents faced a particularly hard challenge when faced with an inflexible employer. Whatever your employment situation, the medical and psychosocial staff will help in whatever way they can. You may ask them to write a letter to your employer to describe your child's diagnosis and the treatment and extent of hospitalizations your child may need. They can also describe additional expenses you are likely to incur. If useful, a psychosocial clinician would likely be happy to add a supporting letter that describes in more detail the emotional burden of the treatment on your child and the importance of your presence at certain, often unpredictable, moments.

10. Advocate for and participate in periodic assessment by your psychosocial clinician or a researcher of your current financial situation during your child's treatment. The more financial hardships are documented (either already existing or precipitated by your child's treatment) and the greater providers' understanding of how they correlate with health outcomes for the children, the more caregivers will advocate for additional resources to be made available to compensate for those losses. Some researchers are already advocating that financial hardship be considered as a risk factor along with certain biological markers in designing an appropriate treatment plan for a particular child.

Summary

Given all you are contending with as your sick child enters the medical world, you may find it hard to focus on what you have already accomplished, on the fact that each day you and your child probably know the hospital and the people in it a little better, and the medical language that seemed incomprehensible at first is becoming more familiar. You may have already handled some of the problems at home that initially seemed insurmountable. You may have begun to assess your financial situation and reached out for support. Still, the situation remains extremely challenging and will require you to continue to mobilize your strengths and to take care of yourself, the subjects of the next chapter.

CHAPTER 2

· · · · · · · · · · · ·

How You Cope
in the Hospital

I t's hard to anticipate how you will respond when your child becomes
seriously ill. After all, few parents imagine that their healthy child
may one day end up requiring such care. And yet this is what you are
now facing. Your family situation, your values, your family's medical
history, and your coping style will all influence how you respond when
your child gets sick. Cultural differences and parenting styles contrast-
ing with those that predominate in the hospital can lead to additional
stressors. This chapter suggests how you can take the best care of yourself in the hospital and still be an effective advocate for your child's
care.

· ·

YOUR FAMILY SITUATION

If You Have a Partner or Spouse

If you have a partner, you are already familiar with dividing tasks to
accommodate new responsibilities involved in having a child. You've
already taken on particular tasks in your roles as parents. Maybe one of
you is in charge of packing school lunches, while the other takes care of
the carpool. Now you will be sharing even more new responsibilities in
looking after your sick child and your other children. It can be difficult
to rethink and reassign new and different roles in the current crisis. For

instance, one parent may be more assertive and comfortable in dealing with professionals but the other parent may be the one who is actually staying in the hospital, so that parent has to become his or her child's spokesperson in relation to the medical staff. Some parents move quickly into these new roles, while others find the transition quite hard. Ideally, you and your partner can talk with your other children about the needed changes in your family's routine.

If you find yourself reacting differently from your partner, don't worry. In fact, differences in style and approach can have benefits. For example, one of you may be more comfortable being with your child during medical procedures, while the other prefers to speak to the medical team about your child's progress. Other differences may need some negotiation. Some people like to have a lot of medical information to feel reassured, while for others, the more information they have the more confused and anxious they feel, so they ask for only the essentials and want the doctors to do what they think best.

If you and your spouse have different styles, you might benefit from talking to a psychosocial clinician and figuring out ways in which the partner who wants more detailed information can meet separately with the medical staff. Some people are helped by talking about what is bothering them; others prefer to distract themselves. Some people prefer to act rather than talk—perhaps to become more involved in outside projects to avoid the emotional stress or to do things with their child. If talking about feelings is stressful for one partner, ask your medical team if there is someone available with whom the more verbal partner can talk.

You may need to share tasks with your partner—for instance, some of the household jobs you usually do. Try to be patient when the task may not be done the exact way you like or the way you would do it.

You and your partner may have hardly any time together for yourselves. Try to make time to be alone together outside of the hospital, even doing something as simple as taking a brief walk outside the facility. Perhaps later you can take advantage of the opportunities sometimes provided by the hospital or outpatient program that allow couples to get away for an evening—maybe a friend or family member could stay at home while you go out.

You need to make sure you are both getting the updated medical information you want and need. One parent may be working and unable to go to your child's regular medical appointments. It is easy for that parent to feel out of the loop. Perhaps you can plan some meetings with the medical team outside the usual medical rounds time that the second parent could either attend in person or be included by telephone.

The important thing is that you are both getting the information you need and are cooperating as best you can based on your particular styles and strengths.

If You Are a Single Parent

As a single parent you are handling a great deal. Between making major health decisions, dealing with practical issues, raising your other children, and shouldering the financial burden, it can feel overwhelming.

You may need to use friends, relatives, colleagues, or community members you respect as sounding boards for particular questions if you do not have a close friend or relative nearby. Other parents or the psychosocial staff in the hospital can be good resources for useful information and emotional support. There will probably be a parent group that you can join in the hospital. This is a time to ask for help, even if it conflicts with the independence for which you may have worked hard. Your employer may need to make adjustments to your work schedule. Colleagues may suggest they share your workload. Try not to be shy about accepting their offer so you can have more time with your child. You can assign tasks—for example, someone else to organize people to come to the hospital when you need to be at work. You may need to remind yourself that you would want to help someone who was in your shoes and that the help that is offered is intended to aid your child as much as or more than to aid you.

It is no easy thing dealing with this situation as a single parent. Remember that the medical and psychosocial staff may have information about resources and supports that could be useful, some of it specifically targeted to what you need. And if there is no one available from outside to be with your child when you need to leave, work with the staff to figure out ways to have volunteers and activities available for your child in your absence.

If You Are Divorced

If you are a divorced parent, you will likely face additional negotiations with your ex-partner and other family members. Depending on your relationship with your ex-partner, you may be able to predict how easy or difficult it will be to make the medical decisions required in joint custody situations. If you have a contentious relationship, you may need to meet separately with the doctors. In case of serious disagreements, you may need to both agree to abide by the doctor's recommendations. If your ex-partner cannot come in for your child's regular visits, the doctor can brief him or her on what has happened. In extreme situations, it may be helpful to bring in a copy of the legal documents regarding custody and decision making so there will be no confusion about the legal situation. Make sure you know where to find these documents should the need arise. Always plan carefully to avoid conflict that might disturb your child later.

If the two of you have worked flexibly and easily before in adjusting schedules to fit each other's needs, so much the better; you may save time and improve communication by meeting with the doctors together.

Try to avoid situations that will confuse or overwhelm your child. If you are unsure how your child will react if you and your divorced spouse visit him together, you can ask your child or have a staff member ask him.

Children often hope their divorced parents will get back together again, so be careful not to set your child up for disappointment if this is not going to happen. If you are worried about this, you can always say something like, "You know Mommy and Daddy both love you even though we do not live together anymore. We are here together now to talk with the doctors and see you are doing okay."

If you are very likely to get into arguments with your ex-spouse, it may be better for your child that you do come in separately. It would likely cause your child additional and unnecessary stress to witness you fighting with each other.

The same is true for other family members. If you know some ex-in-laws fight, take steps to ensure their visits do not coincide. One option is for each family group to come to the hospital on alternate days. If there are hostile exchanges either within your child's hospital room or on the floor, you will quickly find a psychosocial clinician or a member of the medical team asking you to make a schedule for visiting where warring factions will not overlap. The team's priority is to see that your child faces no additional stress.

HOW TO MAINTAIN YOUR VALUES IN THE HOSPITAL

Your Spiritual and Cultural Values

Your spiritual and cultural values will influence how you respond to your child's condition, to the recommendations of the medical team, and to being in the hospital. Often a deep religious faith and membership in a religious community provide support and comfort to parents.

However, sometimes the diagnosis can trigger a spiritual crisis and doubts about your faith. Hospital chaplains are wonderful people with whom to share such questions and the anger and fear that may accompany such doubts.

Sometimes spiritual or cultural beliefs and practices clash with the recommendations or practices of the hospital or your medical team. Here are a few issues you may be dealing with:

- Lack of privacy in the hospital, making it difficult to practice a religious ritual, such as prayers or meditation.
- Gender roles in your community being different from those in the hospital.
- Difficulty complying with a normal dietary rule in the hospital.
- Your religious beliefs conflicting with a medical recommendation.

If you bring up your particular dilemma with the psychosocial staff or the medical team, accommodations can almost always be made. For example:

- Space may be offered to provide religious privacy (hospitals sometimes have nondenominational chapels).
- Family meetings can always be scheduled to include both partners.
- Dietary constraints can be addressed by nursing staff and a special place made available for you to keep your food.
- If the medical team's recommendations clash with your views or values, unless the team or clinician think it is vital to your child's best interests, they would likely defer to your wishes. They will try to offer compromise solutions and may suggest you speak to religious leaders in your community to try to gain their support for the recommended treatment plan. Only as an absolute last resort should you worry that they will pursue the extreme option of going to court to ask the court to appoint a temporary guardian for your child specifically to get permission to give what they regard as lifesaving treatment. They would warn you well in advance if they were considering such a course—and would continue to work to find opportunities for a compromise and any accommodations they can make.

Your Parenting Style and Discipline

Parenting in the hospital is parenting with an ever-present audience (as one father said, "It is like parenting in a fishbowl"). It is extremely challenging to keep regular parenting practices amidst so many medical procedures, doctors and nurses popping in, and outside visitors dropping by. Usually you will find that the staff is accepting of a range of parenting styles, but if you discipline (or do not discipline) your child in ways that differ greatly from the expectations of hospital staff about appropriate child-rearing practices, you may feel that you are being criticized or judged. It may also feel confusing if individual nurses have somewhat different expectations about what they want you to do. However, at minimum, a nurse will likely expect that you will prevent your child from hurting her in any way or being verbally abusive. She will hope you would cooperate with her in encouraging your child to take scheduled medications or to have necessary procedures like dressing changes or blood draws. She may have certain expectations about how much you should be in the hospital, which for various reasons you may not be able to meet, and your relationship with her may be eased if you explain those reasons. A nurse will probably understand if you find it difficult to physically restrain your child and, if staff are available, will likely ask them to help her instead of you. It is possible your child will protest more if you are in the room, sensing how hard it is for you to see him in such distress. So if the nurse asks you to leave the room, consider doing it or, if you prefer, tell your child you will have to leave the room if she has not cooperated by the time you count to five. And if she has not complied by the time you get to five, you should make good on your word and leave.

Nurses will be uncomfortable if you slap your child if he disobeys or does not do what you or his nurse asks. The nurse would probably ask you to manage your child's behavior in some other way. A nurse is mandated to report any physical abuse or neglect of a child that he or she observes to the local department of family services. Parents may have different views about what constitutes physical abuse or neglect than nurses. A parent might maintain that, in his or her view, a quick slap does not constitute physical abuse or that back home her child is used to roaming freely around the neighborhood, so why should he not do the same in the hospital. Hospital staff may have a different perspective. Many hospitals have a child protection team that would be consulted before the nurse would take any action. The team would likely have staff members who would also want to discuss alternatives to slapping as a method of discipline.

It is difficult to say no to a child who is sick, particularly your own child, so do not be surprised if you find yourself relaxing some previously firmly held rules! A few parents do keep to much the same expectations of behavior they had before their child got sick. I asked one mother how she managed to maintain firm but fair limits through hospitalizations and in the face of her child's sickness. She replied, "I don't want him to have turned into a little monster by the time he gets better." At the other extreme, some parents dramatically change expectations during the hospitalization. Funnily enough, this can be alarming for a child. If you notice you are one of those parents, consider that a child who is suddenly allowed to demand, whine, or hit other people when this behavior was not permitted before can feel something must be seriously wrong—not at all the message you intended. Many parents take a middle ground and relax some rules and expectations but not others. There is a difference between hitting and biting a nurse and playing more video games than is permitted at home. Some medications, like the steroid prednisone, may affect your child's behavior. Ask your doctor if you are concerned that a change in your child's behavior might be linked to a medication.

If you keep roughly the same expectations and rules for your child about his behavior that you had previously, your child gets a consistent and positive message. If you relax some of your other past rules, for example, regularity of nap times, amount of TV watched, or video games played and so forth, you are giving your child some control back when he has lost so much control in other major ways. As one wise parent reflected, "It helped to learn to let the little things go and not fight every battle, since the biggest battle gave us all plenty to deal with. And it was important to let him win a few battles here and there, since he had so little control over things." Allowing your child to control the areas he can is giving your child a valuable gift.

Your Family's Prior Medical History

Your family's medical history will influence your reactions to a medical crisis. This history may be recent or it may go back several generations. Perhaps your grandfather spent a month in the hospital as a child alone with polio and repeatedly told you what a terrible experience that was for him. Or your aunt had a serious illness and had a doctor who tried out a new treatment that was successful, or a cousin recently had a routine surgery that produced horrible and unexpected complications. Or perhaps you yourself had a bad time as a child having an emergency appendectomy. That medical family history may trigger in you unexpected and strong reactions when your child's doctors tell you something that reminds you, consciously or unconsciously, of that past history.

Notice if you are having a strong negative emotional reaction to something the doctor has said that seems out of proportion to the content. Ask yourself whether there is an obvious explanation from your family's medical history. If you immediately see the connection, discuss it with the doctor, who will hopefully help you recognize the difference between the past and the present situation. If you are having a hard time remembering any distinct past event, check out your reaction with other family members, friends, or your psychosocial clinician to see if they can shed any light on your response and help you sort out the best way to deal with it.

Similarly, other family members who have their own unique medical family histories may have emotional reactions to what is happening. Sometimes relatives or friends will have very strong opinions about the right way to do things and which treatments your child should get that are based more on their past experiences than on the current medical realities. Although you may want to be sympathetic, you do not want your limited energy to be used reassuring, say, one of your parents, whose fears are based on past, not present, realities. It may be a good idea to ask the doctor or your psychosocial clinician to meet with that parent to understand and to address her concerns—which will, hopefully, get you out of the loop. You may need to tell your parent directly that it is not helpful to you to hear these worries and get another family member, or perhaps a therapist, to be available to talk with her.

Your Attitude

Whether you are an optimist or a pessimist or somewhere in between, and what you are saying to yourself about the situation is likely to affect your reactions. I discuss this further in chapter 6.

■ Are you imagining the situation to be worse than it is? Make a list of the assumptions you are making and check them out with the doctor. You could be making yourself feel worse than you need to. If, on the other hand, your assumptions are correct, you will know you understood correctly and you will know what you may be facing and can plan for different contingencies.

■ Are there accurate but more positive statements you could make to yourself that might help you feel better? Imagine you have just been told by your doctor on your child's day of discharge that your child has developed an infection and will need to stay in the hospital to be treated with a course of strong antibiotics. You notice you are saying to yourself, "We are never going to get out of here." Would you feel better if you said to yourself, "Thank goodness they found this out while she was in the hospital and we did not get home and have to come right back"? The latter statement will probably make you feel better than the former one does. As with many things in life, reframing the situation can help you manage your negative emotions.

Taking Care of Yourself in the Hospital

Many parents have a hard time taking time for themselves in the hospital. They may feel guilty leaving their child even briefly and/or they may be afraid they will miss a doctor visiting the room. Many parents miss exercising but cannot figure out how to work out at the facility. Other parents may miss a more solitary mind-calming activity like reading, meditating, or praying but find it hard to find a place or time to do these things. But remember that neglecting to take care of yourself is a recipe for burnout.

What has helped you relieve tension in the past? Exercise? Venting? Meditation? Writing? Listening to or playing music? Taking breaks? Think about how you can access these activities in the hospital. If you need a break, ask someone to come in and relieve you for an hour or so each day. If you need to vent, talk to a psychosocial staff member or with friends on the telephone (outside your child's room). If you want to meet other parents, there is often a weekly group for parents in the hospital where you can share your reactions, questions, and ideas. A nurse or psychosocial clinician will tell you when and where it meets. Some parents are helped by writing—on a website, in a journal, or by emailing friends.

Consider if any of the steps below would make taking time for yourself easier:

♦ Remind yourself that the better the physical and mental shape you are in, the better able you will be to deal with what is going on. If you are able to exercise or spend some peaceful time by yourself, you are likely to return to your child's hospital room in a better mood and frame of mind than when you left. If you do not feel able to take a long break, even a few minutes away can help.

♦ If you are worried about leaving your child alone, arrange for a relative, friend, or volunteer to come at the same time each day or for a few days each week. Or ask your child's nurse to check on her more frequently than usual and tell your child she can call you if she needs to. You can also see that she is doing something she enjoys when you leave. Be quite specific about when you will be back and always let your child or her nurse know if you are delayed.

♦ An interactive good-bye ritual for a young child can be helpful. Try whatever method for saying good-bye that you used at home or develop a special hospital sequence. For example, use the same sequence of good-bye kisses each time or even the same rhyme:

  ▸ Parent: See you later, alligator.
  ▸ Child: In a while, crocodile.

♦ If you are worried about missing the doctor, go at a time when the doctor is unlikely to come—say, after morning rounds—or leave your cell phone number with your child's nurse.

WAYS TO SQUEEZE IN A LITTLE EXERCISE

■ Make sure the clothes you are comfortable exercising in are with you in the hospital.

■ Find attractive places to walk or jog. Perhaps the hospital information desk can suggest options. Ask if there is a room in the hospital or an adjoining building where you could exercise should it be too cold to exercise outside. A few hospitals may be affiliated with a gym.

■ Walk up the stairs rather than taking the elevator.

■ Ask if your hospital offers drop-in exercise groups.

■ Ask if there is a place where you can form a yoga group or simply do yoga exercises by yourself each morning.

TIME BY YOURSELF—TO READ, TO MEDITATE, TO PRAY

■ Find a peaceful place in the hospital where you can go. Some hospitals have nondenominational chapels, others have gardens, others have a communal area for activities or even waiting areas with comfortable chairs.

■ Ignore other people who may be passing by or sitting near you. (You may need to bring earphones in case other people's conversations distract you.)

■ Give yourself permission to do whatever it is that gives your mind a break and your spirit comfort—be it reading, meditating, praying, listening to music, or even taking a nap away from your child's hospital room.

Hydration and Healthy Eating

Eating and drinking adequately are key ingredients for mental and physical health. Eating or drinking healthfully is a challenge in the hospital. Many parents find it easier to drink than to eat. Unfortunately, coffee (with high caffeine) and sodas (with high calorie and sugar content) are usually the drinks most easily available. Most people are aware that we all should drink much more water than we do. It's easy to get distracted in the hospital and to forget to drink enough water, resulting in mild dehydration, which can make you tired and hazy. At least try to add two or three glasses of water to your daily intake. Medical staff generally prefer you go outside the hospital if you want to have an alcoholic drink, and are likely to ask you to leave the hospital if you appear intoxicated.

Many parents have a hard time eating regular meals or eating at all in the hospital. They will often nibble off the tray of food ordered for their child, and that will constitute their food intake for the day. Parents say it is hard for them to eat because:

♦ They don't feel like eating (they are too worried).

♦ They do not have much appetite because they are sitting around all day.

♦ They do not want to leave their child alone while they get food.

- The food costs too much.
- The food is not good anyway.

Occasionally parents will say they are eating more than usual. They even may be putting on weight in the hospital. All of these are understandable reactions, but they are not good for you or your child.

So how can you persuade yourself to eat healthy food regularly because this will keep you in good shape?

- Remind yourself that it is important to eat regularly and well regardless whether you feel hungry or not.

- Start with one healthy meal a day when you go down to the cafeteria. Select a nutritious option and either eat the meal there or take it back to your child's room.

- If the cost of the food is an issue, check whether the hospital has any free meal vouchers for parents. Often there are discounts even if there are no vouchers for patients' families.

- If it is the taste of the food you dislike, ask friends or family to bring in some home-cooked food. Most hospitals have a refrigerator where patients' food can be kept. Make sure it is clearly labeled and dated, or it may be thrown out by the cleaning staff.

Smoking

If you are a regular smoker, this can be very challenging. Many parents point out that they smoke to relieve stress and provide comfort and this is hardly the moment to give up smoking. Hospitals have understood this, and our hospital tried various methods over the years to discourage but not forbid parents to smoke. First, smoking was banned from all areas of the hospital except for a special parents' smoking room situated near the cafeteria. However, the smoke-filled atmosphere and congested space was so clearly unhealthy that a special outdoor space was instead allocated where parents could smoke. Many hospitals have experimented with versions of this approach.

However, you are placed in a tricky position. Even young children are aware of a connection between smoking and cancer, and your child will have a hard time understanding how you can do something that increases your own risk of cancer while expecting her to get extremely unpleasant treatment to ensure she gets rid of the cancer in her body. She may well lobby you to give up smoking. So what can you do?

Perhaps the most straightforward approach is to say you will try to give up smoking—and try. You can investigate some of the programs described later and see if there is one that is home-based, perhaps app-based, that appeals to you. If you suspect that at the moment you will not be able to give up smoking completely because of the stress relief it provides, then can you commit to your child that you will try to cut down on the number of cigarettes you smoke each day? The inconvenience and frequent discomfort of having to go outside to smoke and the fact of having to leave your child to do so may make this easier. You can even keep track of the numbers to show her you are trying and making some progress. If you are not progressing, you can tell her you will try again when things are calmer.

Getting Better Sleep

Adequate sleep is another key ingredient for mental and physical health. Unfortunately, it is very difficult for many parents to get much sleep in the hospital. So what can help?

- ◆ Exercise during the day or take a short walk before going to sleep.
- ◆ Listen to music or a relaxation app on your cell phone or iPod.
- ◆ Use earplugs and an eye mask.
- ◆ Bring in a white-noise machine.

Even if you do not sleep well, you can give yourself some down time when you let your mind and body rest. Often parents say they want to be alert and easily awoken to be sure their child is all right, but let's remember it is the nurse's job to check on your child every few hours. A good night's sleep will help you think more clearly and feel less emotionally vulnerable.

ADVOCATING FOR THE BEST MEDICAL CARE FOR YOUR CHILD

As a parent, you naturally want your child to get the best medical care possible. You want your child to get the best treatments available and your child's medical care team to be people you trust and can communicate with. Your first priority is to be sure you have full and accurate medical information about your child's diagnosis and treatment from the medical staff. Whether your child has cancer, cystic fibrosis, a heart condition, juvenile diabetes, or an immune deficiency disorder, there will be several medical terms that will be useful for you to know. These will likely be relevant to the treatments your child receives and are described in the boxes that follow.

CLINICAL TRIALS

There are four phases of clinical trials designed to answer separate research questions.

Phase I looks at the safety, dose level, and side effects of a new drug or treatment given to a few people, often healthy volunteers except in the case of some anti-cancer drugs.

Phase II looks at the efficacy, side effects, and safety of the new drug or treatment with patients. It may come up with a proposed dose level range that is safe to use with larger patient groups in Phase III trials.

Phase III looks at the efficacy, safety, and side effects of the new drug or treatment compared with the current standard treatments given to the clinical population it is designed to help. A phase III study can have several experimental arms. Ideally, patients will be randomly assigned to each group and patients and caregivers will not know which treatment the patient is receiving (a double-blind study). However, this is not always possible.

Phase IV occurs after a drug is licensed and studies long-term and other effects of the new drug or treatment compared with standard treatments in extended groups.

The most likely clinical trial your child would be invited to participate in would be a phase III clinical trial, in which the doctors test a standard treatment protocol against a new protocol that they think has some advantage. In other words, doctors want to compare the best current treatment with treatments they hope are even better. Doctors may think one of these treatments might have an even better survival rate or have fewer side effects than the current standard treatment. This benefit has not been conclusively proven, though, which is why there is an ongoing clinical trial. The doctors will explain in great detail why these treatments are being compared and what the possible advantages are for the newer treatments compared with the more standard treatment. As soon as one treatment shows better results than the others in the clinical trial, that treatment will become (or will remain) the standard treatment given.

If you agreed, your child would be randomly assigned to one of several treatments. Examples of such trials for children with cancer could include:

- Different combinations of treatment—say, chemotherapy with or without radiation or different levels of chemotherapy.

- The same level of chemotherapy but given in different forms—say, either by an injection or via an infusion through a central line.

- The same treatment given at different intervals—for example, the same level of radiation given in one or two doses each day.

If you are not comfortable with the random assignment, you can choose to have the standard treatment and not participate in the clinical trial.

A PROTOCOL AND THE INFORMED CONSENT FORM

A PROTOCOL

- A protocol describes the detailed treatment plan for a standard treatment, a clinical trial (e.g., of a drug or medical treatment), or a medical research study. For example, it will list the drug or treatment amounts and the tests required for each stage of treatment and will include a timeline. In a clinical trial, the protocol offers detailed treatment information for each arm of the trial.

■ There are different versions of a protocol. You may initially be given a short version for daily use and a longer version with more detail. In a clinical trial, the protocol describing all treatment arms of the study may include the preceding investigations that led to the new treatments being considered and might be very long. Whether you want to review the complete protocol will depend on your style and the extent of your wish for information.

Please keep in mind that almost no child follows the outlined protocol exactly.

INFORMED CONSENT

You will be asked to sign an informed consent form for whatever treatment or procedure your child will receive whether it is part of a clinical trial or not. The form is intended to document the fact that the doctors have discussed with you all the realistic treatment options for your child as well as the risks and benefits of each, and that you have chosen a particular treatment having this knowledge. The purpose is to see that you, the parent, are fully informed about what you are agreeing to allow the doctors to do with your child. It can be scary reading, because almost every possible known side effect is listed, even those that are truly rare.

The informed consent form and the protocol can also be extremely difficult to understand, because they often include many unfamiliar medical terms. To increase your ability to ask the doctors important questions relevant to your child's best care:

■ Go back to medical staff at your child's institution—your child's doctor or nurse or a research nurse—and ask them to go through the form again and explain anything that is not clear to you.

■ Ask to meet with the attending doctor, the supervisor of your child's primary doctor or nurse practitioner, who may have more experience in knowing the different treatments or can explain the content of the protocol and the informed consent form more clearly.

- Enlist anyone else you know in the medical field to do the same.

- Send the form to your child's pediatrician and ask to meet with him or her to review the form.

- Look on the Internet for definitions of some of the medical terms used. For example, the Children's Oncology Group (COG) website[1] at www.childrensoncologygroup.org does have a broad overview of treatments commonly used for particular diagnoses but may not list information on the latest and newest experimental protocols. Information on experimental protocols will likely be found on the websites of the institutions doing them.

- If you do find information online about experimental protocols, discuss the protocols with your child's doctor, who will certainly look into them and probably get back to you with information about the risks, benefits, and feasibility of use in the United States.

UNDERSTANDING YOUR CHILD'S CANCER TREATMENT

If your child has cancer, there are some facts about the treatment that will be useful to know:

- Few children get cancer. Therefore sharing of information between treatment centers is vital.

- Hospitals across the United States and Canada and in other countries have formed clinical research groups to better understand childhood cancers, including very rare ones, and to increase the medical community's ability to evaluate treatment outcomes. The biggest group is called the Children's Oncology Group (COG). More than 90 percent of children in the US with cancer are treated in institutions affiliated with COG. Several other such groups have been formed across the world.

■ Most children with a similar diagnosis throughout the US will receive treatment based on the same treatment protocol.

■ The Children's Oncology Group (COG) has spearheaded much of the research that has resulted in the enormous improvement in treatment outcomes for childhood cancers.

■ This progress has often occurred through a series of clinical trials.

■ You may be asked if your child will participate in a clinical trial.

BUILDING A STRONG RELATIONSHIP WITH YOUR CHILD'S MEDICAL CAREGIVERS

You need to feel comfortable with your child's medical team, and most important, with your child's primary medical provider. In our hospital, that person could be a fellow or an experienced nurse practitioner. The attending doctor in charge of your child's particular diagnosis would supervise the fellow or the nurse practitioner and would also meet frequently with you.

Imagine you do not initially feel comfortable with the person who is assigned to be your child's primary provider. You may feel he or she is not a good match with you or your child for various reasons. You may think about changing him or her. You may have met another doctor in the hospital whom you like better than your assigned doctor, or you may think your child should have a doctor, not a nurse practitioner, as her primary care provider. Discuss your concerns with the attending doctor. You will probably find that he or she will listen carefully but will be pretty reluctant to change your provider. The attending doctor's preference will likely be that you and your child's provider try to work out any differences. If relevant, the attending doctor may well point out that the nurse practitioner has had many years of experience treating children with your child's diagnosis. The attending doctor will also likely emphasize that the execution of your child's treatment plan is very much a team effort and that he or she supervises closely what is happening at all times.

There are rare circumstances in which you can reasonably insist on changing your child's primary medical provider. Here are four such situations:

♦ If your provider makes several mistakes in implementing your child's treatment plan or forgets or confuses important issues (i.e., appears incompetent).

♦ If, after several attempts, you really cannot understand your provider's explanation of treatment and care.

♦ If your provider over time seems not to listen to your concerns or respond to your questions.

♦ If your child appears very uncomfortable with the provider (more so than with other medical staff) and this does not improve over time.

You may hear from other parents or acquaintances about a particular specialist who is expert in an area where your child needs a consultation, but your child has been referred to see someone else. What should you do? I would suggest bringing up the issue with your child's principal care provider, who could probably find out how easy or difficult it would be to see your favored consultant or whether it would cause an unacceptable delay. You may even discover that your preferred consultant is already part of the team with whom the other specialist would consult.

If you happen to know directly or indirectly one of the doctors high up in the hospital hierarchy, is his or her involvement in your child's care likely to be helpful? To be honest, a connection in high places can be a mixed blessing. If such a doctor becomes extremely involved, it can make staff nervous and lead to unintended mistakes. Generally, medical staff are working hard for your child and there may already be many doctors providing input into your child's care. To feel they are being overscrutinized may not be beneficial. On the other hand, it may be comforting for you to know you have a knowledgeable advocate within the hospital, and the person may be very helpful to you as a consultant who knows the hospital and the medical issues.

Taking care of your newly sick child in the hospital and getting the best available care for your child is challenging. You will bring your unique strengths and vulnerabilities to this situation. The better care you can take of your mind, body, and spirit, the more likely you are to manage your child's care effectively. Resources and people are available to help. Please make use of them, and for everyone's sake, remember to look after yourself and your relationships with those closest to you as well as your child. You will also be an effective advocate for your child if you understand your child's medical picture and build a strong alliance with his medical team.

CHAPTER 3

· · · · · · · · · · · · ·

Babies, Toddlers, and Preschool Children

Illnesses and their treatments can be difficult even for an adult to understand—and it can be nearly impossible for a young child to fathom what is happening. It's important that you take your child's age and level of understanding into account as you talk to her about her illness.

Long hospitalizations, intrusive treatments, prolonged physical therapy, and health limitations are stressful for children whether they are six months or sixteen years old. The next two chapters describe development, behavior, and the range of reactions you may see in your child depending on his age and personality. I will offer tools to help different age groups and suggest ways to match explanations to the age and character of your child.

· ·

THE IMPORTANCE OF OPEN COMMUNICATION

In US hospitals, most doctors expect to speak honestly and directly with parents and in an age-appropriate and sensitive way with children about their medical condition and plans for treatment. Health conditions and different cultural beliefs, values, and practices may affect what you, at least initially, are comfortable sharing with your child. If you strongly prefer to be told details about the diagnosis and treatment while not in the presence of your child, you should discuss your preferences and concerns directly with your health care team.

Why doctors prefer to tell your child about the disease or condition he has:

- ♦ A straightforward explanation establishes a partnership and mutual trust between you, your child, and the medical team for the long haul.

- ♦ Knowing about his disease can decrease your child's anxiety by allowing him to feel he can ask questions and that he does not need to guess what is happening.

- ♦ Understanding what the doctors hope to achieve may help your child accept why unpleasant treatments are necessary, increasing the likelihood your child will cooperate with treatment.

- ♦ Knowing his diagnosis means your child will not find out on his own or from someone other than you or his doctor and feel betrayed or misinformed.

Although most doctors are unlikely to agree to lie to your child, doctors will generally agree to limit the information that is initially shared if that is your wish.

Babies and Toddlers

A baby or toddler may not yet talk but is gradually coming to understand the difference between herself and others and shows growing preferences between people (separation anxiety from parents usually appears between six and nine months of age). Your toddler is probably increasingly mobile, is eager to explore, is likely showing increasing interest in the outside world, and has little impulse control and minimal awareness of danger. More and more, your toddler can sense the emotions of others close to her. She may begin to understand simple words and be beginning nonverbal or limited verbal communication (such as "No" or "Oh, oh" when something breaks). Your toddler may also develop visual and associative memories that can trigger anxiety—so seeing a nurse who gave her a shot or returning to a room where a painful procedure occurred can lead her to cry or to resist.

Despite the basic similarities in developmental milestones, striking individual differences (in startle response to noise, in time taken to calm down after getting upset, at delaying a response, in reacting to separation, in activity level, in empathetic reactions from a very young age) are already evident. These differences will affect the intensity with which individual babies and toddlers respond to being in the hospital.

Stressful factors for most very young children about a long hospitalization

- A baby's routine and surroundings change dramatically.
- A baby or toddler can sense his parents are upset.
- Many new people appear unexpectedly in this new world.
- A baby or toddler has to do new, sometimes unpleasant things as part of his medical care.
- Things hurt (like needles) or his body may feel uncomfortable.
- A baby or a toddler does not understand what is happening or why.
- A baby or toddler may have unpleasant associative memories of people or places in the hospital.

What to say and do right away

- Although your baby may not understand many of the words you say, she will respond to your tone and manner of speaking both to her and to others in her presence. Speak as calmly and reassuringly as you can.
- Use simple words to describe what's happening when it is happening ("The doctor is giving you a shot/ouchee").
- Use what has comforted your infant or toddler previously (rocking, holding, singing, patting, pacifier, blankie, or other transitional object) to soothe him when he is upset. Tell medical staff so they can use the same methods if you have to be out of the room.
- If your conversation with the medical team is likely to be upsetting for you, ask to have it in a separate room while someone familiar stays with your baby so your emotional reaction will not upset your baby.

Reactions in Infants and Toddlers

Some infants and toddlers will show little disturbance, but others will regress (stop doing things they have just learned to do) or show quite dramatic reactions. Almost any reaction your baby or toddler has is understandable under the circumstances. Don't be surprised if your child's disposition appears to change from that of a happy, loving, and easygoing baby to that of a baby who is irritable, demanding, or withdrawn. This alarming but very normal change in behavior is nearly always a temporary reaction to stressful circumstances. When everyone, including you, becomes more used to what is happening, when a new routine is established, and when some appropriate interventions are made, these behaviors will likely moderate if not completely disappear. But initially some infants and toddlers may:

♦ Withdraw
♦ Have tantrums/cry intensely
♦ Appear extremely afraid of medical staff
♦ Actively resist procedures or treatment
♦ Refuse solid food or a bottle
♦ Have difficulty sleeping and be clingier at bedtime
♦ Be more dependent on you

A toddler may, in addition:

♦ Stop crawling or standing up
♦ Forget toilet training

How to Help Your Baby or Toddler Adjust

Your presence and the presence of familiar and loved figures doing what is familiar will be of most comfort. To help your baby or toddler feel things are more normal, you can:

♦ Advocate with medical staff for effective pain management (for example, ask that Emla cream, a numbing medication, be put on well in advance of a shot to numb the injection area).
♦ Advocate that no painful procedures are done in your baby's bed and that he not be woken up abruptly for a procedure, so that he experiences his bed as a safe place.
♦ Arrange your child's bed to reduce the likelihood the pacifier, blankie, or stuffed animal will be lost.
♦ Ask other familiar figures to visit if you have to leave.
♦ Try to establish as much of a routine as you can in the hospital.

- Advocate for as much consistency in nursing staff as possible.
- Consult with medical or psychosocial staff to see if they have any concerns about your toddler's behavior and to see if they have any suggestions.

A CHILD'S STORY—MARK

Mark, a two-and-a-half-year-old who had been seriously ill for a long time, was calm only when watching a particular car video. He became inconsolable if any attempt was made to turn off the video to get him to eat, play, or interact. The video had become his security blanket and his protection from the real world. We gradually helped him change his behavior by encouraging his parents to pause the video rather than turn it off while he ate or played for a few minutes and then they restarted it when he had had a little to eat or had played for a little while. Gradually, his parents were able to lengthen the time the video was paused before starting it again. He was also shown how to turn it off and on himself, which he did with pride.

Preschool Children Aged Three to Five Years

Children at these ages use play and their imagination to handle new situations and to make sense of the world around them. You, the parent, know your own child better than anyone else and you are therefore the key to helping him or her. This includes helping medical staff figure out how to help your child cope with the stress of hospitalization and necessary medical care. You are vital in explaining to the staff how your child reacts in new situations and what is likely to cause stress or provide comfort.

Preschoolers are gradually becoming more verbal and more social. They are literal, egocentric, suggestible, and impulsive with limited judgment, sense of time, or ability to distinguish fact from fiction. They often have wonderful imaginations.

Despite these developmental similarities, preschoolers can still be hugely different from one another. One three-year-old can be inconsolable when his mother leaves; another can become immediately absorbed in an interesting task and turn to an alternative adult for help, if necessary. One four-year-old always wants the same stuffed animals next to him at night, while another will change his "friends" frequently.

One five-year-old will quietly struggle for five minutes to complete a puzzle, another will ask for help or move on after thirty seconds. These differences can hugely affect how your child experiences being in the hospital.

Stressful factors for most three- to five-year-olds about a long hospitalization

+ A young child's routine changes dramatically.
+ His parents and family members are upset.
+ Many new people appear in his life and make demands of him.
+ Things like shots hurt and his body may feel uncomfortable.
+ The young child feels confused. He has a hard time understanding what is happening and why.

What to say and do right away
In talking to your child you can:

+ Be simple, direct, and clear.
+ Deliver information in small portions.
+ Repeat information often and then check that your child has actually heard it as you or the doctor meant.
+ Give simple, accurate, and developmentally appropriate explanations. "You are here right now because . . ." "The doctors need to find out what is wrong. We will go home when they tell us it's okay."
+ Have a matter-of-fact attitude: "We have to do this because . . ." "It will be quick and then we can . . ."
+ Limit the time and content of conversations with the medical team in front of your child—saving the complicated questions for meetings when you are alone with the medical team.
+ Make clear to your child that he or she did not cause the illness or catch it from anyone else.
+ Give information to your child only as it will affect him or her immediately or in the very near future, since your child has little idea of the meaning of words that describe time.

- If your child's doctor has already explained to your child what her illness or condition is and what the treatment will be, you may want to check with your child how much she understood, clarify any misconceptions, and, if necessary, ask the doctor to repeat the explanation more simply on his next visit.

If you choose to tell your child yourself about his condition or what will happen, below are some suggestions for simple explanations:

If your child asks, "How/why did I get it?"
"No one knows."
"Nothing you did or said caused this to happen."
"You did not catch it (and it is not catching)."

If your child has leukemia:
"Your blood is not working right and the doctors need to fix it."

If your child has a solid tumor:
"A lump is growing in your _____ and the doctors need to make it go away."
"You are getting this medicine to make the lump get smaller."

Ways to describe causes of illness, surgery, treatments, and/or side effects

Three things to remember when talking to your young child about treatment:

- As mentioned earlier, children this age have a limited grasp of the concept of time, so it's usually best to tell your child about a forthcoming procedure very close to the time it will happen, maybe a day or even just a few hours in advance. Telling your child about a major surgery one day ahead can be enough time, provided you let your child ask as many questions as he wants and you listen carefully to what his worries are. "We will tell you what the doctors need to do. Let's see if you have questions about it." Sometimes you may want to wait until the morning of a particularly stressful procedure.

- Young children are very suggestible and some side effects (like nausea and vomiting) may or may not occur, so you do not want to predict a side effect that may not happen in case that precipitates the reaction. After the procedure, you can explain the side effect of a treatment if it begins to occur. "The medicine is working—that is why you are feeling sick."

♦ Young children need to be encouraged to ask questions. It helps them feel included. It helps them understand. It also allows you to see what your child understands or does not understand and what is worrying her.

Dealing with side effects

♦ If your child is vomiting: "The nurse will try to help you feel better with some new medicine."

♦ If your child is having tantrums while on steroids: "Sometimes the medicine can make you feel upset and it is hard to control yourself, but we still cannot let you hit people."

♦ If your child's hair will fall out (a common side effect of some chemotherapy), talk with your child as her hair is beginning to fall out. "We hope the medicine will help you get better, but it also makes your hair fall out. Your hair will grow back later." . . . "Would you like us to cut your hair shorter so there is less to come out?" . . . "Some children like to wear a wig when they don't have hair. Would you like to get one?"

If your child had a bad accident:

"The car knocked you into the air. When you landed on the ground you broke three bones in your leg. You will need to keep the plaster on around your leg so the bones can grow back together and then you will be able to walk and run again."

If your child asks how the accident happened:

"The driver of the car did not see you. He was not paying attention properly because he was talking on his cell phone. He is very sorry his car hurt you and hopes very much you will feel better soon."

If your child needs surgery to set a bone:

"Now the doctors will help you go to sleep so you will not feel anything. Then they will put the parts of your bone back together so the bone can grow together again. When you wake up you will have a special cast around your leg so you can't move your leg by mistake. When the bone is mended, the cast will be taken off."

If your child needs chemotherapy:

"Right now the doctors will give you some medicine that will [help your blood get better/make the lump in your tummy get smaller]. Do you have a question about that?"

If your child needs radiation:

"Now, you will need to lie still on a special bed while a machine like a big camera shines a special light on your body. You will not feel the light. The light will help [the lump get smaller/your blood get better]."

If your child needs anesthesia:

"The doctors will help you go to sleep so you will not feel anything. You will breathe through a special mask. You can choose what smell the mask has. Do you like the smell of bubble gum or cherries best? Cherries. Great. You can ask the doctors to make it smell like cherries. The doctor will ask you to count up to ten and see how far you get before you fall asleep. When you wake up, you may have a special tube going into your arm that helped your body get enough to drink while you were asleep. You will wake up in a special recovery room where we will be (or will come right away). You may feel a little tired and dizzy at first, but after you have drunk something and eaten something you will likely feel much better. In a little while you will be taken on a special bed with wheels back to your room. You can ask me or the doctor any questions you want."

If your child needs surgery to remove a tumor:

"Now the doctors will help you go to sleep so you will not feel anything and then they will take out what is left of the lump. When you wake up, it will be gone and you will have a bandage over where the lump was."

If a child needs an amputation of a limb to remove a tumor:

"You are going to have a special operation. Do you know what an operation is?" Explain anesthesia and not feeling anything. "During the operation while you are asleep the doctors will take off the bottom part of your leg, the part with the lump in it. They have to do that because they hope it will stop lumps growing anywhere else in your body." Encourage questions. Give a simple description of a prosthesis if appropriate: "A special metal/plastic leg that will help you walk, run, and get around so you will be able to play with your friends."

Your Child's Reaction

Preschool children react to illness in various ways. Some may be relatively easygoing throughout their illness. Others may seem to adjust with little difficulty at first but appear more distressed later. Some may become withdrawn irritable, angry, or anxious. They may become more dependent on you or actively resist treatment, sometimes in quite dramatic ways.

Helping Your Preschool-Age Child

Every parent wants to help his or her child to cope, but it is important that you tailor your help to your child's age and temperament. As mentioned earlier, many young children cope with external stress through play and their imagination. For other young children, routine, consistency, and familiarity may provide the most comfort.

Play

Let's begin with play. Play has multiple purposes for a developing child. It allows the child to express feelings, to absorb difficult experiences by acting them out over and over again, to try out new ideas, to take on different roles (the child becomes the aggressor instead of the victim, the big guy instead of the little guy), to have fun, and to have a break from the real world.

Most young children identify with animals, stuffed animals, and puppets. They will speak with an animal or puppet in a way they will not speak with an adult, even their parent. So for many young children in the hospital, introducing a new puppet or stuffed animal friend or using a current favorite animal from home may help your child to:

+ Have his worries/feelings named by someone else
+ Feel less alone
+ Express his feelings directly or through identification with the puppet
+ Hear suggestions made to the puppet
+ Be in charge of something
+ Practice coping strategies with the puppet
+ Have fun

Following is an example of how a puppet can be introduced to a young child. Note that the puppet is shy at first. You want your child to feel stronger and less afraid than the puppet. You want the puppet to have similar worries, likes, and dislikes as your child so she will think of him as like her. If you are not comfortable speaking in a different voice as the puppet, you can have the puppet or stuffed animal whisper in your ear and then tell the child what he said to you. Or you can ask a child therapist to introduce a puppet to your child.

INTRODUCING A PUPPET

DIALOGUE	PURPOSE
PARENT OR THERAPIST: There is someone I'd like you to meet in my bag, but he is shy and does not like hospitals much.	Puppet identifies with child.
PUPPET: Where am I?	
PARENT: In the hospital.	
PUPPET: Oh. [disappears briefly] I don't like the hospital much.	
PARENT: How come?	
PUPPET: Nurses and doctors give you shots. You have to take yucky medicine.	Names child's dislikes.
PARENT: Anything else? [Child can add what he wants.]	
PUPPET: I miss not being at home.	
PARENT: What do you miss?	
PUPPET: My dog, stuffed animals.	
PARENT: [asking Child] What else might he miss?	
CHILD: [can add something]	
PUPPET: How did you know?	Admires child.
PARENT: Because he is in the hospital, too.	
PUPPET: How come?	
PARENT OR CHILD: [explains reason]	
PUPPET: Well, I know I'm here to get better.	Reminds child.
And some of the nurses are nice and the playroom is fun.	Makes suggestion.
(Later, Puppet whispers something in Parent's ear.)	Gets child curious.
PARENT: He says he likes you very much.	Flatters child.
Can he come and see you again?	Gives child control.

A puppet or stuffed animal may be particularly effective in re-engaging a young child who is deeply withdrawn, traumatized, and disengaged, like a patient with whom I had the privilege of working named James.

A CHILD'S STORY—JAMES

James was three when he was diagnosed with cancer. He was in the intensive care unit for six weeks with infections, high fevers, and multiple invasive medical procedures. He arrived in the oncology unit withdrawn and not speaking. He would start shaking when new people entered the room. He was not eating or even playing.

Prior to diagnosis his parents described him as playful, engaged, loving, and energetic. He had loved playing with small trains.

My first intervention was to help him play and eat again.

To begin with, James's mother, a puppet named Charlie, and I played together with toy trains on a hospital tray in front of James. For several sessions James did not respond. Finally, after a few days, he reached out for a train. James tentatively pushed the train. The puppet sent the train back to him. James pushed it back to the puppet.

Over the next several meetings his mother, Charlie, and I played with Play-Doh. His mother made different "foods" from the Play-Doh that she "fed" to Charlie. Gradually, James began to make food, too. He began to feed the puppet. We knew we were getting somewhere when one day he suddenly popped the special Play-Doh banana he had made into his own mouth! Shortly after this he began to eat real food again.

James grew fond of Charlie. When I came into the room he would immediately ask for Charlie. And over the course of James's difficult treatment, Charlie served many purposes. He accompanied James to physical therapy and complained loudly at all the exercises he needed to do (James had become so weak he could not walk). Charlie told James how proud he was when he learned to do something he could not do before. He cheered when James took his first step and told him that he was going to try hard to walk, too. The nurses used the puppet to show James new procedures, and Charlie would tell James whether or not they hurt.

When James's little brother was born, Charlie got a little brother too (a much smaller monkey; we practiced ways to feed him and be quiet around him when he was asleep!). When James finally left the hospital and came into the outpatient clinic for the first time, Charlie was there to greet him and tell him that although the outpatient clinic was a little scary at first, the nurses were nice there, too. He was sure James would get used to it soon.

Charlie and James practiced together ways to be brave even when they were feeling scared. At the end of James's treatment, I wrote a story for James about what good friends he and Charlie had become, all the ways they had helped each other, and how they would still sometimes see each other but not so often as they used to when James was sick. I wrote that Charlie would always remember James and would be glad to see James when he came back to the clinic.

The type of play that is often most immediately connected to the current world your child is living in is, of course, medical play. What could be more natural or psychologically healthy than for your child to play doctor and make his own rules! Medical play allows your child:

- To be in charge (he can be the doctor or nurse, not the patient) to say and do what he wants.
- To repeat in his own way what he is experiencing, thus making it more familiar and less overwhelming.
- To show his emotions (fear, anger).
- To practice new ways to cope.

It allows you:

- To appreciate how he understands (or misunderstands) a medical situation.
- To understand what he is feeling about what's happening to him.
- To give him new information about a medical situation.
- To make indirect suggestions via the puppet about new ways to cope.

A CHILD'S STORY—WILLIE

A five-year-old boy, Willie, hated any medical procedures but was quite connected to my monkey puppet, whom he called Alfred. Alfred was the victim of innumerable visits to the doctor. Alfred emerged from one visit with his whole body covered in tape. Willie's mother and I asked whether we could take the tape off Alfred before Willie went home and were told we could not. When we did finally remove the tape on his next clinic visit, Willie did not seem too concerned when a fair amount of Alfred's hair came off. Willie was in charge and told us he was giving Alfred the treatment he needed to get better!

Often young children in the hospital prefer to play with real medical equipment (tape, alcohol wipes, masks, syringes) rather than toy ones. However, if your child is terrified of procedures, toy equipment is better at first. You can gradually supplement a toy medical kit with some extra real medical supplies. Your child can play with the kits at home or in the hospital. If you observe rather than direct his play, only occasionally asking questions, you will likely learn a lot about how he is experiencing things. Resist the temptation to say after your child has given his favorite teddy bear four shots with no warning, "That is not what the doctor does to you." A comment like "Teddy is going through a lot, isn't he?" is closer to a response that will show your empathy and encourage and not limit your child's play and his free expression.

The Lego hospital set is another vehicle through which a child can play out concerns and work out solutions to problems through medical play.

Other Therapeutic Interventions

Free play, artwork, clay, storytelling and games can also be used with some preschool children and are described further in the next chapter, which centers on school-age children and adolescents.

Additional strategies to help manage pain and anxiety like special breathing, relaxation, guided imagery, distractions, and affirmations for younger children are described in chapters 7 through 9.

CHAPTER 4

. . . .

School-Age Children and Adolescents

The older a child is, the more he needs and can understand a fuller explanation of his condition. Just because an older child is capable of deeper understanding, however, does not mean that a serious illness is any less stressful for him than it is for a younger child.

. . . .

AGES SIX TO ELEVEN YEARS

Children between six and eleven years old generally have increased rational but literal understanding, are learning many new skills, have more self-control, and can concentrate for longer periods of time. They often still have terrific imaginations. They need friends as well as family, and are more likely to compare themselves to peers and base their self-esteem somewhat on that assessment. Although they are becoming more independent, they can easily regress to earlier behavior patterns if stressed.

Although these are general developmental trends, children between the ages of six and eleven, as with the younger age groups, show considerable differences from one another. By this point, children show different physical and intellectual skills and varying levels of confidence and self-esteem. They can be more or less anxious and impulsive and need more or less advance preparation for treatments. They need friends and some will feel more vulnerable than others if excluded. These characteristics will affect how you communicate with your child about his illness. You are the best person to judge the extent of explanation, preparation, and ongoing communication that will be most appropriate for your child and can let the medical team know.

Stressful factors for most children aged six to eleven years about a long hospitalization

+ Can affect learning new skills (intellectual and physical).
+ Can affect what a child learns and how he does in school.
+ Can limit what he can do physically.
+ Can make a child feel isolated and different from his friends.
+ Can lead a child to feel more dependent on his or her family.

What to say and do right away

Here are a few guidelines for talking to your six- to eleven-year-old about his illness:

+ Make the conversations simple, direct, and clear.
+ Have a matter-of-fact attitude.
+ Hold short meetings only with your child and the medical team (extended ones with you alone). Your child can tell you if he wants to be more included.
+ Check afterward what your child has understood about what the doctors said and whether he wanted more or less information.
+ Check for misconceptions your child may have about what caused the illness.
+ Describe the treatment plan in small portions so as not overwhelm your child—although some older children may want a broad overview of the treatment plan with details later.
+ Moderate the extent of advance warning you give about treatment or a procedure with the style and age of your child—some older children may want several weeks rather than several days of advance notice about surgery so they can get questions answered or have more time to prepare themselves for what is going to happen.
+ Allow your child a role in medical decisions where there are simple options so your child feels he is a partner in what is happening to him.

♦ Give fuller biological explanations about the illness and treatment.

Examples of specific things to say:

If your child has leukemia:

"Our blood is made up of red and white blood cells and platelets. Red blood cells carry oxygen (which is like food) to different parts of our body. White blood cells help our bodies fight infections. Platelets are small pieces of blood cells that help cuts heal and help our blood clot so a cut does not go on bleeding. Our bodies need a proper balance of red and white blood cells and platelets to work properly. Your body is making too many white cells, which are crowding out the other cells and stopping them from doing their jobs."

If your child needs chemotherapy for leukemia:

"The medicine we will give you will, hopefully, stop the white cells growing so fast and give the red cells more room to do their job." (If your child has bone cancer, say ". . . will make your lump get smaller.")

If your child needs radiation:

"You will need to lie still on a special bed while a machine like a big camera shines a special light on part of your body. The light is very powerful and it needs to go to exactly the right place and nowhere else, which is why you have to be helped stay so still. ("It will get rid of any cells that might be left over from the tumor" or whatever the purpose of the radiation is.)

If your older child needs a brief overview of the course of the treatment, for example, for osteosarcoma:

"For several weeks, you will take some medication called chemotherapy that will make the tumor get smaller. Then the doctors will help you go to sleep with anesthesia and take out what is left of the tumor. After that, they will give you some more chemotherapy for several more weeks to try to be sure that no new tumors grow."

Encourage questions and ask whether your child would like a fuller description or whether he or she would prefer to be told when things are about to happen.

If your older child could benefit from more information about possible side effects, I would describe in advance only likely side effects, not unlikely ones:

"Some children feel nauseous when they take this medication, but some do not. Let us know what you notice. If you do feel sick, the doctors are able to give you different medications that should make you feel better."

With steroids, say, "Some children feel a little different when they take steroids, are more easily upset or more easily frustrated, but some children do not feel very different. Let us know what you notice."

"Occasionally the medications have a few other effects, so tell us if you notice feeling any different and we will tell the doctors."

If your child was hit by a car and the driver was badly at fault:

I might add to the explanation given on p. 48: "The driver is going to talk to a judge in court and explain what happened. Would you like to know what happens? If the judge thinks he was driving dangerously, he may be punished for what he did (lose his license, pay medical costs)."

If you think your child will benefit from having a role in some medical decisions:

"The doctors can have us come into the clinic on a Tuesday or Wednesday next week. Which day would you prefer to be in school? We can ask to come in the other day."

Your Six- to Eleven-Year-Old's Reaction

Like younger children, school-age children show varied reactions. Some may show positive adjustment throughout treatment. Others may seem to adjust with little difficulty at first but seem more upset later. Some may withdraw or become depressed, irritable, angry, or anxious. They may seem more dependent on you or actively resist treatment. Some school-age children may, in addition, be anxious about school and keeping up with their schoolwork. A few may refuse to go to school or say they feel sick once they get there. Some school-age children may also be upset about temporarily losing strength or skills, which can prevent them from keeping up with friends or even being with friends. Some may feel different from their friends and feel quite isolated. Some children may return to using magical thinking and other earlier behaviors and thought patterns.

Helping Your School-Age Child

You can help your school-age child, particularly the six- to eight-year-olds, by encouraging them to use puppets and medical play (see p. 50).

Free play is also useful for preschool and school-age children who have a hard time expressing themselves verbally. A seven-year-old child in our pediatric oncology clinic would construct battles between the "good army" and the "bad army" that had plenty of casualties on both sides, but the good army always won (as we hoped the good cells would defeat the bad cancer cells). A nine-year-old boy who had a long and extremely difficult treatment and who was normally the most good-natured of souls would register his distress by engineering a massive pileup of his much-loved toy cars.

Art and drawing are very effective therapeutic tools for preschool and school-age children. Children are often able to convey their deepest feelings in poignant and heartfelt ways through their drawings. You can ask your child to create a drawing illustrating something about his or her situation specifically or generally. ("Draw your family before your treatment/illness" and then "Draw your family now." "Can you draw a picture that shows something about what is going on now?")

An older child can be given a specific task combining drawing and talking. ("A mandala is a circle that can be divided into different sections. Draw a mandala that shows your different feelings when you heard about your illness/on the first day you went back to school. Give each feeling a color. Color in the mandala, giving the appropriate size to each feeling, and we can then talk about what you've drawn.")

Stories can be another great therapeutic tool for preschool and school-age children. Stories about animals or children who overcome adversity and stories that use metaphors to convey a message of hope show the benefit of persistence and endurance are great to use with this age group and even younger children. *The Little Engine That Could* is a prime example of such a book. *Bravery Soup* is another. For older children there are many stories where a child succeeds despite adversity or overcomes a health problem to achieve a major goal. You can look at the children's book lists beginning on p. 400 to get ideas for appropriate books to get for your child.

Clay is a great medium for preschool and school-age children. Children can make the object of their fears and then change the feared thing into something they are not afraid of. An eight-year-old sister of a patient who was having a stem cell transplant was having difficulty staying in her own room at night because she thought of "scary things." She made some scary monsters out of clay. I had her change them into friendly animals and then suggested she keep the clay by her bed so she could do the same when she woke up at night. Though she still made occasional visits to her mother in the night, the clay animals helped her to stay in her own room more frequently. You can see how your child enjoys making her own monsters or friendly animals.

Therapeutic games for school-age children such as ShopTalk, a game for children with cancer ages seven to sixteen years, in English and Spanish,[1] or The Angry Monster Machine, for children who appear very angry, can be extremely helpful. You can also tailor a game to suit the situation. These games often allow a child to be more open about their experiences and emotions than if they were asked directly without the protection and distance provided by playing a game.

I once designed questions for a suicide assessment with a ten-year-old child, Jill, using the board from the Thinking, Feeling, and Doing game, which allowed me to ask, "Do you ever think about hurting yourself?" and "Do you ever wish you were dead?" Jill answered yes to both questions, adding, "But I would never do it because Mommy would be so sad." Jill earned tokens for each answer she gave and at one point said, "I know what you are doing, but this is fun." This provided the springboard for more conversations about what was so hard and what else might help her not act self-destructively in her more desperate moments.

For some children and adolescents, certain music is distracting, absorbing, calming, and comforting. For others, it can be a wonderful form of self-expression. I worked with an eight-year-old, Mike, who was a young rapper. Mike held the microphone on my tape recorder while he rapped about how angry and sad he got about his illness, which made him act "mean" to people he loved—and how that, too, made him sad. See how your child responds to the idea of listening to some of his favorite music in the clinic or hospital.

Some children can talk directly about what is bothering them. As I mentioned, they often will find this easier if they are doing some other task at the same time like playing a game or doing an activity like coloring or knitting. So don't be surprised also if your child starts a difficult conversation while she is doing something else. This other activity may give her a little distance from the conversation or a safe place to return to if the conversation becomes too anxiety-provoking. A child can talk about various worries: that the treatment will not work, that she will be stuck in the hospital for a long time; that friends will laugh at her when her hair falls out, that she will not be able to keep up in school, or that her friends will forget about her, as well as her fears about not getting better. Often, sharing the worries helps your child feel less alone and may allow strategizing about whether there are things to do or think that might help her feel better.

Adolescents Ages Twelve to Seventeen Years

Adolescence is a time of upheaval, with bodily changes, emerging sexuality, and emotional vulnerability coming at the same time that adolescents are developing new intellectual and physical skills. Many adolescents are increasingly involved with friends and want more independence from you. They may have mood swings, be self-conscious about their appearance, want more control than you think reasonable, take risks, and be quite difficult to live with—and this is before they get sick.

Stressful factors for most adolescents about a long hospitalization

A long hospitalization or illness can affect every aspect of an adolescent's life:

♦ It sets back his growing independence. He needs you in ways he would not if he was not sick—perhaps to help dress or bathe him or drive him around. It may make you feel closer again, but it may also be challenging for your adolescent.

♦ He is likely to have less daily contact with his friends.

♦ He may fall behind in his schoolwork or be unable to play sports.

♦ His physical appearance may be changed.

What to say and do right away

The doctor will, hopefully, give your adolescent a clear and straightforward medical explanation about what is happening. If your adolescent appears to be confused, you can ask the doctor to go over things again until the questions are answered. It is vital to gain your adolescent's cooperation. If your adolescent takes part in making medical decisions and is given choices where possible, he is more likely to feel he is a partner in a joint enterprise. Sometimes knowing how serious, even life-threatening, his illness is will persuade him to cooperate with a difficult treatment—particularly if the treatments will give him a good chance of cure.

Hopefully the description of the full treatment course will include describing common immediate side effects so he is not taken by surprise. The doctors can truthfully say, "Different people have different reactions to the medicines you are taking. Some people do not have much reaction. Others feel tired or sick or get mouth sores. Tell us what you notice. We can give you medications that we hope will help you feel more comfortable."

If your adolescent could suffer some late effects from the treatment, you can ask if she wants to hear about possible (but uncertain) long-term effects from the treatment now or down the road.

Reactions in Adolescents

Not surprisingly, adolescence is a very hard time to become ill. There are major differences between adolescents in their temperaments and their reactions to illness, but it is invariably challenging. Some adolescents continue their lives in the most remarkable way. Others show little reaction at first but more response later. Some may become

- ◆ Angry
- ◆ Withdrawn
- ◆ Depressed
- ◆ Rebellious
- ◆ Noncompliant with treatment

Helping Your Adolescent

Acknowledging directly or indirectly that you realize that this setback has come at a very difficult time for your adolescent—when she or he was hoping for more freedom, more independence, more time with friends and less with family—may be a useful start. And when you are faced with mood swings, rudeness, or rebellion, perhaps you can remind yourself that your adolescent is dealing with emerging sexuality, physical changes, and hormones churning on top of her medical condition. Be sympathetic if possible.

Encourage your child to join a group for adolescents going through medical challenges, if one exists. In our hospital there were rarely enough adolescents in the facility at the same time for an inpatient group to be feasible. Outpatient groups worked best when they centered on an activity and allowed important feelings to be shared spontaneously. Our staff organized several activities for adolescents: "Look Good, Feel Better" sessions, where girls were helped to use makeup; an Outward Bound day program; concerts with donated tickets; and visits to baseball games or spring training. Serious conversations often occurred during these activities. Occasionally a guidance counselor at an adolescent's school would organize a support group for her friends which she could attend when she was in school. Several adolescents found such a group a welcome support, and it is worth finding out what is available to help your adolescent.

Talking about the experience and its effect on their lives can help an adolescent gain perspective, understanding, and hope. Cognitive behavioral strategies considering how an adolescent is looking at his experience—noticing, for example, if he is catastrophizing or overgeneralizing—can help him shift attitudes and perspectives. Some adolescents are helped by talking with their friends; others feel estranged from their friends. Some will talk with a family member or a therapist.

Writing poems and stories, keeping journals, or writing letters of advice can be wonderful ways for articulate older children to express their feelings. Sometimes a hospital or clinic has a newsletter that encourages contributions from children or adolescents. Encourage your adolescent to send in a contribution if he enjoys writing.

A YOUNG ADOLESCENT'S POEM

I Am

I worry if I am going to get better

I cry when I see people being cruel to animals
I am a funny and happy boy that has AA^2

I understand there is a lot of kids with cancer

I say it's not fair

I dream someday we'll find a cure

I try to fight through it

I hope others will win that battle
I am a funny happy boy that has AA

Adolescents can give very perceptive advice to others in their situation. This letter was written by the same boy. He had to have a stem cell transplant and wrote a letter of advice for other kids who might have to have a transplant one day.

AN ADOLESCENT'S LETTER OF ADVICE

Dear Kids,

I know how you must be feeling and I'm writing to help you. I know you must be worried about some things . . . I'll tell you some new thoughts I've learned to help cope.

You Look Different and People Will Stare

Looking different will go away. You'll get used to differences. You can always wear a hat and no one will know the difference. Also people may stare because they are curious and don't understand, not because they are having mean thoughts.

Your Teacher or Your Friends Treat You Differently

They may treat you differently because they don't know. They do care for you, though.

You Also May Not Know the Questions in School

But I bet you do know some. Study or ask questions for the others.

It Also Might Be Weird Going Back After Being at Home or the Hospital for So Long

You can take it little by little. Meet friends at school for lunch or recess and have them over. Also visit with your family members. Also you may end up being relieved to go back to what you have.

You Might Not Want to Be Overcrowded with Questions

The school visit will help with questions. You can always ignore questions, walk away, or say you don't know.

You Might Not Want to Be the Center of Attention

But you can still find a way to keep things private. You can say you don't want to talk about it to people. Maybe you can talk about it to your parents, teachers, and good friends and explain to them how you feel, and they can be the ones to explain to people how you feel and that you don't want to talk about it.

Lastly, It Might Be Scary Because You Have Got So Used to Being Home

It's normal and it's OK to be a little scared. Soon you will be used to being away from home again.

Sincerely,

A kid who had a transplant too

Sometimes a school project can offer a great opportunity for an adolescent to acquire knowledge, assume control, and achieve mastery. Several adolescents chose to report on their illness and treatment as part of required science projects. However, you need to be sure this is his choice without outside pressure. If an adolescent does such a project, he gets the triple benefits of increasing his knowledge of his own illness and treatment, gaining perspective on what is happening, and sharing his experience with peers. If you think this could be a valuable outlet for your adolescent and he seems enthusiastic, you can share the idea with his teacher.

Art, collage, and drawing can also be a valuable means of expression for an adolescent (see page 59). An adolescent can use the mandala to express mixed feelings about various difficult subjects like seeing friends again or having a relapse. You can give her a sketchbook and give her the freedom to draw what she wants, which she can share with you or not as she chooses.

Music can be a wonderfully absorbing or distracting therapeutic tool. Rapping, songwriting, and composition can be forms of self-expression. An adolescent can bring earphones to the clinic or the hospital and an iPhone or iPod filled with his favorite tunes.

You may already know the medium through which your adolescent is most likely to express himself. You can supply the tools, make suggestions, and be encouraging whether or not he wants to show you what he has done.

The next chapter describes the stresses and possible reactions of your other children and simple ways to help them. Then chapter 6 describes circumstances where you, your partner, or a child of any age may benefit from help from consultation with a psychosocial staff member.

CHAPTER 5

· · · · · · · · · · · · ·

Your Other Children

Your other children are hugely affected when their brother or sister has to go to the hospital for a serious medical condition. The more worrisome the condition, the greater is the impact. Your life has been turned upside down, and their life probably feels turned upside down, too. You may be upset, infrequently at home, and unable to pay as much attention to them as usual. Their brother or sister is away in the hospital, and even when they visit, he or she may seem different. Their routine has changed. Depending on their age they may feel left out, confused, or angry. They may worry about him or feel their teachers and peers do not understand. They may need to miss outside activities and even some school. Over time, despite your efforts to be even-handed, your other children may feel the child who is ill is getting special treatment. From your other children's perspective, the situation may not improve even when he comes home from the hospital. School friends and/or family may continue to ask about him and bring him presents. He may have a tutor at home instead of going to school, and there may be fewer expectations about his behavior. One sibling told me, "I was the littlest and got spoiled. Since he got sick, he's the one who gets spoiled." Even if there are good reasons for all these circumstances, it is very difficult for your other children not to feel aggrieved.

Many studies have looked at the effects on children who have a brother or sister with chronic health conditions. The results have been variable, and sometimes contradictory. Overall, many siblings appear to have long-term positive adjustment outcomes, although subgroups have some negative findings.[1] Positive effects included more maturity, a greater capacity for empathy, and increased sensitivity.[2] A significant number of siblings go into caretaking professions. The most recent analysis of these studies found more internalizing and externalizing symptoms[3] and somewhat more negative self-attributes amongst siblings (though less true of younger siblings) when compared with their peers.[4] It also found that these effects were strongest if the chronic health condition was life-threatening and/or greatly interfered with the family's daily life. One well-designed study found older siblings and girls were more adversely affected and hypothesized this was because they were more involved in their sibling's care and thus their lives were more disrupted.[5] Researchers are also trying to tease out the impact of coping styles and family functioning on long-term sibling adaptation and how to recognize and intervene with those siblings who are most at risk.

The good news is that you can make a big difference to your other children's experience depending on how you respond to them. But first let's look at the understandable reactions of brothers and sisters.

YOUR OTHER CHILDREN'S REACTIONS

The pictures and the words of siblings show the impact better than any attempt at description.

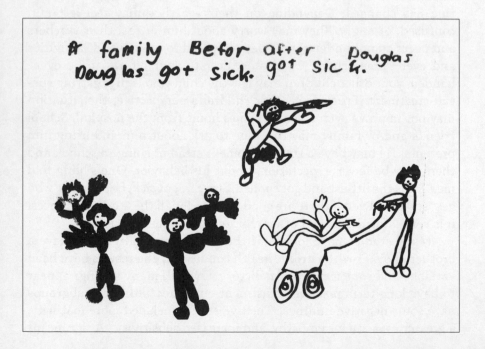

Prior to her brother's illness, six-year-old Jessica imagined she had one parent to herself, and that her brother had the other one. After the illness she draws him in the center of the picture; she is to the side on a parent's shoulder screaming! She has noticed her family's life now revolves around him and she does not like it.

A collage assembled by one family at Sibling Day in the outpatient clinic made the same point differently. Families were asked in whatever way they liked to show how the illness had affected the family. This family drew its members forming a pyramid. The parents were on the bottom, the well siblings were on their shoulders, and the child who was ill was on the shoulders of the siblings. They saw the whole family's current task as supporting the child who was sick.

Older brothers and sisters are more likely to understand that their brother or sister has something seriously wrong and to feel guilty if they feel mad. Some brothers and sisters feel they cannot upset their brother or sister because he or she is ill or hurt. The sister who drew this picture did not feel so constrained even though her brother was in a wheelchair!

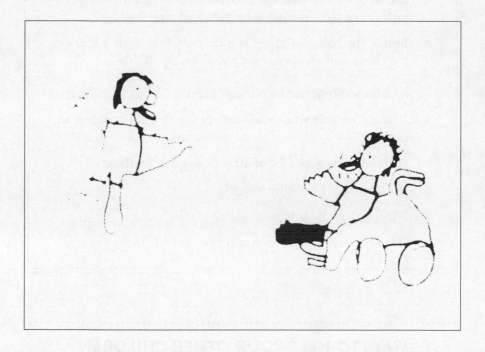

SIBLING REACTIONS

Here is a sampling of the reactions written by siblings:

- "If I'm mean to him, then I feel bad because he's sick."

- "We haven't argued since she got sick. I try to keep her happy."

- "Sometimes he's mean to me. He can get away with it because I feel okay and he doesn't."

A brother drew three balloons.

- Inside the first balloon he wrote, "Too much . . . Mad, Sad, Upset, Angry, Jealous, Envy."

- Inside the second balloon he wrote, "Too much" and drew pictures of balloons, flowers, and presents.

- Inside the third balloon he wrote, "Too much" and drew pictures of pills, medicine bottles, and a syringe.

- Beside the balloons there is a cartoon face with a tear on the cheek and an open mouth exclaiming, "Ohh!"

A sister wrote after the phrase "I feel":

- "Uncomfortable when she and my family gets upset, mad, sad, etc."

- "Left out. She gets a lot of attention, gifts, cards, etc."

- "Sad, for she is my only sister."

- "Happy that she is in remission."

- "Mad because it splits our family up for a little."

WAYS TO HELP YOUR OTHER CHILDREN

How can you help your other children when you are feeling overwhelmed and pulled in a million directions?

These five words can be a guide:

♦ Empathize
♦ Explain
♦ Include
♦ Listen
♦ Delegate

When you **empathize** with your other children about what is hard for them (that you are away, that they have to miss an extracurricular activity or can't meet up with friends), you are letting them know you understand and are sorry about it, too. They are not alone in their disappointment.

When you **explain** to them in age-appropriate ways what is wrong with your other child and why you need to be with her, you are removing the mystery from the situation. At the same time, you can make the point that if one of them had got sick, you would be doing the same for each of them.

When you **include** your other child in your child's care (be it visiting the hospital, meeting the medical staff, seeing the hospital playroom, or if the hospital is too far away, talking to your sick child on the telephone or Skyping, sending cards or emails, bringing home your sick child's homework), you are allowing your other child to feel useful and included.

When you **listen** to your other child—on the telephone, by Skype, Facetime, or face-to-face—you can learn a lot. You can get hints about what is on her mind from what she says and from what she does not say. She may tell you directly what is worrying her or she may avoid discussing a subject that you know must bother her and may need your help to bring it up. She may show you directly what she understands or misunderstands about what is going on or she may need you to ask. After your child gets home from the hospital, you will see how all your children are dealing with one another and will know whether you need to intervene. Are your other children being mean or too nice to your sick child—or are they treating one another as roughly as they did before the illness or accident? Maybe you will need to let a brother know that it is not okay for the sick child to hit him, and reassure him that the reason his sister is being so mean is not because of anything that he has done but because she is feeling sick and fed up. Assure your other child that you too regret how things have changed and you appreciate the sacrifices that he has had to make (missing after-school activities, staying with grandparents, whatever the sacrifices may be) in the process, by saying whatever you need to to let him know you understand that this is hard for him, too.

When you **delegate** to others what you are unable to do on your own (having your other children do a weekly activity with a special friend, having them join SuperSibs through the Alex's Lemonade Stand website,[6] or getting someone to bring them to the hospital for sibling programs or to meet with a psychosocial clinician), you are showing your other children that you care about them and they are special too. Your other children can benefit greatly from learning they are not alone and that other siblings are being faced with similar challenges.

SCHOOL AND COMMUNICATING WITH TEACHERS

School is an important part of your children's lives. School and friends can provide a sense of normalcy when family life has been disrupted. It is also a place where a child may show feelings and behavior that he is deliberately not showing at home. This makes it particularly important that you communicate with your children's teachers. Make sure they understand that you want to hear from them about any concerns they may have.

Your child's teacher should keep you updated. Ask the teacher how your child is keeping up with her work, how her performance or behavior has or has not changed, and, possibly, how her friends are reacting. You can explain to the teacher how brothers and sisters can be adversely affected by such an upsetting family event. It is reasonable for you to ask the teacher to give your child some extra support and attention.

You may want to discuss with the teacher and your healthy child what the teacher will say to classmates. Families have very different attitudes about this. Some parents and children like information to be shared; others do not. You will have your own perspective. The school principal may have a policy about how and what information is shared with parents if a child becomes ill. The advantage of some clear communication from the school to other parents even if your sick child is not in the school is that unfounded rumors are less likely to spread that might have negative effects on your other children. For example, you do not want parents to fear that your children are being exposed to an infectious disease and therefore they should be avoided. You also may want to ask the teacher to let you know if she develops any concerns about your other children down the road.

Circumstances in which you might want any of your other children to have a consultation with a psychosocial staff member in the hospital or clinic are described in the next chapter.

··

SIBLING GROUPS

It is extremely useful for children over the age of three to get together with other siblings who have brothers or sisters with medical challenges.

At Dana-Farber many years ago, we started a special day held once a year for the brothers and sisters of our patients. It began with a puppet show starring brother and sister animal puppets. One animal was sick, the other was not. The animal who was sick started by saying how he has been in the hospital, how everyone quite rightly has been paying him lots of attention, and that he will be happy to tell the audience all that has been happening to him, which is he is sure why they have come. He is then gently told by the puppeteer that actually this day is for the brothers and sisters of children who get sick. Then the animal who was not sick described all the things that have been hard for him and how everything at home has changed since his brother got sick. He mentioned not seeing his parents every day, seeing everyone pay lots of attention to his sick brother and give him presents. He told the brothers and sisters present how happy he was to see them and he hoped they would have a good time talking to one another. Then the children divided into groups for age-appropriate activities and conversations that related to having a brother or sister with medical difficulties. Reactions to the puppet show started the discussion. Each age group got a tour of the medical clinic and got to see and use some of the medical equipment. At the end of the day, they met up with their parents for a joint family activity. Most siblings and parents found the day very valuable, but many said they wanted something for brothers and sisters more than once a year.

A few years later, a senior social worker and a sibling specialist greatly improved what we offered brothers and sisters:

- They organized a monthly group for siblings in the hospital to which siblings of children who were outpatients could also come.
- During one school vacation week, siblings were encouraged to come to the clinic with their brother or sister, to meet

with the doctor, and then to take part in a special sibling activity. Parents were encouraged to have siblings bring in questions for the doctor.

♦ Another school vacation week was called Sibling Week. Siblings accompanied their brother or sister to clinic for the day. Activities included music or art projects in the morning and focused activities in the afternoon where they shared their experiences and gave advice to other brothers and sisters of a child who was sick.

♦ Once a year, several athletic psychosocial staff members accompanied a group of adolescent siblings to an Outward Bound program in Boston. Siblings surmounted various physical challenges like completing a ropes course, helped by Outward Bound staff. The staff reported that the informal conversations between the siblings during the day were moving and illuminating.

The staff also raised money to make a sibling video called "Sibling Voices" that features children whose brothers and sisters were being treated at Dana-Farber. The siblings discuss frankly what it is like having a brother or sister who is ill. You can watch the moving reactions of siblings on YouTube and can decide if your other children might benefit from seeing it.[7]

The availability of these kinds of programs will depend on the circumstances and the available staff and resources in your hospital or clinic. Ask a psychosocial staff member what your hospital offers. You can point out that having a week where siblings are encouraged to visit the clinic, sit in on your child's clinic visit, and look around the clinic would take very little extra staff time. (The clinic tour could even be given by your child!) Find out if it is possible to have some special sibling activities during that week and point out the benefits of such activities. Find out if there are any Outward Bound programs nearby and either contact them directly or see if a psychosocial staff member would do so. You would also need to find out whether there might be any potential funds to pay for a day of sibling activities. An ongoing program for siblings, although extremely useful, usually requires a staff member with designated time to organize, run, and maintain it. If there are limited resources and staff time, sibling events that occur during regular clinic hours once or twice a year may be more possible.

•••

TOOLS FOR YOUR OTHER CHILDREN

There are several excellent activities to which your other children can be introduced when they are with other siblings. My favorite group sibling exercise for children between five and twelve was called the Emotion Ocean. The children draw and color a rough sea complete with sea creatures on a large white piece of paper pinned to the wall. Afterward, they write on sticky notes what has been hard about having a brother or sister who has been sick. A staff member makes the analogy that having a sick brother or sister is like being in a very rough sea. Then children build rafts of tongue compressors, on each of which a child has written something that has helped him or her stay afloat. (For example: Talk with my dad/Play in my room/Listen to music/Being with family/ Talk/Cry/School/Walk/Read a good book/Make a gift/Make a friend/ Doing my best.)

This exercise is appealing because it allows brothers and sisters to express their feelings, find constructive solutions to deal with the challenges, share feelings and ideas, and combine them together "to float." Brothers and sisters learn from each other and can share ideas as they go along.

At the end of each day, the Emotion Ocean posters were pinned on the passage walls that led to the clinic. Brothers and sisters could explain to their parents and their sibling who was sick what they had written down and why, and that sibling also had a chance to look at the ocean and comments.

You could do this activity with an individual sibling or with more than one of your children, and talk about what has been created with your child who is sick.

Another good therapeutic tool is to provide a special journal for brothers and sisters in which they can write or draw about what is going on. An example is shown on page 76.[8]

Each page asks questions related to having a brother or sister with a difficult medical condition and what strategies help, with plenty of space for siblings to fill in their own answers. One page asks what advice the sibling has for other brothers and sisters in similar situations. Children love giving advice—and it is often very good advice! The book can be used with one child or can be used by parents or clinicians with a group of brothers and sisters who can then compare their answers and learn from one another. Prompts can include "I feel mad when I think . . ." "I calm down when I think . . ." I feel happy when . . ." "I feel helpless when I . . ." "I like it when . . ." "I don't like it when . . ."

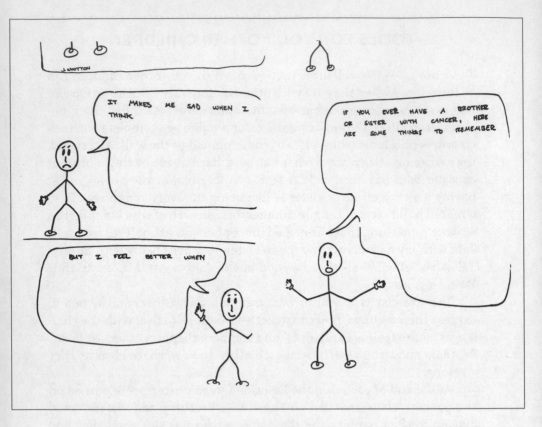

Another workbook, "Brothers and Sisters Together," is free and you can get it from the National Cancer Institute (NCI), where it is available in Spanish and English.[9]

Because children can often express so clearly what they feel in drawings, you can offer them the opportunity by suggesting:

- Draw our family before and after the illness/accident happened.
- Draw some of the feelings you have about your brother or sister's illness (or accident).
- Put together a collage that shows something about us as a family after your brother or sister's illness (or accident).

These drawings can give you lots of information about how your other children are experiencing things that you would be unlikely to learn if you asked them the questions directly.

If you have younger children at home, you might make up an interactive story about two animal siblings in which one gets sick and has to go to the hospital. You can begin a narrative about what happens to the other animal. You can always start with some of the points that our puppeteer made at the beginning of our puppet show described earlier, but if you ask your child what else the sibling animal puppet might say about what has happened in her life, you may get some surprises. Or you and your child could make your own book about what happens to an animal brother or sister when their sibling gets sick.

If your hospital runs sibling programs, I encourage you to use them. I cannot overemphasize how valuable group activities are for brothers and sisters—and how many brothers and sisters I have seen helped by their participation. Brothers and sisters go through a hard time, too, and even though you may do your best to empathize, inform, include, and listen, delegating some of the work may be invaluable. Delegating to individuals and groups who are skilled in providing brothers and sisters with opportunities to share with each other, to express themselves, to brainstorm about what helps during this tough time for the family, is a great gift you can give your other children.

And if such programs do not exist in your hospital, you can advocate for them, while trying to keep in mind the financial and staff constraints that may exist. You can always enroll your child as a SuperSib through Alex's Lemonade Stand.[10] Perhaps you can see if you can adapt some of the ideas developed here to your own situation. Perhaps you can make your own Sibling Week during your other children's school vacation weeks and you or a friend or relative can bring them into the clinic on your child's clinic day for their special time to meet with your child's doctor and look around the clinic. You can also help them plan special questions to ask the doctors or nurses. By doing such things you will help your other children feel included and recognized.

CHAPTER 6

· · · · · · · · · · · · · ·

When to Consult with a Psychosocial Clinician

Sometimes, despite your best efforts to help your child and your other children adjust to the circumstances, you or other family members may hit emotional roadblocks. It might involve you and your partner, your ill child, or one of your other children. In this case there are specially trained psychosocial professionals whose role it is to look at the situation, to help out, and to support you and your family in whatever way you need.

You might consider a consultation in any of the following situations. If your toddler or young child:

♦ Appears withdrawn, depressed, anxious, agitated, or angry over several weeks.
♦ Is head-banging or having prolonged, inconsolable tantrums.
♦ Is having particular difficulty with procedures.
♦ Is refusing to take all medications.
♦ Is behaving very differently from before diagnosis, over several weeks.

If your older child or adolescent:

♦ Appears withdrawn, depressed, anxious, or angry over several weeks.
♦ Is refusing to go to school or speak with friends.

- Is refusing to take medications.
- Is having serious difficulty with procedures.
- Is using alcohol or nonprescribed drugs.
- Is taking major risks like staying out late at night or ignoring doctor's orders.
- Seems very different from before diagnosis.

If your child of any age:

- Appears very depressed or gives any hint of suicidal thoughts.
- Is so anxious that his or her ability to make use of any coping strategies is severely limited.
- Is so out of control during medical procedures that he could hurt himself, you, or a staff member.

If any of your other children:

- Shows dramatic changes in behavior or mood (positive or negative) that have continued over several weeks and are getting more pronounced rather than slowly improving.
- Has major changes in sleeping or eating patterns.
- Makes repeated statements that suggest a serious misunderstanding of your sick child's condition or serious ongoing concerns about his or her own health.
- Shows major changes in behavior or school performance as reported by teachers or in his or her peer relationships that have continued over several weeks and appear to be getting worse rather than abating.
- Demonstrates increased reluctance to go to or stay in school.
- Has increasing and serious separation anxiety when not with you.

If you and your partner or ex-partner:

- Are having serious difficulties with each other, with the medical team, or in dealing with your child.
- Feel depressed, are very anxious, or have other concerning psychiatric symptoms or behaviors.

Other times to consult with a psychosocial clinician:

♦ If your child gets worse and your family is experiencing considerable stress and conflict.

....

PSYCHOSOCIAL CONSULTATION

If the psychosocial staff member is not part of your medical team, you will need to tell your child's primary doctor or nurse that you want a consultation. If the medical staff are requesting the consultation, they will have explained their reasons and whom you will be seeing. If a psychosocial clinician is on your medical team, request a special meeting. The clinician will likely meet with you before meeting with your child to discuss your or the staff's concerns. You can prepare yourself for the meeting by making a list of your own concerns and what you have done so far to address them. You can also think about how your child has reacted in previously stressful situations and what has helped in the past. Say what you think is contributing to the worrisome behavior. Describe to the clinician what you see as your child's strengths and his interests before his illness. You can discuss positive and negative interactions with medical staff and how you think the medical staff could help in the current situation. If your concerns relate to you, your partner, or your other children, again describe how you have tried to address them. Be sure to tell the clinician of any past family history that is contributing to current stresses. Find out which in-hospital supports there are for other family members or whether the clinician could help find an appropriate community resource. Sometimes an in-hospital psychosocial clinician would be available to meet for one or two sessions, but not on an ongoing basis.

Infants and Toddlers

Usually a psychosocial clinician would limit her consultation to speaking with you and observing your baby or toddler while you are in the room and when his nurse is interacting with him. She might then give you specific suggestions about the particular issue of concern—for instance, how to respond if your toddler is hitting you or the nurse, or how to reduce his anxiety going into the treatment room.

Preschool Children Age Three to Five Years Old

After meeting with you, the psychosocial clinician will meet with your child (with you or alone if your child can tolerate it). Do not expect your young child to tell the clinician what is bothering her—she probably has not put it into words! Through playing and talking with a child over time, a psychosocial clinician can hopefully get hints about your child's concerns and can plan with you how to help.

You could say to your child before the meeting something like "Someone is coming by who plays and talks with kids who are in the hospital." Or you could be more indirect if your child has become quite resistant to meeting new people—"Someone is coming by with a special friend (an animal puppet) who has been in the hospital a lot and wants to meet you."

School-Age Children Six to Eleven Years Old

After meeting with you, the clinician will meet with your school-age child. He will give you his recommendations after a few meetings. If the concerns relate to family issues, he may suggest family or couples therapy either with him or with an outside therapist. If the concerns relate to your child, he may recommend continued meetings with him with specific goals for the sessions such as reducing procedural anxiety and offering coping strategies.

Before the initial meeting with the clinician you could tell your child, "Someone is coming by to play and talk with you. He knows lots of kids who have had to be in the hospital/have lots of shots/feel ill/ have to do lots of PT/miss school/miss friends, etc. Maybe you and he can come up with some ideas that can help us all."

Adolescents

After meeting with you, the clinician will meet with your adolescent. The clinician will discuss confidentiality rules and their limits with you and your adolescent beforehand. You and your adolescent should know that what your adolescent tells the clinician is confidential unless he threatens harm to himself or others, which clinicians are legally obligated to report. Your adolescent is very unlikely to be forthcoming unless he knows that what he says is confidential.

After several meetings, the clinician will make recommendations that might include individual therapy for your adolescent and finding a separate therapist for you. Due to confidentiality constraints, it is often difficult to have the same therapist working with you and your adolescent. However, if the clinician is concerned about what the adolescent tells him—for example, that he is regularly not going to school—and thinks everyone would benefit from being informed, even if it does not involve safety, the clinician can explain his reasons to the adolescent. In my experience most adolescents will agree (and may even be relieved) that the information will be shared with his parents.

To introduce the idea to your adolescent, you might say, "What you are going through is hard. There is someone here who has talked with lots of older kids who have gotten very sick/had a bad accident. Why don't you meet with her a couple of times and see if you find it helpful? Sometimes it's good to have somebody outside the family to talk with about what's going on. What do you think?"

Your Other Children

After meeting with you, the clinician will likely suggest you bring in your child to meet with her. Depending on the age of your child, the clinician will probably discuss directly or indirectly the impact of a sibling's illness on a family and on the brother or sister in particular, describe typical sibling experiences, and find out if any of them resonate with the child. Two clinical examples follow of a consultation with a younger and an older sibling. In the first example, the sibling is suffering from the belief that many younger children have that they caused their sibling's sickness, particularly if they have had a competitive or combative relationship with the child who is sick.

A SIBLING'S STORY—SARAH

Sarah was six years old. Her sister, Joy, aged eight, had recently been diagnosed with a brain tumor. Since Joy's diagnosis, Sarah's behavior had changed dramatically. Previously she had been an easygoing, fun-loving child who got on well with her sister most of the time. Now she was clingy, crying a lot, having considerable difficulty getting to sleep, and waking up with nightmares. She refused to go to school, which she had previously enjoyed.

Sarah was friendly when she came with me to my office. During the interview, she drew her family doing some of their favorite activities. We chatted about Joy and what the two of them had done together before she got sick. I asked her about her sister's illness and whether she had had any thoughts about what might have caused it. Sarah immediately said, "I did. We were playing, I knocked her over. I think I caused it and I feel bad inside." I was able to reassure her she did not cause her sister's brain tumor. Sarah agreed I could tell her parents what she had been thinking. We also organized a meeting with Joy's doctor so he could explain again to Sarah that although we did not know exactly what had caused Joy's tumor, we did know for certain that it was not caused by Sarah's knocking her over. The doctor also told Sarah the tumor had been growing since Joy had been quite little.

Sarah's behavior greatly improved. She remained somewhat clingier than she had been (which is not uncommon), but her nightmares stopped, she cried less, and she began to enjoy school again. I continued to meet with her periodically and would check in with her regarding how she was viewing Joy's condition. Sarah was able to say firmly that she now knew she had nothing to do with her sister's diagnosis.

So be sure when you explain your child's illness to a young brother or sister to say explicitly that even if the doctors do not know exactly what caused the condition, they do know that nothing that anyone did or said to him in the outside world caused it. If your hospitalized child had an accident and your other child could reasonably see himself as implicated (if they were playing in the road together when the accident occurred, for example) then it may be very important to get professional help to figure out how best to confront this so your other child does not go through life carrying a burden of guilt.

Older siblings can show major behavior changes and may benefit from a psychosocial consultation in some circumstances.

A SIBLING'S STORY—JACKIE

Jackie was fourteen years old. Her younger brother, Jeff, age eleven, had recently been diagnosed with cancer and was receiving chemotherapy in the hospital. Jackie was close to and protective of Jeff. She had become angry and uncooperative at home, her grades were plummeting, and uncharacteristically, she was getting into physical fights in school with her peers. Her parents brought her in to meet with me. After several meetings, it was clear that Jackie felt angry, concerned, helpless, and isolated from her family. She could not concentrate on her schoolwork and felt her classmates and teachers did not understand what was happening.

Her parents, her teachers, and the school counselor made the following changes: Her parents altered their schedules so they could take Jackie to the hospital more often. They arranged for her to meet with Jeff's doctors and helped her prepare a list of questions. They shared with Jackie their own anger, sadness, and helplessness at the situation. They accepted Jackie's offer to be the liaison with Jeff's teacher. Jackie's teacher became more understanding of Jackie's circumstances and agreed, with Jackie's permission, to tell her classmates about it. Jackie agreed to meet with the school counselor weekly to focus on peer relationships and with me periodically. She and her teacher agreed she would try and do much of her homework in school, where she could focus more easily.

With these interventions Jackie became a wonderful member of Jeff's care team, her schoolwork improved (though not to the level it had been), and she stopped having physical fights with her peers.

Depending on what transpires in the meeting with the sibling, the clinician may make a referral to a local therapist or school counselor. Most likely he will suggest your other children participate in whatever sibling programs are offered by the hospital or outpatient clinic so your other children will have the invaluable experience of sharing and learning with other siblings who have a brother or sister who is ill.

SUMMARY

Long hospitalizations and difficult treatments are hard for a child who is sick and for his brothers and sisters, in different ways at different ages, and this process is harder for some children than others, regardless of how old they are. Strong reactions can occur in children of all ages and in some instances may warrant consulting with a psychosocial clinician. There are many ways in which children can be helped to cope with what is happening, and the sooner these tools and strategies are introduced into your child's life, the sooner she is likely to start feeling better. The next four chapters describe how special breathing, relaxation strategies, distractions, guided imagery, and affirmations may help your child.

CHAPTER 7

. . . .

An Introduction to Coping Techniques

For many children, the most challenging parts of hospitalizations, treatments, and rehabilitation are not just the medical procedures, but also the anxiety, discomfort, and pain involved. The interventions I describe in the next four chapters are designed to help a child feel greater mastery of his experience in the moment.

Most of these tools and strategies are designed to reduce anxiety and the immediate experience of pain. Some address negative attitudes or mood. They can be taught separately or can be combined with one another as part of a more comprehensive plan to manage pain and anxiety. While they can be used to manage acute procedural pain, these same strategies can also be used to help children coping with chronic pain conditions such as headaches, abdominal pain, muscle pain, joint pain, or nerve-related (neuropathic) pain that can sometimes occur after radiation, chemotherapy, surgery, or other procedures. Most important, many of these strategies can also help an adult, adolescent, or a child cope more easily with the challenges of a prolonged hospitalization and a variety of other illness-related stressors that may arise from a child's treatment.

. . . .

WHY OUR PERCEPTION OF PAIN IS MALLEABLE

If we accidently touch a hot saucepan with our bare hand, nerve receptors in the hand will send signals through the peripheral nervous system into the central nervous system up to the brain. The brain is then responsible for producing the actual sensation or experience of pain. In other words, the experience of pain is not directly produced by the tissues, muscles, or bones in an affected area but rather by what is going on in the brain when it registers the sensation.

Because the brain produces the sensation of pain, we can often use brain-based interventions to reduce both the intensity of pain (how much it hurts) and pain duration (how long it hurts). Interestingly, there is not one special area of the brain that is solely responsible for producing pain sensations. Rather, pain sensation is produced by a complex interplay of many areas of the brain and is influenced by individual factors, such as age, gender, and genetics, including pain susceptibility and pain-related memories. Pain sensation is also directly influenced by emotional factors such as fear, worry, and sadness. This is true whether the origin of the pain is from internal or external damaged tissue (nociceptive pain) or from damaged or malfunctioning nerves (neuropathic pain). Pain medications can act on the local site or within the central nervous system (the spinal cord and brain) to lessen or block pain sensations.

Thus pain intensity can be altered by changing the messages that travel between the place in the body where there is pain to the brain and back again. We can often modify or change pain sensations by changing what we choose to do about the pain and how we think about the pain. For example, if we bump our forehead going through a low doorway and rub the affected area, we likely reduce the sensation of pain because we have activated competing sensations (through our sense of touch) that override or diminish the pain messages. If we catastrophize the extent of the injury ("Perhaps I've got a concussion and will need to go to the hospital"), the sensation of pain will likely increase. In contrast, perhaps you remember a game of tag when your child was playing, fell down, got up, continued playing, and did not notice his knee was badly skinned till the game ended. This is an example of how the distraction of the game minimized the attention to the pain and thus reduced, indeed eliminated, the actual pain sensation.

This is all good news for us, parents and clinicians alike who are trying to alleviate a child's perception of pain. In many cases, pain can be greatly diminished by the use of medications. However, it is important to understand that because pain sensation is processed in the brain, we can often also reduce pain intensity, pain duration, and pain-related fear or anxiety with the use of nonpharmacological strategies such as slow or fast breathing, relaxation, imagery, self-hypnosis, distraction, thought restructuring, and education.

It is also important to note that sometimes a child can develop a cycle of chronic or recurrent pain that can disrupt day-to-day functions such as sleep, social relationships, and the ability to attend school or participate in activities. Persistent pain can also impact mood and increase anxiety. When pain has gone on for a long time, it often requires a multidisciplinary approach to ameliorate. A recent book by Rachael Coakley outlines the combination of factors that can contribute to a chronic pain problem and beautifully describes multidisciplinary interventions combining cognitive behavioral, physical, and pharmaceutical methods to improve a child's functioning and help the family manage the pain more effectively.[1] If your child is suffering from chronic pain, I strongly recommend you read her book.

There are many ways in which these interventions can also help with acute procedural pain. Different strategies can be useful before, during, and after a particular procedure. They can be included as part of a behavior plan in which a child is rewarded for using them and for not doing other things like biting or hitting. A younger child may be taught these interventions directly, or they can be taught to a puppet or stuffed animal while the child initially listens and hopefully joins in later.

The drawing below illustrates a child's experience of getting a shot.

The child is tiny compared to the adults. His mother's face appears a cross between a devil and a monster, the doctor has a mean face. The needle is bigger than the child, who is defending himself the only way that appears possible—by running away. Our hope is if he learns some of the strategies described in the next few chapters, he will feel less fear and isolation and more efficacy. He would then draw a rather different picture!

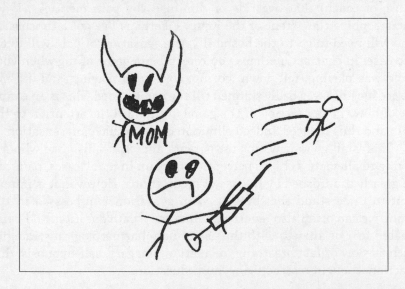

....

HOW PARENTS CAN HELP

You play a vital role in helping your child cope with medical procedures.

♦ You know your child best and what his style and temperament is, so you can help choose the strategies that will help him most.

♦ You will likely be with your child during most procedures.

♦ Your support is necessary for any interventions to work. Your child will look to you for encouragement and will also note your reaction and your attitude.

Because of this last point, it might be better in some circumstances, at least initially, for someone else to be with your child during medical procedures. If you recognize yourself in the following list, your presence during procedures may inhibit rather than help your child:

♦ If you are needle phobic or hate the sight of blood

♦ If you feel acutely anxious during the procedure

♦ If seeing your child hurting is truly unbearable

♦ If you suspect you will not be able to stick to an agreed-upon plan if your child gets upset

♦ If you are angry with the medical staff and are proud of your child when he resists

♦ If you seriously doubt any of these interventions will help your child

In any of these circumstances your child will probably have a better chance of learning and using these coping tools and cooperating with treatments if someone other than you is with him during procedures. If you are gradually able to watch and see that those interventions do help your child, you may feel different about them. You may then find it easier to be in the room with your child and to work with the medical staff. Talking to a psychosocial staff member may also help.

Children may show more distress overall when their parents are in the room; however, most children want you there and most parents want to be there.[2] Being with your child while he undergoes painful procedures is extraordinarily hard, so it is important to find ways to make it a little easier for yourself. Study after study has shown that children can use behavioral strategies effectively to reduce their anxiety and manage pain, and that the effectiveness of these interventions is well established.[3] Studies have also shown that a child is extremely attuned to a parent's emotion, and that the more anxious a parent is during a procedure, the more distress a child is likely to show.[4] Therefore, the calmer you can be, the better for your child.

Here are some suggestions for ways in which you can help your child if you choose to stay with him:

◆ Get to know the details of the procedure beforehand so you do not get blindsided by something unexpected happening.

◆ Remain calm (practice slow breathing for yourself).

◆ Show a matter-of-fact attitude and a positive expectation. ("It will be quick and you can do it.")

◆ Focus on your child versus chatting with the nurse or doctor. Your child needs your undivided attention.

◆ Work with your child's style. If your child is distractible, distract him. If vigilant, ask him focused, matter-of-fact questions that you have thought of in advance.

◆ Doing something with your child will likely let you feel less helpless and more focused. Practice relaxation techniques like slow breathing (for yourself and/or your child) in advance.

◆ Gently remind your child about or model the technique— taking slow breaths, for example. Do not insist that your child does something or criticize him for not doing it.

◆ Give your child limited choices such as which arm to use, NOT when to start the procedure!

◆ Set and keep to time limits. ("If the sand runs down in the egg timer and you are not still, then your nurse will help you stay still.")

◆ Work with the medical team and support their efforts. Notice what helped your child briefly stay still or recover more quickly and build on that next time.

◆ Think of something positive and truthful you can say to your child afterward that will encourage him for the next time. ("The procedure was quicker this time. Next time maybe we can see that it goes even faster.")

Recognize that what you are doing is very difficult. It is very hard to be in the room and watch your child suffer. One of the bravest parents

I knew was needle phobic. She could not sit beside her son while he was getting a spinal tap, but she remained seated at the far side of the room where he could see her. Do not expect that using these strategies will miraculously improve things right away. Usually they work slowly, over time, with practice, and the improvement comes in fits and starts with some backward steps, but with your child gaining greater control and confidence. Please believe that these strategies will help your child. In twenty-five years of experience working with young children going through invasive medical procedures, I did not meet one child who could not be helped a little in one way or another.

DIFFERENT PROCEDURES HAVE DIFFERENT DEMANDS

There are different sensations and emotions your child will have before, during, and after a procedure. Before a procedure, your child may be anxious; during a procedure, your child may experience pain and anxiety; and afterward your child will remember his experience in ways that will influence his attitude when he has a similar procedure again.

WHAT TO EXPECT DURING SPECIFIC PROCEDURES

- A **port-a-cath insertion** is a short procedure involving insertion of a needle into a port-a-cath that then allows blood to be drawn or medication given easily. (The port-a-cath will have been previously inserted surgically with anesthesia under the skin, usually on the left side of the chest.) If Emla cream, a numbing medication, is applied half an hour beforehand, your child should experience minimal to no pain sensation. However, some children can become acutely anxious during the needle insertion whether or not Emla cream is applied. Some parents prefer not to use the numbing cream because putting it on alerts the child that his port will be accessed and his protests start half an hour earlier than they would otherwise.

■ A **shot** or a **blood draw** causes a brief experience of pain unless Emla cream is used.

■ Happily, most US hospitals now do **bone marrow aspiration** and **spinal taps** under brief anesthesia, which has made a huge difference to children's well-being. However, when the procedures are done without anesthesia, they require considerable preparation and will cause painful sensations as the needle is inserted and when the bone marrow is withdrawn. After the insertion of the needle for a spinal tap, the child must remain completely still while the spinal fluid drips out. Here management of pain as well as anxiety is required.

■ **Radiation treatment**, a **CAT scan**, or an **MRI** cause no pain but require the child to remain still for varying lengths of time. The MRI also requires that your child tolerate a loud and unpleasant repetitive noise.

■ **Stereotactic radiation** requires the child's head to be placed in a specially fitted mask that is secured to the bed for the duration of the treatment.

■ Some **scans** require drinking preparations beforehand that are unpalatable to most children and can contribute to feelings of nausea and anxiety.

■ **Physical therapy (PT)** after an injury may be uncomfortable, at least initially, as well as physically challenging. PT often requires treatment several days per week for several weeks or months.

■ **Setting a bone** may require complete immobilization and be anxiety-provoking as well as painful.

PLANNING INTERVENTION STRATEGIES

Your plan or intervention needs to be suited to the particular procedure or condition and to address the sensations your child will experience. Anxiety can usually be significantly reduced before and during a procedure by using one or several of the following interventions: preparation, medical play, rehearsal, distraction, breathing, relaxation, and/or guided imagery. For example, a nurse can prepare a child by demonstrating a dressing change on a puppet or doll and the child can be asked if he would like to try it as well. Rehearsing going through a stressful procedure like an MRI can also help reduce a child's anxiety. A London hospital uses a model MRI machine complete with noise to prepare successfully children as young as three years old to have an MRI without anesthesia. We often rehearsed with a young child who was about to receive radiation by having the child practice lying still in the treatment room and talking to her parent on an intercom.

Managing acute pain or neuropathic pain may need more active strategies like rapid breathing, squeezing something, or an imagery or self-hypnotic technique that can shift how pain is experienced. Practicing breathing or imagery ahead of time develops a skill to the point that it can be used in stressful situations when pain is experienced. And a behavioral plan with rewards may increase your child's willingness to practice and use the strategies. Breathing and relaxation are described next. Distraction, affirmations, guided imagery and self-hypnosis are the focus of the later chapters.

CHAPTER 8

....

Coping Techniques

Breathing and Relaxation

....

THE FIGHT-OR-FLIGHT RESPONSE AND THE RELAXATION RESPONSE

Let's start by thinking about what happens to our bodies when they are relaxed and when they are not. Let's think how our bodies function. The peripheral nervous system includes the somatic nervous system, which is responsible for how we move our muscles and for how we experience the world through our senses, and the autonomic nervous system, which controls vital functions of our bodies like our breathing and our heart rate. Our autonomic nervous system operates most of the time without our conscious awareness.

The autonomic nervous system also controls the ancient reaction of the body to a perceived threat by automatically mobilizing the body's ability to respond quickly—our hearts race, adrenaline increases, our breathing gets faster, and our muscles tense. This is sometimes called the fight-or-flight response. When our bodies are in this state—hearts pounding, muscles tensed, breathing racing—they will be hyperalert to pain sensations. And tight muscles themselves can cause pain.

Occasionally the fight-or-flight response does not turn off, perhaps as a reaction to trauma or to repeated exposure to perceived painful events, in which case pain sensations will continue to be more intense. To counteract this fight-or-flight response, we can train our bodies to relax. This is sometimes called learning the relaxation response. If our muscles are relaxed, the pain sensation is lessened. Using slow, deep breathing and relaxation exercises are the most usual ways to bring on the relaxation response, which helps slow our heart rate, decreases our blood pressure, and reduces our muscle tension, among other benefits.

••

BREATHING AND BREATH CONTROL

There are many different ways you can help your child to use his breath to slow his body down and to feel calmer and more relaxed. It may help you too in facing the hassles of daily life. The important thing is to develop a slow, deep, rhythmic way to breathe that is practiced and calming and that you and your child can use when you want.

Indeed, special breathing and control of breath have a very long tradition and have been incorporated into spiritual practices, sports, and natural childbirth, and for chronic and acute pain and anxiety management. If you are not familiar with special ways of breathing to handle tension, you will likely find that you will benefit and feel calmer when you teach them to your child.

Children can use slow and fast breathing in age-appropriate ways. Here are a few ideas about how to begin to use breathing tools in enjoyable ways with your child age three years or older:

■ **Blowing Bubbles:** Most young children love blowing bubbles, so you can say something like this: "Let's blow some bubbles." After you have blown a few, say, "You are good. Now take a big breath in. Fill up your tummy so you have lots of air to blow out. Now blow out very slowly. The slower you blow, the bigger a bubble you make. Let's try it together. Wow, that was a great bubble. Let's do it again." (Repeat until your child gets the hang of it. Sometimes the bubbles pop, and sometimes they get so big you may be amazed, too!) Then you can ask, "What do you think would happen if you take a big breath in and breath out with some short, sharp breaths? I wonder if the bubbles will get smaller. Let's try." You can try it too and see whether the two of you can vary your breathing rate and the bubble size. Then you can say, "Notice how your body feels when you blow fast and when you blow slow. Which way helps your body feel calmer?" If your child says that she feels calmer when she blows slowly, you can tell her that is what you notice, too. And tell her that maybe you can both blow bubbles slowly when you want to feel calm.

> ▶ In the treatment room later, you can both blow real or imaginary bubbles while your child is getting his shot. If it goes well, you may

want to say something afterward like "Isn't it great that when you are doing something fun like blowing bubbles, you have less time to worry about getting a shot?"

■ A **pinwheel** is another wonderfully portable tool that can easily be brought into the treatment room. You can introduce a pinwheel and suggest to your child, "Can you blow and get the pinwheel to move? Great. Now take a deep breath in and then see how long you can keep the pinwheel spinning as you blow out. Wow, that was very long. Let's try that again. You are getting good at keeping it going for a long time. Now let's see if you can make it stop and start. That's neat. How do you feel when you blow it fast and when you blow it slowly?" You can add, "I notice when I blow it really slowly, I begin to feel calmer inside."

■ A **party blower** is another fun tool; your child can experiment with blowing it, starting by taking a deep breath in. Then you can say, "Let's see how quickly you can blow it out. Wow, that was quick. Now how slowly? If we bring it into the treatment room while you are getting your shot, will you promise not to blow it at the nurse giving the shot? I'll hold my hand up and you can see if you can reach it." This technique uses both breathing and distraction.

■ **Blowing out "birthday candles"** is another engaging blowing game: "Let's pretend my fingers are imaginary birthday candles. On your next birthday cake, how many candles will you need? Four? And maybe one for luck? Do you blow hard or soft to blow out a birthday candle? Hard, that is right. Let's practice. [Hold a finger out.] Deep breath in and blow. And now one big blow for each candle. Do you think you can blow them out before the nurse finishes doing the shot?" You can always bring up the other hand with more candles to blow out if the nurse has not quite finished.

■ **Balloon breathing** is a way to teach your child slow and rapid breathing by suggesting, "Take a deep breath in. Count 1, 2, 3, 4, and now as you let it out, make a noise like a slowly deflating balloon or a hissing snake. Take a deep breath in. Pause. *Sssssssss* as you breathe out. Great." Repeat several times until your child seems comfortable and does it at a regular pace. "Now let's take another deep breath in and maybe this time the air comes out just a little at a time. What would that sound like? *Hiss-s-s-s-s.* Great." Repeat until your child can do it and the sound resembles a controlled, repeated pant.

Once you have both chosen the special breathing to use, practice it with your child. For a younger child, start with only a few minutes of practice. In my experience, the slower breathing helps you and your child relax and stay calm; the more rapid breathing is useful if short procedural pain occurs. You want to avoid very rapid breathing, which can lead your child to hyperventilate. Have your child plan a special word or image to remind him to start his special breathing. For an older child, remembering or being reminded of the prop he uses may be all that is needed. The younger your child, the more he may need the actual physical prop.

Breathing Scripts

There are several terrific scripts for older children that teach breathing and combine breathing with mindfulness, yoga, and relaxation that are well written, child-friendly, and practical.[1] You can also use some of the props we described in the previous section to teach the breathing in these scripts.

DIAPHRAGMATIC BREATHING FOR RELAXATION

Deep and slow diaphragmatic breathing relaxes our bodies and calms our minds. When we inhale deeply, filling up the available space in our lungs, tummy, and rib cage, we counteract our tendency to breathe rapidly in a shallow way particularly when we feel tense.

You might say:

"If you breathe slowly and deeply, it will help your body to relax and feel calmer.

"I will count out loud to help you slow your breathing down and you can count in your mind with me: breathing in—one two, three, four; out—one, two, three, four.

"Now sit back in a comfortable chair (or lie on the floor).

"Let all the air out of your lungs.

"Breathe in deeply and slowly through your nose into your lungs, your belly, and your ribs.

"[Count slowly out loud] One, two, three, four."

Pause.

"Slowly breathe out through your mouth, one, two, three, four. Let all the air out of your lungs, ribs, and belly. Let your body relax at the same time."

Pause.

Repeat this four or five times until your child seems comfortable doing it. You can tell her: "Notice how your body feels a little calmer and more relaxed with each breath you take."

You can practice taking deep, slow breaths several times a day in different situations to calm down and compare notes about what you each notice.

You can substitute words like "calm" or "relax" for the numbers on the in-breaths and out-breaths depending on your and your child's preferences.

Some children may be helped by a concrete reminder that they are breathing deeply. These children may find it useful to place their hands on their tummies and to watch their hands rise and fall as they breathe in and out. Some children—indeed, some adults—prefer to focus on the movement of their hands rather than on their breath.

A longer exhale may be particularly useful when you want to encourage your child to release tension, worries, or negative emotions. We breathe in oxygen, which our bodies need, and breathe out carbon dioxide, a waste product our bodies do not need. You can easily suggest to your child that he is breathing in warmth, energy, and strength to the count of four, and he is breathing out the tensions and worries that his body does not need to the count of five.

RELAXATION TECHNIQUES

Progressive muscle relaxation (PMR) is a common way to teach relaxation. PMR involves either actually physically tensing and relaxing (active PMR) or imagining (passive PMR) relaxing your muscles sequentially in small muscle groups. In active progressive muscle relaxation, the idea is to tense (not strain) each muscle group for approximately ten seconds and then release for ten seconds. Repeat the exercise for each muscle group before moving on to the next one. Over time and with practice you can group the muscles together to achieve total body relaxation rapidly. With a young child, you may want to start with fewer muscle groups to avoid losing your child's attention.

ACTIVE PROGRESSIVE MUSCLE RELAXATION SCRIPT

"As you sit comfortably in the chair, take a slow, deep breath in through your nose into your lungs and your stomach. Slowly let the air out through your mouth. (Repeat several times.) And notice as you take each breath and slowly release it that your body feels more and more relaxed.

"Now stretch out your legs and feet, point your feet away from your body, and tense your feet muscles: 1, 2, 3, 4, 5, 6, 7, 8, 9, 10, and now relax them. Let all the tension go as you let your feet sink comfortably to the floor: 1, 2, 3, 4, 5, 6, 7, 8, 9, 10. Notice the difference between the tension and the relaxation and enjoy the relaxed feeling in your feet. (Repeat.)

"Next, stretch your feet toward your legs as you tense the muscles of your lower leg: 1, 2, 3, 4, 5, 6, 7, 8, 9, 10. And now relax them. Let all the tension go as you let your legs go back to resting peacefully on the floor with all the tension gone: 1, 2, 3, 4, 5, 6, 7, 8, 9, 10. (Repeat)

"Next tense the muscles in your upper legs, your powerful thigh muscles: 1, 2, 3, 4, 5, 6, 7, 8, 9, 10. And now relax them. Let the tension slip away: 1, 2, 3, 4, 5, 6, 7, 8, 9, 10. Notice how your legs now feel warm and comfortable, perhaps a little heavy, as they relax, and appreciate the difference between the tension that they did feel and the relaxed state they are now in." (Repeat.)

Repeat two cycles for each of the following muscle groups: hands, lower and upper arms, lower body, upper body, head and neck, and face, including the forehead, cheeks, and jaw.

"Now you have done a wonderful job of relaxing your whole body. Take a minute while your mind scans your body for any remaining places of tension. If you find tension anywhere, take a deep breath and let the remaining tension go. When your mind has completed its body scan, you can notice and enjoy the feeling of relaxation and comfort that your body now has."

After a few minutes say, "And know you can return to this comfortable relaxed state whenever you want by breathing slowly and deeply and tensing and relaxing your muscles. I will now count back from five to one, and when I reach one, you can be aware how refreshed, alert, and relaxed you feel."

If the exercise is intended to help sleep, the ending can be altered to "When I reach one, you can drift off into a deep and comfortable sleep."[2]

Useful information and adult and adolescent scripts for progressive muscle relaxation can be found online.[3] Some scripts have audio downloads, or you can record the script for yourself or your child. The Comfort Ability is the newly opened Pain Treatment Service Website of Boston Children's Hospital, and it will shortly include relaxation exercises, scripts, videos, and other useful resources for parents.[4]

For a younger child you can combine several muscle groups: feet and legs; hands and arms; lower and upper body; neck, head and face. Asking him to stand on his tiptoes, stretch up his arms, and tighten all the muscles is a good way to let him feel tension all over his body and then to notice the difference when he lets his whole body go floppy. You can also ask him to clench his fist and then relax it while using the tip of a pencil to gently touch the area of his hand below his thumb and index finger to show him how much softer the muscle is when relaxed. You can make learning PMR more interesting for your young child by including appealing concrete images in a script.

- ♦ "Squeeze your hands as if each hand had a lemon in it and you were squeezing out all the juice. Now drop the lemon and feel all the tension go out of your hands as you continue to breathe slowly and deeply.

- ♦ "Hold your arms (legs) out straight and stiff like uncooked spaghetti. Now let them become soft and relaxed and bendy like cooked spaghetti."

- ♦ "Make your tummy stiff and hard as the shell of a turtle that is hard enough to protect you from anything that wants to sit on it. Now the turtle can let himself feel soft and comfortable under the shell and you can let all that tension out from your tummy."

♦ "Wiggle your nose and your mouth to get rid of an annoying fly that you want to get rid of. Now it's gone, and your nose and mouth can relax."

You can find other examples of progressive muscle relaxation scripts for younger children online.[5]

You can record a customized script, making whatever alterations you think might appeal to your child. For example, if your child has a particular floppy stuffed animal she sleeps with, you can include him in the script. Your voice is likely to be appealing for your child to listen to. The memo device on many cell phones is an easy way to record a script. Practicing tensing and relaxing the appropriate muscles with your child is likely to help her to focus and to stay with the exercise.

Passive progressive muscle relaxation may be better to use if you or your child find it uncomfortable to tense muscles, or if your child dislikes tensing muscles. Passive PMR requires less physical effort but more imaginative effort. Passive PMR may make it harder for a younger child to recognize the difference between tension and relaxation.

PASSIVE PROGRESSIVE MUSCLE RELAXATION SCRIPT

"As you sit comfortably in the chair, take a slow deep breath in through your nose and let the air fill your lungs, then flow into your stomach. Slowly let the air out through your mouth." (Repeat several times.) "With each breath, notice your body feels more and more relaxed.

"As you continue to breathe slowly and deeply, imagine a warm light from the rays of the sun moving slowly over your body starting with your feet and your ankles. You can feel the warm light slowly moving from your toes up your feet toward your ankles, releasing any muscle tension as it moves. It covers the top and bottom part of your feet, which begin to feel warm, relaxed, and perhaps a little heavy. You can enjoy the feelings of relaxation in your feet as you continue to breathe slowly and deeply.

"And now the warm light moves up your lower legs, releasing any tension there. Your leg muscles begin to feel relaxed, warm, and perhaps a little heavy. Notice what a pleasant feeling that is as you continue to breathe slowly and deeply.

"Now the warm light moves up your upper legs, releasing any tension allowing your powerful thigh muscles to feel relaxed, comfortable, and perhaps a little heavy. You can enjoy the feelings of relaxation in your legs as you continue to breathe slowly and deeply."

[Repeat the instructions as you describe the warm light moving over each of the following muscle groups: hands, lower and upper arms, lower body, upper body, head and neck, and face, including the forehead, cheeks, jaw.]

"Now have your mind gently scan your body and let the warm light move over any part that does not feel completely relaxed and comfortable and release any remaining tension. You have done a wonderful job of relaxing your whole body. Notice and enjoy the feeling of relaxation and comfort that your body now has. And know you can return to this comfortable relaxed state whenever you want by breathing slowly and deeply and imagining the warm light relaxing your muscles.

"I will now count back from five to one, and when I reach one, you can be aware how refreshed, alert, and relaxed you feel."

(Or if the exercise is to help sleep, the ending can be altered to "When I reach one, you can drift off into a deep and comfortable sleep.[6])

Another script of passive muscle relaxation is available at the Guided Meditation Site.[7]

Passive progressive muscle relaxation for a younger child may include more concrete images. You can suggest to your young child that he feels soft and floppy like a rag doll or calm, relaxed, and comfortable like a purring cat. Or you can ask your child to imagine that she is painting a soft, soothing color slowly over her body, and as she paints each part of her body, that part becomes soft and relaxed.[8]

Other approaches combine relaxation with mindfulness strategies. More information about meditation, mindfulness, and relaxation is available online,* and several meditation scripts can be downloaded.†

Many children and adults find that soft music or sounds of nature,

---

* the-guided-meditation-site.com/more-on-meditation.

† www.the-guided-meditation-site.com/guided meditation downloads.

like ocean waves, in the background enhance relaxation. Children may want to choose their own favorite sound as background.

Breathing and relaxation are very effective strategies for dealing with the pain and anxiety associated with medical procedures. They can be taught in age-appropriate ways to even very young children. They help your child to stay calm so hyperarousal, tension, and anxiety do not exacerbate the sensation of pain. They also provide something for your child to do that can keep his attention away from the pain and they may lessen the perception of the pain itself. The more your child practices special breathing and relaxation, the better able your child becomes at using the strategies automatically in situations where he feels pain and/or anxiety. These will also be invaluable skills for facing stressful circumstances throughout his life.

CHAPTER 9

. . . .

Distraction and Affirmations

. . . .

DISTRACTION

Another simple tool to use to help a child going through medical procedures is distraction. You probably already try to distract your child if she is hurting. I am suggesting you consciously select those distractions you think will work best with your child. The distractions can be visual, auditory, tactile, or mental. A distraction can be a game for a playful child or questions about the procedure for a vigilant child.

DISTRACTIONS

	PRESCHOOL CHILDREN	SCHOOL-AGE CHILDREN
Visual	Pop-up books, egg timer	Visual focus, hypnotic wheel
Auditory	Songs, modified screams	Favorite tapes, conversation, jokes
Tactile	Squeeze hand, hold stuffed toy	Squeeze object, hold hand
Mental	Cartoon quiz, knock-knock jokes	Quiz, Pokémon, trivia questions

At our clinic, we kept boxes of enjoyable distractions in rooms where children had procedures. The boxes were filled with toys like pop-up books, light wands, superhero figures, squeeze balls, and sand timers that parents and children could use and return after the procedure. If your hospital does not have such boxes, bring favorite books or toys from home.

Distractions can help keep a child occupied and calmer before a procedure and allow a child to recover faster afterward. During a procedure, the best distraction is often squeezing someone's hand or a squishy object that can directly counterbalance a pain sensation. If you know the treatment will be painful, you might want to try both distracting your child and suggesting she use special breathing.

GETTING THROUGH A PROCEDURE USING DISTRACTION

Imagine a curious four-year-old child who becomes very frightened when she has to get a shot but wants to watch what goes on. She will soon be five, so we have been practicing blowing out five imaginary birthday candles, one at a time. She has had Emla cream put on her leg where she will get the shot. We choose a bug pop-up book that we will read in the treatment room. I start reading the book with her in the waiting area. When she is called by her nurse, I say, "Oh, good, we can go on reading the book in the examining room," and lead the way. When she is sitting on the examining table, I continue to speak in order to divert her attention away from the upcoming procedure:

"So how many bugs are under here? How did you know that? Whatever are they doing? Let's see how many bugs we can find before Annie (the nurse) is ready for us. She'll tell us when she's nearly ready. Now, how many bugs do you think are under here? Annie looks ready for us, so she will clean your leg. Now it's really clean. I wonder how the bugs would do if they were getting a shot. You could tell them Annie will count one-two-three, you'll blow one, two, three, four, five candles out and then it will be done. Notice carefully because with the Emla cream, wouldn't it be neat if you didn't even know you'd had the shot and you could tell the bugs that? Annie, go ahead. One, two, three . . . blow, one, two, three, four, five. Did you blow out all the candles? Great, it's done. So, let's see what the bugs have been up to since we last looked."

For vigilant children, it may be useful to ask them to pay close attention to certain aspects of the procedure such as "Notice exactly what it feels like so the nurses can be sure to tell the other children correctly" or "Notice what you feel this time because we put the Emla cream on a little earlier." Having a question to focus on will help your child to consider her answer rather than her anxiety.

For a child who does not need to watch what is happening, it is less necessary to refer to what the nurse is doing. I would ask the child beforehand, "Do you want Annie to count, 'one, two, three' before she puts in the needle, or would you rather she just does it while we are looking at the bugs?" And Annie and I would follow her preference. At the end I might say, "My goodness, you did such a great job looking at everything in the bug book, you hardly seemed to notice getting your shot. Is that right? Isn't it amazing when you are thinking hard about one thing, you hardly notice other things, like getting a shot?"

AUDITORY DISTRACTION

If you're coming up with things to say, sing, or play for your child, make sure you match the distraction to your child's temperament and interests. See the examples given below.

MARY

A three-year-old child, Mary, who had to go through many spinal taps and bone marrow aspirations without anesthesia was most comforted by having the entire medical staff and her mother sing her favorite nursery rhymes to her. Interestingly, the singing had a calming effect on the staff as well and changed the atmosphere in the treatment room from tension to one of relaxation and humor. Although Mary still cried briefly as the needle was inserted into her back, she quickly became calm as the singing resumed.

Some children like to choose a song to listen to, and adolescents can bring an iPhone or iPad with their favorite music on it. Earphones may enable a teenager to increase the volume while not deafening everyone nearby! Musical tastes differ considerably, so it is important that a child chooses music that will hold his attention most. Even young children may know absorbing songs, like those from the musical *Hamilton*, and might benefit from singing along while they listen.

Conversations on subjects that interest an older child or even telling jokes are obvious auditory distractions. However, a thirteen-year-old once told me he did not like too many jokes being made in the treatment room because it made it hard for him to do his breathing. (He had a doctor who had an inexhaustible supply of jokes!)

A child who is screaming (which may be a strong auditory distraction for the child as well as an effective protest) during a procedure can be asked if he could change the scream a little. The noise, however justified, may rattle the staff doing the procedure and make it harder for them to do what they need to do. One child I worked with managed to modify his earsplitting yells to "owee, owee, owee" which had the dual benefits of allowing him to see he could control his reaction and helping the staff do their job more easily.

TOUCH

Everybody is familiar with the benefit of squeezing something when experiencing something painful. Ask your child to squeeze a hand or an object to show what he is feeling. A strong adolescent may be given a squeeze ball or putty rather than his parent's hand. (Several parents reported suffering considerably from the strength of their teenager's squeeze!) A gentle touch from you can be a cue for a child to remember an intervention plan. For example, I had practiced a freeze game with a twelve-year-old child who had great difficulty in not moving when the doctor was trying to insert the needle for a bone marrow or spinal tap. We would practice in my office remaining completely still in different positions when I touched his arm and said the word "freeze." His mother and I used both cues effectively with him in the treatment room.

MENTAL DISTRACTIONS

Helping your child to become absorbed in something they are interested in—whether it's Legos, car videos, or Harry Potter—is a wonderful way to turn their attention away from the procedure.

Here are two examples:

JAMIE

Jamie, an intelligent, highly verbal ten-year-old, liked being in control and was acutely anxious getting chemotherapy. He would begin vomiting as soon as the chemotherapy started. Anti-nausea medication was not helping, and he complained about how it made him feel. He loved baseball quizzes and was a Red Sox fan, following each game avidly. I read my sports pages and prepared questions for him. I began asking the questions just before his chemotherapy began, and we continued talking baseball and the Red Sox for at least another fifteen minutes. This contained his anxiety sufficiently for his vomiting to reduce dramatically, and I would leave him with a series of baseball cards to look at.

JEFF

A seven-year-old boy, Jeff, could not tolerate his port being accessed. He cried, he told his mother he hated her and that he thought she hated him. He said he wanted to die, which was of course very painful for her to hear. His tears dropped onto his chest, which meant that his chest had to be cleaned several times before the needle could be inserted. He needed a nurse to hold him and insisted on watching everything the nurse was doing, including the needle insertion. He described the needle as feeling acutely uncomfortable and walked bent over until it was taken out at the end of his clinic visit. He was inconsolable. His mother alternated between sympathizing, reasoning, bargaining, and threatening. It was clear there was something extraordinarily upsetting to Jeff about the experience of a needle going into his chest. His behavior was particularly striking given the fact that he tolerated spinal taps without getting upset (a more challenging procedure for most children). He selected books for his mother to read to him during the spinal tap and remained focused on them throughout. The difference, perhaps, was that he could not see the needle going into his back.

Jeff was understandably depressed and angry—with the world, with his parents, and with what he had to go through. His mother was feeling helpless and worried at Jeff's behavior, but not optimistic that either she or I could do much about it. *"When we first met I was very overwhelmed and preoccupied, so I was pretty wrapped up in my own distress."* . . . *"We were so frustrated it was hard to see things from his point of view."* Despite his depression and anger, Jeff loved playing one video game in the clinic and liked demonstrating his considerable skill. Having to leave the video game and go into the treatment room was what began his protests. His mother confirmed that control, skill, and winning were important to Jeff, and we decided to use the video game as a way to distract and reward him and to bring the positive mood and associations he had with the video game into the treatment room.

So I sat with Jeff before he was called into the treatment room and watched the game he was playing. I made up quizzes about the characters and different levels of combat, etc., and let him know I'd be asking him questions as soon as we got into the treatment room, so he had better be paying close attention to the game. When we were in the treatment room, I reminded him that the quicker his port was accessed, the sooner he could get back to the video game. I asked some questions and he took pride in invariably getting the answers right. When he began to cry and make his deeply negative statements, his mother and I ignored the content but acknowledged how hard it was for him to get his port accessed. Seeing the needle escalated his protests further. I reminded him that the quicker we were done, the quicker we could get back to the video game. Over his tears, I asked a question about the game that Jeff answered. I also commented that a few of those magic powers or weapons might be useful right now and wondered out loud which power would be most useful. His mother was pleased when she succeeded in getting Jeff to look at her so his chest did not need to be cleaned twice.

Jeff continued to dislike having his port accessed, but it was done more quickly and less painfully for all concerned. My knowledge of the video game increased dramatically, and I saw to it that the video game was always waiting for him after his port was accessed.

The qualities that led many young children to protest so strongly at what they were going through often served them in good stead later. In this instance, Jeff has applied the qualities evident during his treatment—determination, focus, persistence, motivation, and endurance—positively to pursue academic studies and to achieve other impressive goals.

Distraction is a very useful tool to help children tolerate procedures more easily. It can counteract anxiety before a procedure and help a child recover afterward, but additional strategies will likely be required during the procedure itself, particularly if pain is involved.

. . . .

SELF-STATEMENTS AND AFFIRMATIONS

What your child says to himself or herself—and what you, as a parent, say to yourself—about what is happening in the hospital or about a medical procedure will affect how your child—and you—feel. An event—or a picture—can often be interpreted accurately in different ways. In the picture that follows we can accurately see either a duck or a rabbit.[1]

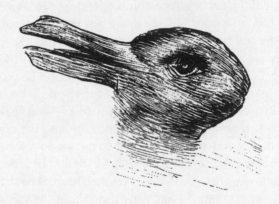

Sometimes different interpretations have different emotional impacts. If your child's interpretation is positive, the words can generate feelings that will help her surmount the most difficult of circumstances. If negative, the words can generate feelings and actions that can lead to major difficulties for your child, the doctor, and you.

DINA

Dina, normally an easygoing, friendly, responsible, and thoughtful ten-year-old girl, came in every three weeks for regular chemotherapy treatments that made her very sick. For the last several sessions she had been quite calm in the car coming into the clinic. She appeared calm when her blood was drawn on arrival, but when the doctor told her that her blood count was high enough that she could get her chemotherapy, she became completely hysterical. Her parents and the medical staff were mystified by her behavior. After she attempted to run out of the clinic into the street, I was asked to meet with her. It turned out she deeply hated the chemotherapy and how it made her feel. She had kept herself calm on the way to the clinic by repeating to herself over and over again, "I won't get chemotherapy today, I won't get chemotherapy today, I won't get chemotherapy today." When her blood levels came back high enough to get chemotherapy, she felt completely overwhelmed, betrayed, out of control, and desperate and her only defense left was to run away.

We discussed what in particular she hated about getting the chemotherapy. She said it reminded her each time how sick she was and all the things she was missing. We took several steps to improve the situation for her. Her mother arranged to have her blood tested the night before a possible session so they would have to come into the clinic only if she could get chemotherapy. Her doctor prescribed a small amount of Ativan to relieve some of her anxiety. We brainstormed what else she could say to herself on the way to the clinic that would be comforting but would not set her up to be upset. She came up with "I will get home after the chemotherapy and watch my favorite video." She used this phrase as a mantra to stay calm on the drive in. I also taught her progressive muscle relaxation to help her stay calm while she was waiting for and getting her chemotherapy.

Over time we also explored what she was saying to herself about her illness and treatment and its effect on her life. It turned out she was saying negative things like "I'm never going to catch up with the work I've missed." We thought about whether there were other things she could say to herself that would be accurate but would be less negative and make her feel less discouraged. She came up with "It's going to be a challenge to catch up, but the teachers have all said they will help me." She became increasingly able to catch herself thinking negatively and to reframe her thoughts in a more positive but accurate way.

The insight Dina gained during our sessions and her impressive personal qualities helped her do well during the rest of her treatment despite some health setbacks, and she was soon back in school working hard and catching up. Later these same qualities helped Dina became an adored teacher of children with special needs and the beloved mother of a little girl.

Encouraging positive statements or affirmations can help some parents and children during medical procedures. Many young children know the story of *The Little Engine That Could*. "I think I can, I think I can, I think I can" is a great affirmation. You can ask your child if he can think of anything he could say to himself that would help him do something really difficult just like the Little Engine did. The affirmation can be a simple statement or a line of a prayer or a poem. It needs to be short, repeatable, positive, and accurate (not like Dina's "I won't get chemotherapy today," when in fact it was likely she would). It can also function as a chant or a mantra to contain anxiety.

Examples of encouraging statements or affirmations that you could say to yourself if you are feeling anxious are:

♦ "Just keep breathing."
♦ "Stay calm."

Or you can repeat a selected line of a prayer or poem.

With a younger child, you could make up a phrase to say together, such as:

♦ "We can do it."
♦ "You can do it/I can do it."
♦ "Keep it up."
♦ "Keep us safe."
♦ "It will be over soon."

Older children may make up their own phrase. For example, one highly vigilant ten-year-old boy was terrified of getting an IV inserted, and often the staff made repeated attempts before it went in correctly. He kept himself still and in control by saying loudly and repetitively, "Let it go in, let it go in, let it go in, let it go in." Once the needle was in, he changed it to "Let it stay in, let it stay in, let it stay in," which he said continuously until the medicine was running.

This may be the moment for you reflect on what you are saying to yourself about your child's medical situation. Are there any areas where you could, without kidding yourself, usefully switch your attitude to a more positive one? Compare "She is never going to go back to the way she was" with "She is going through an extraordinarily difficult time— we don't know yet how it will turn out or how she will be affected, but we are all doing our best to help her get through it." Imagine the difference you would feel depending on which statement you are making to yourself.

What you and your child are saying to yourselves about what is happening can indeed alter how you feel. If you think it would help, come up with a few brief, comforting phrases you or your child can think of as mantras to use while your child is undergoing procedures. Such phrases can offer hope and lessen anxiety. And as we all know, hope is a beacon of light that can lead us through the hardest times.

CHAPTER 10

Imagery and Self-Hypnosis

We all move between different levels of awareness of our surroundings, depending on what we are doing and what we are thinking about. When we are watching an absorbing television show or reading an interesting book, we will notice less about what is going on around us. Someone may need to ask us a question twice before we hear it. Children playing a game may not hear their names being called. Some children who injure themselves when they are actively enjoying an activity will not notice they are bleeding or that anything hurts until they stop playing.

Children have terrific imaginations and can switch easily between fantasy and reality. For sick children, guided imagery can help them to relax before a procedure, to remain calm and absorbed during a long procedure like an MRI, and/or to reduce the experience of pain during a painful procedure like a spinal tap or bone marrow aspiration. Imagery can also provide a comforting break for a child who is generally feeling ill, depressed, or going through a long hospitalization. Imagery can help with sleeping difficulties, anxiety, and other problems. Parents can use guided imagery in age-appropriate ways with children aged three and older.

Using imagery, we relax our bodies and focus on internal images (what we see, hear, feel, smell, or experience). We are deliberately distracting ourselves from what is otherwise claiming our attention to experience something we are imagining in our minds. Sick children can use imagery to turn their attention deliberately away from an unpleasant experience—say, of pain or the sensations that accompany having an unpleasant medical procedure—to more pleasant internal images like doing a favorite activity. This can help to change the unpleasant experience into a more enjoyable one. Some adults and some children have remarkable talent at doing this, and children in general are more imaginative and receptive to suggestion than adults.

BILL

Four-year-old Bill was becoming distraught when blood had to be drawn from his hand. I met with him and his father before the procedure and asked if he had ever seen a leaf frozen in ice. He said he had. I said to him perhaps if he thought very hard about that leaf, perhaps he could imagine that his hand was just like a leaf frozen in ice because then it would be numb—and did he know what "numb" was? He said he did. I said if he imagined his hand was numb, perhaps he would not feel anything when the needle went in. To be honest, I was not expecting this to work. His father went with him into the accessing room, noticed Bill was beginning to get upset as he held out his hand, and said to him, "Remember the leaf." Bill stopped crying, looked thoughtful, and held out his hand, to the astonishment of the nurse, who then drew the blood. Bill commented to his father, "That didn't hurt."

LUCY

Five-year-old Lucy was very afraid getting spinal taps. We had made an extensive plan for how to make the experience more tolerable for her, which included her doing special breathing and imagining hugging her dog, Snowy, while looking at some pop-up books. During the spinal tap, I coached her through the breathing and showed her different pop-up books. She was relaxed and still. When it was done, I remembered I had never mentioned Snowy, so I said to her, "Oh my goodness, we were so busy, I forgot to mention Snowy," to which she replied, "Don't worry. I was lying on Snowy all the time!"

INTERACTIVE STORYTELLING FOR YOUNGER CHILDREN

Interactive storytelling and/or asking questions about a favorite activity is an age-appropriate version of guided imagery for younger children in which the back-and-forth interaction with a trusted adult may hold a young child's attention. Choose a subject that will interest your child, like a favorite activity or TV character, and begin talking about it. Ask him to fill in some details as you go along and see how much he wants to participate in making up the story. Examples follow.

A CHILD'S INTERACTIVE STORY—WILLIE

The mother of a highly imaginative six-year-old boy named Willie who, she remembered, "fought every medical procedure tooth and nail" became expert at using interactive storytelling with her son during his spinal taps. She began a story and asked Willie questions as the story progressed. One story I remember her telling was how Willie had just learned to jump into the pool holding his legs so he made a cannonball (the position in which he was now curled up to get his spinal tap). She wondered if Willie could see himself running to the side of the pool. Willie nodded. "Are you ready to take a big jump?" "Yes." "I hope you remember to hold your nose as well as your knees as you jump way, way up into the air. And now what's happening?" "I made a giant, huge, enormous splash [big grin], everybody got wet [bigger grin]." While this was going on, the doctor was numbing the area on his back where the spinal tap would be done and beginning the insertion of the needle, which Willie hardly seemed to notice.

You might like to tell an interactive story about an activity your child enjoys. A nurse practitioner in our hospital described leading a four-year-old in a delightful interactive story about getting ready for a snowball fight as a way to overcome his acute anxiety about having a procedure.[1] Or you can tell an interactive story about your child's favorite fictional character (maybe he is holding a small model Batman) in the treatment room. If your child is easily absorbed in fantasy, it might be better if the story is unrelated to the current context. If your child is vigilant, perhaps you could wonder aloud what Batman would be doing if he was getting his blood drawn. If your child likes Curious George, you can have some fun discussing with him all the trouble Curious George would likely get into in the treatment room. "Probably all the nurses would be trying to chase him out of the room and they'd forget all about having to give you a shot. Wouldn't that be nice?"

Interactive storytelling can also be an excellent therapeutic tool to use if a young child is exhausted, sick, and perhaps depressed during a long hospitalization.

TESSA

One of our psychology interns recorded an interactive story she created with a four-year-old girl, Tessa, going through a long stem cell transplant. The story was about two naughty dolls who got into all kinds of trouble at home and outside. The intern began her story with a brief relaxation instruction. "Take a couple of deep breaths and let your body feel calm and ready to begin our next adventure with Jill and Jane. I wonder what they are going to get up to this time?" Tessa would choose to be more or less involved in creating the story plot depending on how she was feeling that day. In one story, the intern described the dolls bouncing up and down on their parents' bed before sliding down the banister to go and make delicious-smelling cookies in the kitchen. The dolls made an awful mess and did not do too good a job of clearing it up, which made Tessa laugh. Tessa looked forward to and enjoyed sharing in these stories. Her mood appeared improved after the sessions.

GUIDED IMAGERY FOR OLDER CHILDREN

You or a clinician can introduce your child to guided imagery. If you have not used imagery before, you can download some guided imagery podcasts on your cell phones or tablets, then follow their directions and see whether you think you could teach imagery to your child. Guided imagery exercises usually begin with brief instructions to relax and then focus on a particular image: a trip to the beach, a walk through the woods, enjoying a favorite activity, or going on a special journey.[2] The coach may give the child or adolescent specific details through the imagery or may give more general directions that allow him or her to fill in the details. If you are describing the scene to your child, the more senses you can use in the imagery, the more real you make the picture for him. If you are taking him on a walk in the woods, have him see the trees around him, smell the pines, hear the birds, maybe take a rest by leaning his body against the trunk of the tree and feeling its rough bark against his skin, experience the wind blowing through his hair—and when he finds a boat on a pond, take a ride in it and perhaps suggest he feels the gentle rocking of the water as he lies back in the boat. If it turns out he is able to experience some senses more vividly than others, emphasize those senses. Often the imagery exercise creates feelings of calmness, relaxation, and a sense of well-being. Over time and with practice, the adolescent can imagine the scene or the activity on his own by listening to a recording (either made by you, created by a clinician, or downloaded).

Guided imagery can be used for several different purposes with a child who is sick.

+ To increase a general feeling of well-being in the hospital or at home
+ To lessen or manage acute anxiety
+ To relax
+ To improve sleep difficulties
+ To manage pain

Children may choose to focus on active or passive imagery. What for adults may be calm, relaxing, and absorbing imagery like lying on the beach in the sun may not be as fully engaging for a child as more active imagery such as running through a field. Several teenagers chose to imagine themselves doing their favorite sport while they were having a bone marrow aspiration or spinal tap.

AN ADOLESCENT'S IMAGERY—DAVID

One teenager, David, asked me to talk him through an imaginary basketball game his team was playing during his bone marrow aspiration. I was comforted when he told me it did not matter if I got some of the details of the game wrong. He said it was the tone of my voice he was listening to. I had him coming off the bench, stealing the ball, dribbling it down the court, shooting despite being challenged by the guard, and scoring. His opponents started off with the ball; then he was chasing them back down the court to try and retrieve the ball again. When he felt something from the bone marrow procedure, he would imagine it was one of his opponents running into him. By the end of the procedure David's team had a convincing lead, he had played really well, and the bone marrow was done with minimum acknowledgment from him.

Guided imagery can also be designed specifically to alter the sensation of pain—to change its color to a cooler, more soothing shade, to alter its shape to blunt its edges, or to find the pain center in the brain that controls the sensations we feel and turn the volume down.[3]

Imagery can also help a child having an unpleasant though not painful procedure. Some years ago children undergoing an MRI were told to imagine themselves on a space mission and to pretend that the MRI machine was their spaceship. The blastoff made a lot of noise, but they needed to focus to keep the ship on the right path. This intervention combined reducing the anxiety associated with the procedure, incorporating the unpleasant noise of the MRI, and giving the child a sense of control.[4]

Nancy Klein's book *Healing Images for Children* includes several guided-imagery stories combined with relaxation that are intended to reduce a child's experience of pain, and can be used for a range of other purposes like managing nausea or the anxiety that accompanies waiting for medical appointments.[5] One pain management imagery involves using a soft paintbrush first to paint a favorite color and then a numbing paint over the area that is hurting. Another suggests taking a hot air balloon ride, leaving behind a suitcase with the pain or worry inside it on the ground.

Many imagery scripts for older and younger children are also available online.[6] You can review them and see if there are some you think would appeal to your child. Or having listened to them, you can ask your child or adolescent which subject he would choose for his guided image and do it with him. Based on his feedback, record it for him so he can use it when he wants.

Remember:

+ Start with a few relaxing breaths.
+ Choose a subject that interests him and will absorb his attention.

- Remember that the imagery can be either active or passive.

- Speak slowly and calmly.

- Use as many senses as you can to make the imagery as real as possible for him. Incorporate sight, touch, smell, hearing, and taste into your images. If he tells you he finds a particular sense easier to imagine, emphasize that sense.

- Give him choices where you can. Saying things like "You can choose to walk a little farther or just stop here and rest" or "You will know what you want to eat first from your picnic box" will increase your adolescent's sense of control.

If you use interactive storytelling, you can create your own stories based on your knowledge of your child's interests and reactions. If you already make up stories with your child, this might be a natural and enjoyable activity together.

· ·

SELF-HYPNOSIS

When a child learns to use self-hypnosis, his or her sense of control and mastery often increases. I strongly encourage you to have an open mind as you consider whether self-hypnosis could benefit your child. Self-hypnosis is a powerful tool with a greater range of purposes and potential for more remarkable outcomes than imagery. It can also have unintended effects if not used carefully. Self-hypnosis needs to be taught to a child by a trained professional.[7]

A recent article summarizes much of what we know about hypnosis with children and adolescents, and if you are interested in learning more about hypnosis, I strongly recommend you read it.[8] When we use self-hypnosis we narrow our attention and focus more intensely on our internal images and sensations. With practice, we can learn to alter these images and sensations. There is often a more specific goal with self-hypnosis than with imagery. You might look for a therapist to assess the potential benefits of learning self-hypnosis in the following situations:

- If your child is experiencing considerable distress during procedures that have not been alleviated by other strategies including antianxiety and pain medications.

+ If your child needs a painful medical procedure in which the usual pain medications cannot be used (perhaps your child has an adverse reaction to the medications) or you or your child do not want them used.

+ If your child is suffering from neuropathic pain or chronic pain and discomfort that other interventions including imagery have not alleviated.

Self-hypnosis can also be used to help with a variety of problems that children or adolescents may have—pain management, insomnia, teeth grinding, bedwetting, trauma, or getting to the cause of a phobia.[9] It can also improve a child's confidence, impulse control, sense of mastery, and self-esteem. Self-hypnosis has been used effectively with children to manage painful medical procedures.[10] Specifically, it can help your child who is sick to:

+ Learn to counteract the sensation of pain

+ Learn to change the sensation of pain

+ Learn to distance the pain

So what would be involved in your child learning self-hypnosis? You and your child would meet with a therapist experienced in teaching self-hypnosis to children. Initially, the therapist would ask what challenges your child or adolescent is facing and ask some questions about your child's medical, emotional, and school history. Learning self-hypnosis might not be a wise course to pursue if your child has ever experienced hallucinations, has had major mood swings, or has a diagnosis of attention deficit hyperactivity disorder (ADHD) or post-traumatic stress disorder (PTSD)—unless the treatment of the trauma was the goal. The clinician might give you a preliminary opinion about whether self-hypnosis could help your child with his or her particular challenge. She would likely meet with your child or adolescent alone to assess his motivation to learn self-hypnosis, his style, and his absorbing interests. She might take him through some self-hypnosis exercises and see how he does. If your child appeared motivated and was willing to practice at home, the therapist would likely give some homework assignments for him to practice before meeting with her again. She would then review with him how the practice had gone and give him further suggestions and homework assignments. Over time, your child or adolescent would hopefully learn how to bring himself into a quiet and focused state, quickly and in different settings. He would develop ways to regulate what his body was experiencing and what his mind was focusing on, giving him more control and more choices.

AN ADOLESCENT'S EXPERIENCE WITH HYPNOSIS—JANE

Sixteen-year-old Jane underwent frequent bone marrow aspirations, and she strongly disliked the way the short-acting anesthesia used during the procedure made her feel. She had read that self-hypnosis could help manage pain and wanted to learn it. Jane received three training sessions from a trained clinician where she learned how to go into a hypnotic state through visual focus, slow breathing, and suggestion. She practiced deepening the state in the way she had selected, remaining focused on the place where she had chosen to go in her mind, and bringing herself back to her normal state of consciousness when the procedure was over. She ended each session by reminding herself that she could return to this comfortable state whenever she wanted through self-hypnosis. The therapist worked with her during her first bone marrow aspiration without anesthesia, gave her brief prompts during the second one, and Jane managed the third one on her own. She reported experiencing minimal pain on each occasion.

Self-hypnosis is a powerful tool. It should always be taught by a qualified professional and can be hugely helpful and empowering to your child as a means to manage pain and discomfort as well as a host of other stressors while increasing self-confidence and self-control.

CHAPTER 11

Making Plans to Manage a Procedure

When you are considering what strategies your child should learn and making plans to handle a particular procedure, relevant factors are:

- The demands of the particular procedure
- Your child's temperament and style
- The level of distress your child is showing and its causes

· ·

THE DEMANDS OF DIFFERENT PROCEDURES

The interventions you choose need to be suited to the demands of different procedures and the style and behavior of your child. If fear and anxiety is involved, distraction, relaxation, imagery, medical play, and rehearsal may be good strategies to consider. If pain is involved, more active strategies, like breathing, squeezing, active imagery, or self-hypnosis and practicing the techniques may be needed. A behavioral plan can help motivate your child to practice and use the strategies in any procedure.

. . . .

YOUR CHILD'S TEMPERAMENT AND STYLE

You need to consider your child's style and her interests when figuring out what is likely to help her.

Children have different characteristics, and are likely to benefit from strategies that match their style:

+ A child who is vigilant will likely benefit from focusing on the procedure using distraction in a way that includes and refers to the procedure.

+ A child who is playful and imaginative will likely benefit from a range of techniques.

+ A child who is anxious will likely benefit from calming interventions.

+ A child who is inflexible will likely benefit from establishing a routine and a clear plan.

+ A child who is impulsive with a short attention span will likely benefit from active participation in the strategies used.

+ A child who likes control will likely benefit from having an active role in planning the techniques to use.

+ A child with good sense of humor will likely benefit if humor is incorporated into the strategies.

You want to devise a plan that suits your child's personality. If there has been a major change in your child's behavior and personality during the hospitalization, address his current behavior but keep his past interests in mind when planning interventions. It also may be necessary to combine several interventions like special breathing, puppet play, distraction, and a behavior plan to intervene effectively.

Additional factors to consider:

+ Try to offer distractions or imagery that reflect your child's interests—whether it is dolls, animals, soldiers, pop-up books, imaginative play, videos, or TV shows—in your intervention plan. But limit what you bring in with you to the hospital or treatment room, because too many objects can interfere with the medical procedure itself.

+ If something previously helped your child in a stressful situation or, better still, in a medically challenging situation, consider adapting it to use now.

♦ Use what motivates your child in planning rewards for a behavioral plan (mini Lego kits, time to play a video game).

· ·

YOUR CHILD'S LEVEL OF DISTRESS

Minimum Distress

If your child is showing minimal distress and has to deal with shots, blood draws, and/or port-a-cath access, then breathing techniques and distraction may be the first strategies to try. Remember you want to match your child's style with what you are offering.

IF YOUR CHILD LOVES . . .	TRY . . .
blowing bubbles	using the bubbles first to teach breathing. If she can blow the big and small bubbles, see if she can blow imaginary bubbles. Ask if she would like you to bring real bubbles into the procedure room. Also check with the nurse if that will be all right or in the way. If she has any difficulty blowing bubbles, move to a pinwheel or party blower.
being read to	using pop-up books as a distraction during a procedure
stuffed animals	asking if she'd like to hug one in the treatment room
moving around (not sitting still)	introducing the Freeze game
mental challenges	coming prepared with riddles, jokes, or quizzes on subjects in which he is interested
music	songs or bringing in her favorite music from iTunes or another streaming or download service
watching what is happening	mixing your distractions with focus on the procedure (questions about the procedure itself is another way of distracting your child). With a vigilant child you may also want to combine distractions with special breathing during the procedure.

Experiment to see which types of distractions appeal to your child most and vary them over time. (Use different pop-up books, come armed with new jokes.) If you are reluctant or don't feel ready to try these strategies yet, you can request that a psychosocial clinician or child life specialist use them with your child first while you watch, and you can take over later. If your child is doing well during procedures, it may not be necessary to make a specific intervention plan with him, but you can check with him afterward to see if he liked the distractions and breathing strategies you offered.

Most young children (ages three to five), even if they are showing only minimum distress, will also benefit from having a designated stuffed animal or puppet and medical supplies for medical play at home or in the hospital. This allows them to feel greater control and participation in what is going on in their lives.

If you know your child will have procedures that require remaining still for any length of time, brainstorm with him for ideas (such as slow breathing to relax, a video game or video, or talking on the intercom with a parent) to help him to stay motionless and calm, and consider having him practice in advance. Check with him how it went afterward and modify what happens next time based on his feedback.

Medium Distress

If your child is showing a medium amount of distress about painful procedures, consider showing your child the breathing strategies combined with distraction based on your child's interests. If your child is less than seven years old, puppet play and medical play can be added to those interventions. If no improvement occurs, or your child's distress gets worse, consider consulting with a psychosocial clinician and introducing a behavioral plan. You can include your child in its design, notably in planning the rewards he will earn. Ask your child what is particularly difficult about the procedure and what he is saying to himself about getting the procedure. See if the statements could be positively reframed. Consider having the psychosocial staff or child life specialist work with him during the procedure while you watch (allowing you to see if a style different from your own appears helpful to your child). You can review the intervention plan with your child before the procedure begins and change it based on his feedback afterward.

If longer procedures are scheduled, you can have your child plan and practice with you what to do during the procedures in advance, and you can both alter it later if necessary.

If you suspect your child's medium level of distress is more associated with how long he has been in the hospital and general feelings of depression and distress rather than with the procedures themselves, consider whether play therapy with a psychosocial clinician would be helpful for your child. If your child is older, consider whether talking with a therapist or using imagery for relaxation and to create peaceful interludes in his day might be useful.

Considerable Distress

If your child is showing considerable distress or is actively resisting treatment, and seems very different from his pre-diagnosis self, consider consulting with a psychosocial clinician and strategize with him or her about possible interventions. These could run the full gamut of strategies coupled with a behavioral plan that includes personally appealing rewards: breathing and relaxation, appropriate distractions, cognitive behavioral interventions including reframing, puppet and play therapy, medical play, talking therapy, and, depending on your child's age, interactive storytelling or imagery and self-hypnosis. A psychiatrist could be asked to assess if medications might help. Sometimes, for example, an antianxiety medication can lessen a child's anxiety sufficiently enough that he is better able to use the intervention tools. Again, the intervention plan can be reviewed with your child before the procedure and amended as needed afterward based on what he says. Expect gradual, not rapid, improvement. And remember to pick out something that went positively for which to praise your child.

If your child needs long procedures and has difficulty staying still, you might consider rehearsing, using imagery, or getting a referral for self-hypnosis. The intervention plan can be reviewed with your child and changed based on his feedback. Again, make sure to pick up on any positive change.

If your child seems very depressed in addition to his distress at medical procedures, consider asking for a meeting with a psychiatrist to assess whether antidepressant medications might help over time, as well as considering cognitive behavioral therapy.

A CHILD'S STORY—SUSIE

Susie was three years old when she was diagnosed with leukemia. She had a difficult hospitalization lasting several months. She became increasingly withdrawn and actively resisted any procedures. She fought the nursing staff, occasionally hitting and biting them. Susie had long negotiations with her mother and struck bargains that she invariably broke. She eventually had to be restrained by nursing staff for any procedure to occur. It took her a long time to calm down afterward. She became less interactive and responsive with her parents and hid under the covers anytime a new person entered her room.

Prior to diagnosis, her parents described her as a playful, sociable, outgoing, imaginative, determined child with a great sense of humor; she was "a control freak," occasionally anxious, and highly sensitive to pain—although if she was playing she might not react until she saw blood. She loved dolls, imaginative play, and certain videos. When she was an infant, being held or rocked would calm her. When she became a toddler, being given space and time on her own was more helpful.

Susie was highly vigilant during procedures and needed to watch everything.

Her parents were loving and devoted. They believed in giving Susie choices, reasoning, negotiating outcomes, and respecting Susie's independence and wishes. They did not always carry out threatened consequences such as time-outs for undesirable behaviors. It was extraordinarily hard for them to witness Susie being restrained and forced to do something against her will. Her parents and I worked together to come up with strategies to help Susie, which included an agreement that if Susie could not cooperate after a specified time, the nurses would help her get the needed procedure.

Using Susie's many strengths (imagination, humor, determination, wish for control), we introduced coping strategies, planned interventions, and made positive suggestions that would help her manage her anxiety and help her get the necessary treatments more positively and less traumatically for her, her parents, and the medical staff. We introduced a puppet, Ned, as an ally who would help Susie to counteract her pain and anxiety. We showed Susie how Ned got a port and did not like getting it accessed. He needed to practice special breathing using bubbles and a pinwheel to help stay calm. Susie helped him practice. Ned received Emla cream and said, "I didn't notice when I was accessed because I was blowing and didn't feel it." Ned told Susie she can use the bubbles and pinwheel too, and that she should let him know how it goes.

We made a chart for Susie so that she could earn a sticker for completing each difficult task, such as walking into the room by herself, climbing onto the bed by herself, not hitting anyone, and using her special breathing.

••

SUSIE'S BEHAVIORAL PLAN

BEFORE ACCESS

♦ Walk into the room by yourself (1 sticker)
♦ Climb onto the bed by yourself (1 sticker)
♦ Use special breathing (1 sticker)

By prior agreement, the nurse came in after Susie was on the table.

DURING ACCESS

♦ Susie stays still and is accessed before an egg timer runs out (two stickers)
♦ "Helped" (restrained). Accessed before the egg timer runs out twice (one sticker)
♦ No kicking, hitting, or biting (one sticker)

Six stickers earn Susie a prize.

Each time Susie needed to have her port accessed, we played with Ned beforehand and went over the behavior plan. As it was being accessed, her mother and I reminded her of the ways she could earn stickers, and modeled the special breathing we had practiced. Afterward, we focused on what Susie did well and noted the number of stickers she had earned.

Over time, Susie was able to cooperate, and any occasional setbacks would be brainstormed with Ned. Her general state of mind became much less depressed. Ned became a friend, an ally, and a key figure in gaining her cooperation with treatment. She also pretended that she was *his* doctor and in charge of his treatments.

Two years later when Susie needed a stem cell transplant following a relapse, Ned got a thorough wash so he could keep her company in the isolation room where she received her successful transplant.

A wide array of strategies can help your child deal with the anxiety and pain often associated with medical procedures or long hospitalizations and recovery. The techniques range from the simple to the more complex. Some techniques you may already be using with your child. You have a crucial role—in modeling calmness and positive expectations to your child and in collaborating with medical staff to design, teach, and help your child use the available and appropriate tools that match his style and the demands of the situation.

Most important, these strategies are gifts you can see that your child obtains—to help him cope, to increase his confidence and sense of mastery, to help him find the positive in what he is enduring, and to build skills and resilience as well as to form attitudes he can use in later life when faced with adversity.[1]

CHAPTER 12

. . . .

Taking Medications

Many childhood conditions that require hospitalization also require children to take medications—sometimes for a long time. Taking medications and following a medication schedule can be a challenging task. Younger children may have difficulty taking the medications, while some adolescents may have difficulty consistently keeping to a medication regime. A few adolescents may refuse treatment or refuse to complete ongoing treatment. In fact, there is evidence of considerable noncompliance with medication and treatment protocols among adolescents.[1] This chapter reviews some commonsense hints to help your child take necessary medications and suggests how to proceed if your child or your adolescent continues to resist taking medications and following the treatment plan.

. . . .

TAKING MEDICATIONS

Medicines come in four main forms: liquids, pills, gel caps, and suppositories (used infrequently). Very young children will almost always get medicines in liquid form. Usually pills can be crushed or gel caps can be emptied and mixed with other food like ice cream or applesauce. You need to check with your doctor, however, because some pills or gel caps have to be swallowed whole to be absorbed properly. Also, some pills or medicine should not be mixed with particular foods, and other pills and medicine should be taken on an empty stomach. Some children dislike swallowing liquid medications; for others, swallowing pills is harder. Nurses are often experienced and inventive in persuading children to swallow medications. Their interventions will often gain your child's cooperation over time. A good booklet titled *Medicine and Your Child* is available from the National Cancer Institute.[2] Your nurse may give you a handout with ideas to help children of different ages take their necessary medications. The one we used at Children's Hospital and Dana-Farber included several commonsense tips. I've summarized them in the following list:

Infants and toddlers

♦ If your toddler is old enough, give him a Popsicle to suck before he takes the medication to numb his tongue so he will taste less.

♦ Use a syringe or a dropper rather than liquid in a spoon to give liquid medicine. It allows more accurate measurement and easier administration.

♦ See that your baby's body is tilted slightly back (with her head still above the level of her body).

♦ Put the syringe into the side of her mouth, not on her tongue, so she will notice the taste less.

♦ Give the medicine in small amounts and wait until you see her swallow before squeezing the syringe again. (Try blowing softly on your baby's face to encourage her to swallow.)

♦ If your baby seems to dislike the taste, discuss with the pharmacist what you could mix the medicine with—for example, orange juice, applesauce, jam, or honey (honey if your child is more than a year old).

♦ Do NOT put medicine into milk or your child's formula (you do not want him to develop an aversion to either).

♦ If your baby or toddler is resisting strongly, you may need to restrain him using the following steps:

  ▶ Cradle him.
  ▶ Swaddle him in a blanket or tuck one of his arms behind your back, which allows you to hold his other arm.
  ▶ Use the hand of your arm that is supporting him to hold his free arm so he will not knock the syringe out of your hand.

> ◗ Give him the medication slowly using the syringe or dropper as described earlier.

For preschool and school-age children

◆ Have your child suck ice or a Popsicle first so she will taste the medicine less.

◆ Your child needs to understand why the medicine is necessary. Explain that it is not a punishment; rather, it is necessary to help him get better.

◆ If your child strongly prefers medicine as either a pill or liquid, see whether his medicine is available in that form.

◆ If your child hates the taste, discuss with the pharmacist whether a different flavor could be added to the medicine or what liquid the medicine could be mixed with to disguise the taste (such as orange juice, apple juice, maple syrup). If a pill has been crushed, consider the texture and flavor most likely to appeal to your child (applesauce, Jell-O, ice cream, peanut butter, Nutella).

◆ Never leave your child alone while he takes the medication.

◆ If your child is playing a game or watching a favorite video, tell him he has two minutes to take the medicine before the game is turned off. Count to ten just before you turn it off. Usually children do better if they focus on taking the medication without distraction, but if your child is able to take it more easily with distraction, so much the better. (Do not, however, allow more than the two minutes!) If you have switched off a computer or TV game, switching it back on as soon as your child has taken his medicine is an immediate reward.

◆ Give him some choices but not others. He can choose which medicine to take first or what to drink after but NOT whether he takes the medicine.

◆ Have the drink he likes available as soon as he has taken the medicine.

◆ If your child is quite resistant, suggest he can earn stickers toward a particular reward (to reduce delaying tactics, have him earn two stickers for taking the medicine within one minute and one sticker within two minutes).

♦ Try having your child hold her nose and perhaps drink through a straw while she swallows (smell can increase taste).

♦ Give her lots of praise and encouragement when she does successfully swallow the medicine.

If your child continues to have difficulty taking the medication or if his resistance increases, consider what is making swallowing the medication difficult for him.

1. Does he hate the taste?

2. Has he not learned how to swallow a pill?

3. Does he get too anxious beforehand?

4. Is he in a control struggle with staff or you, or is he just fed up?

The interventions you try would be different depending on what you think the problem is. Sometimes several factors may be involved. For example, your child may have had a very bad experience taking a pill and therefore has developed considerable anxiety about swallowing pills. (See how Jane learned to swallow pills on p. 137)

Hates Taste

If your child hates the taste of the medicine and you have tried all the suggestions in the commonsense hints listed above, consider using medical play and puppets to help.

A CHILD'S STORY (CONTINUED)—SUSIE

Susie has just started taking a new liquid medication that she has to take three times a day at home. She says it tastes yucky, fights, spits it out, and sometimes throws up. Her parents are negotiating for up to an hour before forcibly giving it to her. She is probably, at best, getting half the prescribed amount. She is showing increasing resistance and anxiety beforehand.

Susie hates the taste, but she also is in a power struggle with her parents and is developing increasing anxiety about taking the medications. So interventions need to address all three elements. Susie needs some say in how the medicine's taste gets changed;

any plan needs to have agreement from her parents and Susie needs to buy into it.

We come up with the following plan:

♦ Susie's parents ask the pharmacist what flavor could be added to the medication. The answer is grape or strawberry.

♦ After consulting with Susie's parents, we agree Ned, the puppet, will get involved. Ned develops a problem taking medications. He complains, "It tastes yucky." Susie is brought in to help him. We ask Ned if he likes strawberries or grapes better. He says strawberries. We tell him the medicine will be made to taste more like strawberries and that will make it much easier to drink.

♦ We also all practice slow breathing before taking the medication so he stays calm.

♦ Ned holds his nose while he swallows it.

♦ Ned has orange juice there to drink right afterward.

Everybody practices each step and Ned does well. Ned tells Susie the medicine was much easier to swallow. He adds, "Wouldn't it be neat if the strawberry flavor worked for you, too, Susie?" Susie immediately says, "I like grapes." Her parents say that they will ask the pharmacist if a grape flavor can be added to the medication.

We also agree that Ned needs a reward for doing something so difficult. So Susie and I decide:

♦ Ned will get two stickers if he takes the medication by himself before the egg timer has run out once.

♦ After that I will help him take it and if he takes it before the egg timer runs out twice and he does not throw up, he will get one sticker.

♦ When he gets four stickers, he will earn a prize.

Ned asks, "Why can't Susie get stickers, too?" I reply, "We'll have to ask Susie and her mom about that." Susie and her mother agree this is a good plan, and Ned suggests we all write it down so everyone will remember.

Two days later I get a call from Susie's mother: "Susie wanted to call Ned to tell him that the grape flavor worked for her. I said I'd ask you to tell him. Thank you very much!"

Unable to Swallow Pills

If your child has never learned to swallow pills, here is one sequence to try:

- ◆ Emphasize that we swallow bits of food every day much bigger than the size of normal pills.

- ◆ Get your child to practice keeping his head straight up, taking one swallow of water followed by several more without anything in his mouth.

- ◆ Make tiny bread pellets or use a chocolate sprinkle for your child to put one at a time at the back of his tongue. He should take one swallow of water to get the pellet or the sprinkle down his throat and two more to wash it down completely.

- ◆ Gradually make larger bread pellets and have your child swallow them till they approximate the size of the pill he needs to take.

- ◆ Only then move to the actual pill.

If the medicine is in a medium-size gel cap, the pharmacist should be able to give you smaller sizes of the gel caps for your child to practice swallowing until he builds up to the actual size. Put something like sugar or a tiny piece of rolled-up bread into the empty capsule so it weighs something and does not get dislodged from the back of your child's tongue too easily. If your child continues to have difficulty with the larger gel caps, the pharmacist usually can divide the medications into the smaller gel caps.

High Anxiety

If your child gets very anxious before taking his medicine, see if you can figure out what makes him so anxious. Did he have an earlier experience in which he choked or threw up swallowing a pill? Is he telling himself he can't do it or that he will throw up again? Is he getting so tense that he is shaking or getting physical symptoms like a stomachache? It is important your child calm down before he tries to take the pill. You can suggest that he take a couple of deep breaths to help himself focus. I've pointed out to children who like sports that this is what athletes do before they make an important play. If your child is telling himself he can't do it, have him choose another phrase to say to himself (something as simple as "relax," "focus," or "I can do it"). If he has a good visual imagination, you can suggest he imagine the pill is like a tiny stick and the water he drinks is like a waterfall that will carry the stick all the way down the river—to his tummy

A CHILD LEARNS TO SWALLOW PILLS—JANE

Jane was an eight-year-old girl beginning a stem cell transplant. She had been unable to swallow pills since she choked on a pill when she was five. Since then, she became extremely anxious if asked to swallow a pill and invariably choked and threw up. Prior to her discharge home, she needed to be able to swallow pills. Moreover, she was now prevaricating, negotiating, and throwing up oral medications that she needed to take to get through the transplant. Her parents were very supportive with different parenting styles. Her father was easygoing, permissive, and calm, while her mother supervised her care closely and was very concerned about these problems. Her father felt his wife should be involved in planning how to help Jane swallow pills.

Jane, her mother, and I agreed that the first priority was to lessen delays and for Jane to become more relaxed in taking and keeping down oral medications. Moreover, Jane had mouth sores that delayed any plan to teach pill swallowing. NEVER teach a child to swallow pills if it will hurt her if she succeeds.

- ◆ Jane learned slow breathing, tensing and relaxing her muscles, and focusing.
- ◆ Jane got a reward for taking oral meds faster and reminded herself of that.
- ◆ Jane used coughing (usually her cue to throw up) as the cue to begin slow breathing.
- ◆ Jane's mother agreed that Jane's favorite video game would be available the moment she swallowed the oral medication. (Jane sometimes continued to work herself up and would throw up several minutes after taking the meds, so the video game would be both a reward and a distraction.)
- ◆ Jane, her mother, and I agreed we would postpone any pill-swallowing practice until her mouth sores were better.

Jane's ability to take the liquid medications with fewer delays and less vomiting improved considerably and she used the strategies effectively. I told her this suggested she would also be able to use the strategies very successfully when she began swallowing pills.

Three weeks later Jane's mouth sores improved, her bone marrow counts rose, and she was getting close to discharge.

♦ We planned a reward for successful pill swallowing: I would teach her a new card trick when she earned five stickers.

♦ We developed a sequence. We started with tiny bread pellets that increased in size gradually. When the pellets were the size of a mini M&M, we switched to M&M's that were the same size as the pill she needed to take.

♦ Jane developed a new swallowing strategy that her father used and she liked.

♦ We suggested she use the breathing and the focus that she employed with oral meds to calm herself before she started. She used the new swallowing strategy and distracted herself with a video game immediately after swallowing the M&Ms.

♦ Jane then succeeded in swallowing the real pills with little difficulty. She was very proud of herself, and her parents strongly reinforced her efforts. She was able to be discharged on time and continued to take the pills successfully at home.

Control Struggle

If your child is expressing her unhappiness regarding her illness and treatment by fighting with you about taking the medications, there are several actions you can take.

■ See if you can remove yourself from the struggle and ask the nurses to help your child take the medication. You can judge whether things go more easily. To the extent that your child is expressing anger at you for not saving her from the situation and at some level wants you as upset as she is, it may be easier for the nurses to deal with the medications for a while.

■ If you cannot remove yourself, have a very clear plan that your child understands in advance about what will happen *and carry it out* with minimum fuss and bother. Let's imagine you have both agreed your child will have one minute on a timer to take the medicine before the nurses will help her take it. If the minute goes by and your child has not taken the medicine, ignore protests and requests for delay, saying once,

"I know this is hard but this is what we agreed to do and we need to get it done, so the nurses will help you take it." Next time you can remind her shortly before the timer runs out that this is what will happen. You can also remind her of the pleasant activity waiting for her after she takes the medicine.

■ Try to find other ways for your child to express her unhappiness. This could involve play therapy or puppet or medical play with a young child. If she is older, talking about her reactions to the upsets in her world, either with you or a psychosocial clinician, could be of benefit.

■ Help her shift her perspective about what is going on. Try to make the medicine an ally in the struggle against the illness rather than the enemy. You may need to use indirect rather than direct suggestions or use a puppet to talk about what is going on.

■ See if you can get her to come up with suggestions about what could help.

Develop a strategy that works for you and your child. For example, Steve refused to take oral medicines during the day without a huge fight. Then his parents adjusted their routine: "One thing that really made a difference for us was when my husband figured out that our best bet for giving Steve his medicine at home was to do it at night when he had been asleep for a bit. That way he was so tired he didn't protest and work himself into a tizzy—he just took the medicine so he could go back to sleep. That was a game changer for us."

REFUSING MEDICATION OR NOT COMPLYING WITH A COMPLICATED MEDICATION SCHEDULE

Teenagers are less likely to have difficulty swallowing pills or to have a taste aversion to medication, but their resistance can take more complicated forms. A few teenagers may refuse treatments completely, and many teenagers can have difficulty following a precise medication schedule. It is easy to think your teenager should be able to manage his schedule—perhaps he says he can manage it and resents it when you remind him—but the evidence suggests he will likely benefit from your help.

There could be several reasons contributing to a teenager not complying with his medication schedule or refusing treatment, ranging from the simple to the more complex:

♦ He is disorganized.

♦ He minimizes the importance of the medications.

♦ He has intellectual or philosophical objections to his treatment, including his medications.

♦ He is being ruled by his emotions (depression, anger, engagement in a power struggle), which are distorting his judgment.

Often a combination of these factors may be at work.

There are some precautions you can take to reduce the likelihood your teenager will miss taking her medications just because she is disorganized.

♦ Help your teenager plan a manageable and easy-to-remember schedule. Can she take the medicine at regular mealtimes?

♦ Have your teenager write the medication schedule down and put it in an obvious central place such as on the refrigerator "to help everyone remember."

♦ Be present when your teenager is taking her medications.

♦ Praise her when she remembers and takes it without prompting from you.

If your teenager appears to be minimizing the importance of the treatment and the medications:

♦ Determine whether she has not heard the information correctly, or if she has heard it and discounted it.

♦ Ask the medical team to explain to your adolescent the reasons for a particular treatment recommendation. Be sure you understand exactly what they are saying so you can repeat it to your child back home.

♦ Be sure your teenager heard the doctor explaining the importance of taking the medicine when and as prescribed. If she cannot repeat to you what the doctor said, ask the doctor to explain it again. You can explain you need to hear it again (and you probably would benefit from hearing it twice).

Intellectual or philosophical reservations about his medications or treatment can affect your child's compliance.

+ Find out what these reservations are. Are they recent reservations (in which case perhaps they are associated with how he is currently feeling)? Or are they long-standing ones? Could he believe the treatment is causing or will cause his body more harm than the illness does?

+ See that you and the medical staff fully understand what is behind your adolescent's reasons for not taking the medications or completing treatment (family, religious beliefs, mood, side effects).

Most often, if an adolescent is not taking his medications on schedule despite your efforts to make it simple, emotional factors are likely involved also. Your adolescent may be clinically depressed or just fed up with everything about his treatment (side effects, isolation from peers, constraints on activities in which he can participate). He may be angry with you and/or his doctors, whom he blames for putting him through this ordeal. He may show his resentment subtly by taking less medication than he should[3] or more openly by actively refusing to comply. In either event you need to work closely with the medical team to gain his cooperation.

+ If you do not agree with his view, explain to him what you do think about it.

+ Ask the doctors to give your adolescent information about the relevant medical outcomes given treatment versus no treatment (published studies showing risk, impact on likely survival, etc.).

+ Read the information and then check whether your adolescent has accurately understood the findings.

+ Suggest that your teenager meet with a therapist. It may be easier for a therapist than for you to point out areas in which he is not thinking rationally and to encourage your teenager to consider how his emotions are affecting his judgment. Is the immediate satisfaction he is getting from exercising control over his medications preventing him from recognizing the long-term harm he may be doing himself by not completing treatment or by skipping medications?

+ If your adolescent relents and agrees to continue treatment, be sure she makes a verbal contract with the doctor to do so. It will make your life easier if your teenager knows you and she are trying to follow the doctor's orders and it is not just you nagging her. You want your teenager to understand the issue is between her and her doctor and not between her and you.

If your teenager continues to refuse a potentially lifesaving treatment that has a high rate of success:

+ You can mobilize other family members, friends, or professionals he respects either from the community or from the hospital who might influence him.

+ You can request that your adolescent meet with a therapist either within the hospital or clinic or in the community so there is a professional outside the family working with your child who may help him shift his perspective.

+ You can ask the medical team whether accommodations that are less risky than stopping treatment completely can be made to meet your adolescent's concerns and wishes.

+ In many hospitals, you can request an ethics consultation to help all concerned to gain perspective or clarify issues, particularly if you feel the medical team is not being responsive to your teenager's concerns.

+ If you are unwilling to force your adolescent to take medicine against his will, theoretically the medical team could go to court if they thought your child's survival is at stake. The court would appoint a temporary guardian (called a guardian ad litem) to give the hospital the authority to administer a particular treatment. However, I never saw that happen in the over twenty years I was at Dana-Farber. The medical team is much more likely to take such an extreme measure if they think you are opposing a younger child's necessary lifesaving treatment (like getting a blood transfusion) than if you are doing your best to work with them trying to persuade an older adolescent to complete treatment.

If the potentially curative treatment has a low rate of success and high risk of adverse side effects, the situation is even more ambiguous. The medical team is unlikely to advocate strongly for such a treatment against the wishes of the family. If you and your adolescent have different views about whether to get a treatment or not, it may help to ask yourself and your teenager the following questions:

♦ Does he understand that the treatment is his only hope for cure?

♦ Can he give rational reasons why he would prefer either to have or not to have the treatment?

♦ Is he relatively mature?

♦ Is he clinically depressed and/or is his judgment being influenced by his mood?

♦ Are you prepared to go against your teenager's wishes?

In my experience, if the treatment outcome predictions were very poor and the teenager appeared to understand the situation and was not clearly clinically depressed, most medical teams and most parents did not, in the end, feel they could give treatment against the teenager's wishes. Giving a treatment with a low likelihood of success to a teenager against his will, even if it offers a remote chance of cure, puts you in an extraordinarily hard position where your hope and wish that your child will survive have to be balanced against his stated wishes.

AN ADOLESCENT'S STORY—JOHN

John was sixteen years old and being treated for a cancer that had a high cure rate with treatment but a low cure rate without it. He was in the middle of a grueling course of chemotherapy. He had refused to come in for treatment for several weeks and said he would not have more treatments. He had suffered many painful and unpleasant side effects. He was also refusing to go to school. John's parents were divorced, and he lived with his mother, who worked every day, but was also close to his mother's father, whom he saw frequently. His mother finally brought him in to our clinic and I met with John.

John was depressed and angry and most reluctant to meet with me. He was at home a lot on his own. He was feeling no control over what was happening to his body. He felt nauseated and weak most of the time. His grandfather, who believed in homeopathic medicine, was telling him that chemotherapy was poison and John believed him. He had not told his mother about this. She did not share John's grandfather's views. John also told me, "I cannot deal with treatment and school at the same time." He was feeling isolated from peers with whom he had had little recent contact.

His mother and his caregivers agreed on the following course of action: His doctor gave him and his mother the research literature on the difference in survival rates for his condition comparing completed treatment versus no treatment. The differences were dramatic.

We then had several family meetings with his mother, his medical team, and John to discuss these results. His mother strongly supported the views of the medical team. Both John's mother and the doctor volunteered to speak with John's grandfather to convey their concerns. John described the side effects he most disliked and his doctor agreed to treatment changes that might reduce them.

John reluctantly agreed to meet with me regularly for the remainder of his treatment. We focused on what he was saying to himself about his treatment and its outcome. I supported his decision not to return to school while he was completing treatment. He agreed to regular home tutoring and to reconnect with his friends gradually. His mother agreed to see John had more company during the day, and finally John agreed to complete treatment with these accommodations.

John did complete treatment. He had home tutors for the rest of the year and returned to school the following year, where he did very well academically and socially.

ADOLESCENTS' PARTICIPATION IN DECISION MAKING

It is not uncommon in the United States for parents and doctors to show greater deference to the wishes of an older and more mature adolescent. Courts can declare some adolescents emancipated minors—that is, someone who is legally entitled to be treated as an adult, and can even sign treatment consent forms. In our hospital, older adolescents sometimes signed treatment consent forms along with their parents whether or not they had been formally recognized as an emancipated minor by a court. In those cases, the doctor presumably thought the adolescent was mature enough to be fully involved in making treatment decisions. And it certainly made the adolescent a full partner in the decisions that were going to affect his life.

Taking the necessary medications and adhering to the treatment protocol as closely as possible are vital. The medication challenges for younger children are often solved by learning the skills to manage the anxiety or anger that has become associated with a particular medication or hospitalization. The challenges for some adolescents are more complicated and may be connected to how they view their role in what is happening. Do they see themselves as partners in a shared enterprise, or as victims forced to undergo a treatment they hate? Helping them shift their perspective can be essential to gain their cooperation with treatment and to persuade them follow their often rigorous medication regimens.

CHAPTER 13

. . . .

A Stem Cell Transplant

A stem cell transplant (SCT) is a complicated medical procedure with considerable risks as well as potentially lifesaving benefits. A SCT involves a child being in a germ-free environment in the hospital, usually for about five to eight weeks, while receiving treatment. Prior to the SCT, the child receives chemotherapy and usually radiation, which effectively destroys her own stem cells and renders her immune system unable to fight infection. This, hopefully, allows her body to accept the new bone marrow, which contains stem cells. She then receives an infusion of new stem cells (either her own or a donor's cells). She has to remain in the hospital while the new stem cells engraft, her blood counts rise, and her new immune system begins to function.

An SCT is the treatment of choice for an increasing number of serious medical conditions including various cancers, some blood disorders, and some immune, metabolic, or neurological conditions. It is the second line of treatment for several other pediatric conditions including some solid tumors and brain tumors. Sometimes it offers a child the only hope for cure. In some cases, there is a high likelihood of success; in other cases the odds are much less good. So the stakes are high, the risks are considerable, the outcome is uncertain, and a parent's anxiety, not surprisingly, is likely to be high. You have good reason to ask many questions before you agree for your child to undergo an SCT.

STEM CELL TRANSPLANTS—THE BASICS

The Function of Stem Cells

Stem cells are found in the bone marrow (the soft material that fills most of our bones). The bone marrow is the "factory" where blood cells are made. The job of stem cells is to create:

♦ Red blood cells to carry oxygen through our bodies

♦ White blood cells that help our bodies fight infections

♦ Platelets that help form clots that stop bleeding

New stem cells may be needed:

♦ If stem cells are not making blood the way they should, as occurs with certain blood disorders

♦ If bone marrow stem cells have been damaged or destroyed. This can occur after radiation or high-dose chemotherapy has been given deliberately to try to eliminate remaining cancer cells elsewhere in the body. This is common in the treatment of some leukemias, solid tumors, or brain tumors. In this case, the transplant may be needed to allow new stem cells to form in the bone marrow.

The Two Main Types of Stem Cell Transplants

■ In an **autologous transplant** your child gets his own stem cells back. The cells are harvested when your child's cancer is in remission, and sometimes they are specially treated to increase the likelihood they will function properly before being given back to your child

■ In an **allogeneic transplant** your child receives stem cells from a donor whose human leukocyte antigen (HLA) typing matches your child's as closely as possible. HLA is a protein that helps your immune system differentiate between your own cells and someone else's. Antigens determine your child's HLA typing. The closer someone else's antigens match your child's, the better the chance for a successful transplant. Genetics dictate that an identical twin will be an exact match, a sibling will have a one-in-four chance of being an exact match, and parents have a low likelihood, because a child receives half of his HLA genes from each parent. More distant relatives have even less likelihood of being a good match. Sometimes a matched unrelated donor (MUD) can be found through the US National Marrow Donor Program or through other registries here or abroad. More specialized testing might soon help identify the closeness of a match even more accurately.

Harvesting Stem Cells

If an allogeneic transplant is planned, stem cells will be collected from the donor. If an autologous transplant is planned, the stem cells will be collected from the patient. In both instances the stem cells will be stored until the patient is ready for the transplant to occur. Doctors can obtain stem cells in three ways:

■ Doctors remove bone marrow from the donor or the patient under anesthesia by multiple extractions, usually from the middle of the hip bone. The extraction process usually takes about one and a half hours. The bone marrow replenishes quickly, but the donor or patient's back can feel sore for a few days. Usually the process involves an overnight stay in the hospital. Sometime later the marrow is infused intravenously into your child's body after the conditioning phase of the transplant is completed—when chemotherapy and/or radiation has been given to prepare your child for transplant.

■ Stem cells are removed from the donor's or the patient's peripheral blood. Peripheral blood circulating in the body has fewer stem cells than the bone marrow, so doctors often give donors or patients a dose of G-CSF (granulocyte-colony stimulating factor) for several days to boost stem cell production prior to the stem cell harvest. The doctors connect the donor or the patient to an apheresis machine that removes the blood from one arm, filters out the stem cells, and pumps the filtered blood back into the other arm. Sessions can last for two to eight hours, and several sessions may be needed to get enough stem cells for the transplant. Occasionally the donor or the patient may feel muscle cramping, tingling, or dizziness or get a fever or chills during or right after the procedure. The donor or patient is monitored carefully throughout the process and symptoms are promptly treated with appropriate medications.

■ Stem cells are collected from umbilical cord blood, which contains many stem cells. Some institutions have been collecting cord blood for years, usually by asking expectant mothers to volunteer for the program. The umbilical cord blood is collected after the baby is born, so the baby is not involved. If parents know their in utero child or his sibling has (or could have) a condition where a stem cell transplant is (or might be) needed, they can arrange in advance for the infant's cord blood to be preserved and sent to a public or private cord blood bank to be frozen and made available for possible future use.[1]

TECHNOLOGICAL INNOVATIONS

Very occasionally, parents conceive another child for the specific purpose of trying to provide a sick child with matched stem cells. Previously, there was only a one-in-four chance that the stem cells of the infant would match the sick child's. Now, with some extraordinary technological advances such as in vitro fertilization (IVF) and preimplantation genetic diagnosis (PGD), it is theoretically possible to ensure the infant's HLA typing will match that of the sick child's. Obviously this could be very expensive, it is unlikely insurance would pay for it, and more stem cells in addition to what is obtained from the cord blood might still need to be removed from the infant later in order to ensure that there are enough stem cells for the transplant. Moreover, the burden and responsibility of caring for an additional child in these stressful circumstances need to be carefully considered. Over time it is likely to be a complicated emotional situation for a child who is conceived for the purpose of saving his brother or sister's life, particularly if the brother or sister does not do well.

The Process of a Stem Cell Transplant

Pre-transplant

■ Before admission to the hospital, your child will need many medical appointments and tests. She will need blood tests, different cultures, X-rays, and EKGs so the bone marrow team is sure she has no infections and they know her body's baseline functioning. She will need a central line surgically inserted if she does not already have one (to avoid the multiple blood draws and tests using a needle that she would require otherwise). Some institutions may do this before her transplant admission, others at the same time.

■ If the treatment could cause infertility and your son is an adolescent, you will want to discuss the idea of sperm banking with the doctors. Some parents prefer a nurse or doctor on the transplant team to steer their adolescent through this process; other parents prefer to be part of the discussion. Banking eggs for adolescent girls is a more experimental and expensive process that you may also want to discuss with your daughter's doctors. Some organizations listed in the resources section have funds available to cover some of the costs.

■ You will also have to sign an extremely complicated and often alarming **informed consent** form[2] that staff will go over with you carefully. The form will list the details of the stem cell transplant and all possible adverse effects that can occur.

■ You may be asked if you want your child to be part of an ongoing randomized **clinical trial**[3] that compares the standard treatment for your child's diagnosis with one or two other treatments that could be intended to reduce side effects or lower relapse rates. You want to be sure you understand the hypotheses being tested with the alternative treatments, and it may be wise to get a second opinion on the pros and cons of each treatment protocol given your child's particular clinical picture. You can choose the standard treatment if you prefer but not one of the alternative treatments.

■ This is also an important time to give your child's medical team **relevant psychosocial information** about your child and your family that could influence how you will all cope with the transplant. If psychosocial staff are not available to explore relevant background information, you may need to volunteer the information to the team yourself. As discussed in chapter 1, the more information the team has in advance about what could be particularly stressful for your child, you, and your family, and what helps you all cope, the better they will be able to work with you.

What Happens After Admission

■ Chemotherapy. Your child gets high doses of chemotherapy to kill remaining cancer cells and/or bone marrow stem cells so they will not fight the new stem cells. At this point, your child has no internal mechanism to fight infections.

■ Radiation. Many children are given radiation treatments once or twice a day for several days.

■ Rest. Sometimes the medical team will schedule a day of rest between the end of chemotherapy and/or radiation and the infusion

■ Infusion. The new stem cells are given through your child's central venous catheter, similar to a blood transfusion on Day 0. The infusion takes one to four hours. It is pain-free, but can cause chills, fever, or a strange taste in the mouth. Your child will be carefully monitored throughout.

■ Engraftment process. Somehow the new cells find their way to the center of your child's bones and hopefully the engraftment process begins. This process is what allows the new stem cells gradually to make new healthy blood in your child's bone marrow. If your child is getting an autologous or cord blood transplant, doctors may give your child growth factor drugs (similar to those given to stimulate stem cell growth in the donor's peripheral blood) to speed up the process of engraftment and reduce the likelihood of infections. Monitoring blood counts checks how engraftment is progressing. The engraftment can take anywhere from two weeks to more than four weeks, and it often takes between three months and six months before your child's new immune system begins to function effectively. So whether you are in the hospital or at home, your child will be more than usually susceptible to bacterial, fungal, and viral infections—hence all the recommended precautions in the hospital and after discharge. Each type of infection requires different treatments, and some centers give preventative medications immediately after the transplant when your child is most vulnerable to infection.

Discharge

■ Initially hospital staff will want you and your child nearby so your child can be checked daily at the outpatient clinic

■ How soon you can go home will depend on how soon your child's blood counts rise, signifying the new stem cells have engrafted; how far you live from the hospital; and what the local medical facilities can offer.

Expected Immediate Side Effects During the Transplant

♦ Tiredness. Your child may benefit from frequent brief naps during the day.

♦ Hair loss. If this is happening for the first time for your child, consider cutting her hair short. If the loss of her hair is bothering your child, consider a wig. The hospital will likely have a referral for you, and if the doctor writes a wig prescription, your insurance should cover it.

♦ Mucositis (mouth sores, intestinal inflammation). Careful mouth care is necessary (your child may have to swill his mouth with unpleasant-tasting liquid and use a soft sponge cleaner). Frequently, children are prescribed pain medication to minimize the discomfort around mouth care.

♦ Difficulty eating. Most hospitals will give your child IV nutrition while she waits for engraftment.

♦ Mood swings. These can be alleviated somewhat by empathy, behavioral interventions, and, if extreme, by medications.

♦ Nausea/vomiting. This can be alleviated by medications.

♦ Diarrhea. This may require dietary restrictions and medications.

♦ Easy bleeding. This can be treated with frequent platelet transfusions.

Possible Complications During the Transplant

■ Infections. Some may be more severe than others. These can be treated with a range of antibiotics.

■ Acute graft versus host disease (GVHD). If your child has had an allogeneic transplant, he is at risk for this type of reaction. Donor cells attack mainly the liver, intestines, or skin, which can produce jaundice-like symptoms, stomachaches, mouth sores, or a rash. Doctors give immunosuppressive drugs to try to prevent acute GVHD and medications like cyclosporine and steroids to treat acute GVHD. About half of the children receiving an allogeneic SCT do not get such symptoms. The children who do have mild to moderate symptoms may gain some protective effect against relapse.

■ Engraftment failure. This is when the new stem cells do not start to make new healthy blood cells—most likely to happen with an unrelated or mismatched donor. Sometimes a child then receives more infused stem cells to try to produce engraftment.

■ Veno-occlusive disease. Restriction of blood flowing through the liver can cause symptoms like fluid retention, enlarged liver, and weight gain. Treatment involves limiting liquid intake, including intravenous nutrition, and giving diuretics and other medications.

Chronic Graft Versus Host Disease (GVHD)

If your child had an allogeneic transplant, he is also at risk for chronic graft versus host disease (GVHD). In this case, symptoms can start several months after the transplant occurred and can cause symptoms somewhat similar to acute GVHD like an itchy rash, odd skin color, tooth decay and mouth dryness, coughing, or shortness of breath. The symptoms are usually treated with similar medication as are used to treat acute GVHD.

Later Cognitive Effects[4]

Many children receiving the current levels of radiation and chemotherapy as conditioning treatment do not show long-term adverse neurocognitive effects. However, those children who had brain tumors, were under six years old, had total body irradiation, had previous cognitive challenges or developed acute GVIID do appear at greater risk of developing these effects.[5] Longer term follow-up and further study of more specific areas of cognitive functioning (especially areas relating to concentration, speed, and organization) are needed before the medical community can sound the metaphorical all clear for most pediatric stem cell survivors. These issues are discussed in greater detail in chapter 17. It is also worth noting that according to a recent report, most pediatric stem cell survivors report functioning well, though a subgroup report poorer quality of life with health, employment, neurocognitive, and financial difficulties.[6]

New Directions in Stem Cell Transplants

+ **Multiple or tandem stem cell transplants** is a technique in which two or three stem cell transplants occur in a series, allowing a child to recover strength between transplants at home.

+ **Mini-transplants** use less intense chemotherapy but more immunosuppressive therapy compared to a full transplant. Acute side effects are fewer, but it may take longer for the immune system to recover.

+ **Haplo-identical transplants** use a parent as a donor. Stem cells need to be manipulated to decrease the risk of GVHD.

+ **Cellular therapy** is used to treat a child's stem cells before returning them in an autologous stem cell transplant to reduce risk of relapse.

+ **Precise assessment of compatibility** of blood types between potential donor and recipient is used to reduce risk of rejection and/or GVHD.

....

ADVICE FOR PARENTS

Talking with Your Doctor

If your doctor suggests your child needs a stem cell transplant, here are some questions you should ask:

+ Is this the only treatment that can cure my child, or are there other options?

+ What are the survival rates for children with my child's condition and history who have undergone a transplant versus receiving other treatments?

+ Why is one type of transplant being proposed rather than another (autologous vs. allogeneic)?

+ If an autologous transplant is being recommended, is this a condition for which an autologous transplant is more desirable anyway? Or would an allogeneic transplant be preferable if a close match could be found?

♦ Are any clinical trials going on for my child's condition? If there are, would you recommend them over the recommended transplant, and is my child eligible?

♦ If an allogeneic transplant is proposed, is my child's sibling a match?

♦ If no relatives are a match, has the medical team searched every available bone marrow registry?

♦ If an exact match cannot be found, would there be a reduced level of match that the doctors would find acceptable—and what are the risks if a less complete match is used? (Normally a mismatch increases the risk of GVHD and non-engraftment. Doctors are exploring ways to use a mismatched donor's stem cells more effectively.)

♦ What is the proposed method of harvesting the stem cells and why? Some institutions prefer to use bone marrow extraction for the donor. Other hospitals are using peripheral blood apheresis to collect stem cells both from the patient for an autologous transplant and from the donor for an allogeneic transplant. You may be told that apheresis avoids the risk of anesthesia and an overnight stay in the hospital for the donor. On the other hand, the bone marrow extractions take less time, may have fewer side effects than apheresis, and have minimal risk of complications from anesthesia.

♦ Check that your child's doctors have the most current information on all transplants being done for your child's diagnosis. Several excellent organizations have websites providing valuable information for parents.[7]

....

INSURANCE

Ask your doctor whether the proposed transplant is likely to be considered experimental or standard treatment by your insurance company. Transplants are very expensive and can cost upward of $350,000. Insurance companies historically have been reluctant to pay for what they call experimental treatments and want to pay only for what they consider standard practice. It is extremely important to work with your insurance company and the medical staff from the start to be sure your insurance company will agree to pay for the procedure. The advances that have occurred in the transplant field often occur through randomized controlled studies that compare the standard transplant with one or two other treatments that could be labeled as experimental by an insurance company.

Sometimes early results of a randomized controlled study will suggest one treatment is preferable to another, at least for your child, but the results have not yet been published. Some parents have had to reapply several times before an insurance company agrees to pay. It may require working with your child's medical team, a resource specialist, and a patient advocate from the National Marrow Donor Program and making several applications before the transplant is approved by your insurance company, particularly if your child has a complicated diagnosis or history and the doctors are trying to individualize a treatment plan. Most medical teams will help in whatever way is needed.

CHOOSING WHERE TO GO

Selecting a stem cell transplant center is an extremely important decision for you and your child, and there are many questions you would reasonably want to ask about the center you are considering. Because some centers have waiting lists, you should start the research process as soon as you can. You can get a lot of information online. The National Marrow Donor Program (NMDP) website offers resources for patients and families to help them plan their transplant and choose a transplant center.[8]

If your child's diagnosis is one that regularly requires a transplant, there are likely many centers that could perform the procedure. If your child has a more complicated diagnostic picture, you may have fewer centers to choose from. But even if the treatment protocol given is similar among the treatment centers you are considering, the other hospital procedures, rules, supports, and follow-up care may differ, and all of these factors might affect your choice. Here are a few key factors to consider:

■ **Experience.** Some institutions have been doing pediatric transplants for years. Others have started very recently or perhaps have pediatric and adult transplants on the same unit. Some institutions may have only just started doing transplants for your child's diagnosis compared with others who have done them much longer. The success rate of a particular institution for the type of transplant your child needs is particularly important. **Remember, some hospitals do riskier transplants than others, so the success rate for the specific type of transplant given for your child's diagnosis is most relevant, not the overall transplant success rate.**

■ **Infection precautions.** You want to be sure that the hospital's infection precautions make sense to you. In the past, children used to be isolated in their room throughout the engraftment process. Now, because of improvements in infection control and in controlling air flow, most hospitals allow a child greater freedom of movement at least within the transplant floor, although the extent of freedom may differ. All hospitals will have strict handwashing rules—required on coming into your child's room or before any contact. Rules about wearing gloves and gowns may vary between hospitals. Different hospitals also have different rules about who can visit. Most transplant units now allow parents to stay overnight, but many do not allow young children, even siblings, to visit. Some hospitals have outdoor spaces where parents and siblings can meet. Because there is so much variation, be sure you find out what the precautions are at the center you are considering and the reasons for them.

■ **Psychosocial support.** The transplant is an anxiety-provoking experience and can be extremely stressful for your child, you, and your family. You will want to know what psychosocial support is provided routinely at the clinic you are considering. You can ask if social workers and/or psychologists are part of the medical team and if someone will be available to meet with you as well as with your child. You should know whether a psychiatrist is available if needed as a consultant, and if the clinic has a resource specialist who will be available to help you with insurance questions as well as other financial needs. Find out if they have a child life specialist who will work with your child throughout the transplant. Different institutions offer different levels of psychosocial support, and you may want to consider this factor as you make your decision.

■ **Rules about discharge and the availability of post-discharge accommodation.** Aftercare and discharge rules are particularly important if you are a long way from home. Institutions may have slightly different rules about when they allow discharge. Usually blood counts need to reach a particular level and your child must be able to swallow any needed medications. Some teams will want your child to be eating some solid food. Almost all institutions will want you to stay close by for several weeks after initial discharge. At first they may want to see you daily or every other day. Then, if all goes well, the visits will gradually become less frequent. Some hospitals have nearby local facilities like a Ronald McDonald House with separate apartments where a family can stay free of charge for some time after discharge. Others have agreements with local hotels where pediatric families can stay posttransplant. In some places it may be hard to find medically safe, convenient, and affordable local accommodation. If you live far from the institution, find out in advance how soon they anticipate you being able to take your child home and how they would work with your local health facility to see that there was appropriate continuity of care. You will want to be able to continue to consult with them if necessary—even if the center is too far away to bring your child in for regular visits. Again, you need to factor these variables into your final choice.

Once you get home, continuing precautions are key, because your child's immune system is not fully functioning yet. Recommendations vary from one institution to another, and will also depend on how your child's body responds to the transplant. Staff in the outpatient clinic will likely discuss precautionary measures with you at length before your child's discharge from the hospital. The most common home precautions are listed in chapter 15. The doctors will also suggest that the house or apartment be well cleaned prior to your child's return. Most institutions suggest limiting visitors to just adult family for the first few months.

If your child has had an autologous transplant, the recommendation for recuperation time before she returns to school could range from three to six months. If she has had an allogeneic transplant, doctors often recommend a tutor at home for up to a year. The list of medications that your child will need after discharge will be considerable regardless of the institution that treated him. The primary purposes of the medications will be to prevent or fight infections and to boost and support the immune system. There could be many additional medications depending on your child's medical picture.

HOW TO HELP YOUR CHILD

Give adequate and age-appropriate information. Once you have decided your child will need a transplant and where she will have it, you can start preparing your child. Your young child may need a simple explanation delivered in small parts:

"You will need to stay in hospital for a while in a special room and get some medicine that will get rid of the cancer cells (or the cells that are not making your blood right). You will get new stem cells through your central line that will help your body stay healthy (will help your blood work better). I will be able to stay with you. You will be able to walk around the floor or visit the playroom sometimes (if this is the case). If you do not feel well in the hospital, the doctors will give you medications to help. When the new cells start working properly, you should feel much better."

Your older child will need a fuller explanation about the transplant process that could be led by the oncologist or the transplant nurse coordinator. The important points to convey are:

+ He will need to stay in hospital for a while in a special room and will initially get chemotherapy (and maybe radiation).

+ The purpose of the medicine (and radiation) is to destroy his current stem cells that are not working right and/or to allow him to get stronger medicine for treatment of his condition.

+ He will then get new stem cells (his own or from a donor) through his central line. Over time the stem cells will hopefully create the proper balance of red cells, white cells, and platelets, so his blood can do its job properly (or achieve the special purpose of his stem cell transplant).

+ You can stay with him while he is having the transplant.

+ The doctors expect that he may not feel well for some of the time he is in the hospital—that is part of the process working—but he will get medicines to help with any side effects.

+ When the new stem cells start working properly, the doctors expect he should feel much better.

+ He should spend time thinking of his own questions to ask the oncologist or transplant nurse coordinator, who can supplement your description of the process.

If your child needs an allogeneic transplant, your other children will need to be prepared for their possible role, from having their blood tested to possibly being the donor if they are a match (see chapter 14, Stem Cell Transplants: Siblings as Donors).

Encourage your child to pose questions both to you and to the medical staff. If you are pretty sure she is wondering about something, you can ask the doctor the question when your child is with you.

Have a positive, matter-of-fact attitude toward the transplant. You can encourage your child while acknowledging that a transplant can be tough to go through. As the time gets closer, you can help her select familiar and comfortable things to take with her to the hospital. (Check with the hospital first to find out what would not be allowed and how objects need to be cleaned. For example, stuffed animals used to be problematic, but a more efficient sterilization program can allow your child to bring them in now.) Remind your child that you or someone else will stay with her, and comment on how much she got to like other nurses on previous hospital visits. Plan for ways to keep in regular contact with the family—this is particularly important if you are going far from home. Even if you are able to switch off with another adult and go home regularly, you may still want a regular time for your child to communicate with everyone at home. Once your child is in the hospital and some of the common side effects occur, you can remind him they are expected and a temporary consequence of getting a transplant.

Keep your own spirits up. Remind yourself that this is the best treatment option for your child, and try some of the strategies recommended in chapter 2, How You Cope in the Hospital., If your partner or a close relative can spend one or two nights a week in the hospital, thus allowing you to go home, it will give you a much-needed break. If you notice you and your child are becoming discouraged by the side effects he is experiencing, remind yourself that these unpleasant side effects are expected and actually mean the transplant is doing what it is supposed to do.

Help yourself and your child feel more relaxed and calm. Use some of the strategies discussed in previous chapters, such as breathing and relaxation exercises and guided imagery. If you use these tools with your child, you may find they also help you feel more relaxed and calm. Starting them before you go to the hospital is a good idea so your child will have already practiced them by the time he is admitted. It is easier teaching a new skill to a child who is feeling well, not sick.

Listen to your child. Your child may tell you how miserable he feels, and the best thing to do is to reflect your empathy for what he is going through. Here you have a challenge—try not allow your child's understandable upset to lead you to feel so discouraged and upset that it is hard to comfort him or yourself. Talk to a psychosocial professional on the team if this is the case. They can help you, and in turn you will be better able to help your child.

Offer activities and distractions. Laughing is a good tonic, so bring any humorous CDs, programs, or movies that you think will appeal to him. Distraction in the form of a card game, board game, or video game may hold his attention but may require more effort if he is tired or feeling ill than watching a program or movie. If he feels up to it, ask if he wants to keep a diary to describe his time in the hospital. This diary can be personal, you can distribute it to family and friends, or it could offer advice to other children who have to get a stem cell transplant. If he does not feel like doing anything active, you can read to him, which offers the comfort of your voice and gives you something useful to do for him. You can record some of his favorite books so he can listen to you reading if you have to go home in the evening. This also might be a time where he could listen to audiobooks or to his favorite music.

Make it easy for him to be in contact with his friends. Suggest to your older child that he call, Skype, or have face time with his friends at a particular time each day. You can leave the room so he has privacy during those times. You can warn his friends that sometimes he may not feel up to talking much and encourage them to take the lead in the conversations on those occasions.

Encourage your child to engage with his medical team. In addition to talking with your child and medical team members about subjects you know would interest your child (about sports, TV shows, etc.), you can find activities that also connect your child and his medical team. For example, you can learn new magic tricks together and then help him surprise or "mystify" the medical staff. Or you can bring in a joke book that you can read to him, and he can choose which joke to tell his current nurse. It will increase his feeling of connection with them and theirs with him. It will also increase his feeling of competence and mastery.

Help increase his sense of control. You can help him write up a schedule and instructions to pin on the door. Include some private time when he has no active medical demands. Sometimes the medical staff may need to interrupt during this time, but let them know in advance that your child will ask them to explain why they are there. He can include simple instructions like "Please introduce yourself and explain why you are visiting me" on the door so everyone who comes into his room knows what is expected and he knows the medical staff respects his wishes.

Work with the psychosocial staff to see that they are providing you and your child with the support you and he need during his hospital stay. Concrete examples of such support could include being a sounding board for you and your child, offering a place where you can express yourself freely, developing interventions like a behavioral plan to help your child cooperate with necessary procedures or swallow unpleasant medications, advocating with the medical team for more effective pain medication or smoothing interactions between you and the medical team, helping your child to use guided imagery more effectively to get to sleep, or suggesting appealing activities that are compatible with his physical condition.

Prepare him for initial discharge from the hospital. You can acknowledge to your child how exciting it is that he is getting out of the hospital, but assure him that it is normal to feel a little anxious about leaving after being in hospital so long. You can encourage the hospital staff to say they will visit your child when he comes to the outpatient clinic so he will know he'll see some familiar people there. (In some centers the aftercare is done by inpatient transplant staff, so this will automatically occur.) Your child needs to know that, most likely, he will not go home right away but will stay somewhere nearby so he can be checked daily at the outpatient clinic. Let him know that after he is discharged he will need to take special precautions to prevent infections, like wearing a mask when he comes into the outpatient clinic.

Ease the transition into the outpatient clinic or other lodging. Be sure you take your child's favorite things from the hospital to your new temporary lodgings while you or your partner can take the less important stuff you and your child have accumulated during the transplant directly home. Once you are both in your new space, make it as welcoming and friendly as possible—put out photos and drawings, place your child's favorite blanket or stuffed animals on the bed—even if it is only for a short stay. Remind your child that this is a necessary stepping-stone to going home. Hopefully your child will enjoy the novelty of a new setting after being in one place for so long, despite the precaution constraints.

Let both of you adjust to your new roles. You may find it a little alarming to be solely in charge of your child's medical care and medication schedule overnight if you have grown accustomed to a nurse checking in with you frequently. Remember that you can always reach the physician on call if you have questions that will not wait until the next day. You can also use this time to encourage your child to do a little more for himself, such as choosing the clothes he'll wear each day and making his bed. He too will need to get used to not having a nurse at his beck and call. If your other children can visit (rules about this may vary from hospital to hospital), prepare them for the infection precautions and the routine handwashing they will need to do when your child gets home. You may be relieved that you are checking in with the doctor daily at first.

Reassure him if things don't go smoothly. If your child has a medical setback, which may even involve his going back to the hospital for a few days, assure him that this is very common. It may even be reassuring to both of you that it is actually possible to get in and out of the hospital in a few days and not have to stay there for several months!

Finally, the doctors will tell you that your child is ready to go home. They will likely make the immediate follow-up appointments your child will need either at their clinic or at the health facility near your home before you go home. The scenarios you will likely face when you and your child returns home are discussed in chapter 15.

CHAPTER 14

. . . .

Stem Cell Transplants

Siblings as Donors

The increasing use of stem cell transplants as treatment for various childhood conditions was described in chapter 13. I noted that sometimes a stem cell transplant is the only treatment that can cure your child. As noted there, if your child's own cells cannot be used and stem cells need to be obtained from another source, the transplant is called an *allogeneic* stem cell transplant. The best chance for a successful allogeneic transplant is if the patient receives stem cells that are a perfect match with his own. These matched cells can be obtained from unknown adult donors around the world, from umbilical cord blood, or, most frequently, from a brother or sister.

When one sibling donates stem cells to another sibling, it often creates a feeling of closeness and a special bond between them. There may even be a new physical connection; for example, the patient may become lactose intolerant like his sibling or develop similar allergies. This connection is sometimes reflected in jokes, threats, or offhand comments like "I wonder if he'll be afraid of the dark now, too," or "I told her if she doesn't let me play with her doll, I won't give her my bone marrow" or "I hope my hair doesn't grow back blond." If the donor is of the opposite sex, both siblings may worry that the new stem cells will make the patient more masculine or feminine. The connection may produce feelings of pride in the donor if things go well or feelings of worry, shame, and guilt if things do not go well. For the more far-out comments, you may want to say something like "I don't think there is any likelihood that will happen, but I will certainly check with the doctor and let you know what she says."

You, the parent, have a key role to play at each stage of the transplant for your donor child.

....

BEFORE THE TRANSPLANT

The three ways of obtaining stem cells were described in the previous chapter (see pp. 148–149). Two methods involve obtaining stem cells directly from a sibling or an unrelated donor, and the third method, using umbilical cord blood, does not. Public and private blood cord banks have indeed increased the availability of umbilical cord blood and in some instances can offer the chance of a transplant for a child without using a sibling or an unrelated donor match. But still, if the doctors tell you that your child needs a stem cell transplant, a sibling will be the most likely match and therefore all your other children will be involved. You will need to explain to your other children that they will all have their blood tested. At this stage, you can tell them that this is necessary to see which of them has blood that most closely matches the blood of your child who needs the transplant. After the tests, doctors will almost always want to use the brother or sister whose blood is the closest match, so you will then need to tell your children who is being considered to be the donor. Sometimes brothers and sisters who are not chosen are very disappointed; sometimes they are relieved. You can always tell them that they will be able to help in other ways. You will then need to explain to the child who has been selected as the likely donor what you hope will happen and why. It is reasonable and truthful to say to your child that he or she is being asked to do something very brave and very important to help his brother or sister. You are neither minimizing the importance of what he is doing nor setting him up to experience a sense of guilt and failure if the transplant is not successful.

If the first method of stem cell extraction is used, your child receives general anesthesia while the stem cells are extracted from his hip bones and he usually stays in the hospital overnight. Your child's back can feel sore for up to a week, and he will have to avoid contact sports for four to six weeks while his stem cells are regenerating and the extraction site is healing. Our hospital required a psychosocial clinician to evaluate any potential minor stem cell donor receiving surgery and anesthesia, following a recommendation by the Joint Commission on Accreditation of Hospitals (JCAH). This requirement also complied with the policy statement from the Committee on Bioethics from the American Academy of Pediatrics that recommended a donor advocate be appointed for each minor sibling donor. For many years, I or another psychologist evaluated potential minor donors between four and seventeen years old. The objectives of the interview were to be sure that:

♦ The brother or sister donor understood in an age-appropriate way what the medical procedure involved and why the patient needed new stem cells.

♦ The brother or sister donor was not being unduly pressured to be the donor.

♦ The brother or sister donor understood the limits of what he was doing—most important, that it would not be his fault should the transplant not be successful.

Many parents were glad their child would see a psychologist before the medical team would agree that the child could be the donor, but some felt differently. For some, it seemed to be just another demand when they were already feeling stressed, overwhelmed, and anxious, and some did not want to give their child the option of not being the donor. There were several concerns that parents or the potential donor sometimes had before the interview or that emerged during the interview, including:

A parent did not want a young child to be seen alone or a younger child did not want to meet alone.

To address this, we agreed that parents could be present. If a parent came into the interview room, he or she was asked to sit back from the table where the child and the interviewer were sitting and, if possible, to leave the room after the child became comfortable.

A younger child had difficulty understanding what was being discussed.

To help the child understand, we used concrete props and play materials like hospital Lego kits or syringes to make the information more concrete and understandable for the very young child.

A parent did not want the patient's possible death discussed, even hypothetically.

Sometimes parents wished to protect their children from anxiety and were determined to remain positive, so they did not want the possibility of their sick child's death to be discussed even hypothetically. We were able to use different words and describe the situation in ways that parents found acceptable. We felt it particularly important to say that perhaps the transplant treatment would not work if the prognosis for the child getting the transplant was poor. We used such words as "Jane has a very serious illness and the medicine might not make her better. We hope it will but we cannot be sure."

If we checked what the child already understood by asking a question like: "What do you think would happen if Johnny does not get your stem cells?" many children answered: "He would die." Children are excellent at picking up information and listening in on conversations, particularly if the adults deliberately lower their voices so the children will not hear!

A child believed he or she had to be the donor to save his brother or sister's life.

At the other extreme, some parents might have told the potential sibling donor that he or she will be saving his brother or sister's life by giving his stem cells. A parent might say this to persuade the child that he should be the donor and to help him understand the importance of his action. These parents were worried that we would minimize the importance of his role and thus he would feel it less necessary to give his stem cells. This was an understandable concern, but it set the brother or sister up to experience enormous guilt if the transplant failed or the patient developed long-term negative side effects.

We told these parents we were trying to walk a narrow line between not generating unnecessary anxiety and fear in the potential donor and not setting him up for a possible later experience of guilt and self-criticism. We emphasized with all donor siblings the limits of their responsibility as the donor while acknowledging the importance of the stem cells to the patient. With an older sibling donor, we might say something like: "You are giving Jane the best chance she has. But other things need to work, too. After she gets your cells, how she does is up to her body and the doctors."

With younger children, we often made an analogy to planting a seed: "You are giving Sarah the best possible present you can. Giving

Sarah your stem cells is like planting seeds. Perfect seeds can be planted in a garden, but they need help to grow. What are some of the things they need to grow?" Even children as young as four years old are likely to say "sun" or "rain." "That's right, the seeds need sun and rain and even good soil to grow well, so perfect stem cells like yours can be given to Sarah, but those stem cells need help from her body and the doctors (who will give her special medicine) to help those new stem cells grow well. If anything goes wrong and the new stem cells do not grow properly, it has nothing to do with you or your stem cells. Do you understand that?" We sometimes gave the lovely little book *The Gift* by Sue P. Heiney and Sheldon Lamphier to share with the child who was going to be the donor.[1]

Complicated family histories

Sometimes complicated family histories involving adoption, legal difficulties, or complicated birth histories can make considering a particular sibling as the donor problematic. In this case it will be particularly important to explore the consequences and ramifications of having a particular sibling as the donor and to make a plan about how to deal with different possible outcomes of the transplant over time.

Psychiatric history

If a child who is the potential donor has a psychiatric history, obviously particular care needs to be taken in the donor assessment, including considering the impact of a poor outcome.

It is important to:

♦ Consult with the child's prior therapist.

♦ Insist that the prior therapist, the hospital psychosocial clinician, and the medical staff talk with one another as well as with the child and parents before any decision is made.

♦ See that the child's current mood and functioning is thoroughly assessed, especially her attitude and wish to be or not to be the donor.

♦ Be sure the child understands the limits of her responsibility as the donor.

♦ Be sure she understands the possibility of her sibling's death even after a transplant.

♦ Discuss with her and her parents how she might react to her sibling's death and what might help her deal with it.

♦ Explore her readiness to resume therapy during the stressful time of the transplant and its aftermath.

♦ Get a commitment from her and her parents that she will return to therapy should there be transplant complications at any point.

SIBLING DONOR INTERVIEWS

Two colleagues and I assessed more than 120 minor siblings between 2000 and 2010. With the types of accommodations, interventions, advance planning, and extra interviews described earlier, no potential donor was rejected. Overall, most parents were receptive to the interview, but some were not. In either case, the assessment was required for any minor who was being considered as the donor. Most children were not deeply upset during or after the meeting. Some children cried, particularly when their brother or sister's uncertain prognosis was discussed. Many siblings discussed fears they had about the procedure, but explicitly stated that they wanted to be the donor anyway. Sometimes the fears were based on a misunderstanding of what would happen during or after the procedure, such as on a fear of needles or medical procedures, or arose out of family concerns. These fears could often be alleviated by arranging a special meeting with a doctor or nurse, by suggesting breathing or relaxation strategies, or by discussing the family concerns with the parents.

DURING THE TRANSPLANT

How can you help during the transplant? The donor and any other brothers and sisters may benefit from knowing that:

♦ One parent will likely be staying with their brother or sister in the hospital because he feels sick and needs support.

♦ Doctors expect their brother or sister to feel sick (get fevers, throw up, get mouth sores). This is part of what happens during a transplant and is normal. These symptoms almost always improve over time.

♦ The donor or the other brothers and sisters can ask if anything unexpected or unusual is going on with the patient if they are worried.

Different hospitals have different rules about brothers and sisters visiting during a transplant. Many hospitals want to keep visitors to a minimum to limit the possibility of infection to which the patient is so vulnerable. If you can organize it, your donor sibling can come to the hospital and meet you in the cafeteria or the garden even if she cannot visit her brother or sister.

If brothers and sisters cannot visit, hopefully you can set up a regular time for the donor and other siblings to check in with you daily. It may help that they understand that sometimes procedures or doctor's visits may mean you can't always talk when they call. Skyping, texting, and using Facebook or other social media may be useful additions to enable siblings to be in touch regularly and for you to arrange a convenient time to talk. You should prepare the sibling donor for the possibility that your sick child may not always feel like talking.

....

AFTER THE TRANSPLANT

Often the donor and your other children may hope that when their brother or sister comes home, family life will return to normal, that their brother or sister will be just the way he was before he got sick, and that you will have lots of time for them again. Moreover, different medical centers may have slightly different rules for transplant follow-up care, which could affect your other children. Before your child comes home, you need to check, for example, what is the posttransplant policy about visitors at home. To prepare your other children and to avoid disappointment, you can tell them:

♦ Your sick child may not feel well or get his strength back for weeks or even months even though the transplant was successful.

♦ Your child will still need a lot of your time—the nurses will not be around to help.

♦ Your child will still have to take lots of medicine and visit the doctors often, especially at first.

- Your child may feel grouchy and not want to play or even talk much for a while.

- Your child might have to go back to hospital (hopefully briefly) if he gets a fever or has other complications.

- You will try hard to do things with them, but plans may still change quickly.

- Based on your child's posttransplant care guidelines, explain who can visit home (close family members only, a teacher, one or two healthy school friends, or whatever the case may be).

Over the years, you need to remember the special position of your donor child. If your child who had the transplant continues to do well, it is likely the sibling donor will continue to be proud of his role in helping. If negative long-term effects quickly or slowly appear, or if your child relapses, pay particular attention to the reactions of your child who was the donor—especially if you suspect that he is protecting you from his negative feelings and worries. If you have concerns, do not hesitate to arrange a meeting with a clinician. Your donor has done something very special and brave and may have had to overcome his fears to do it. He deserves protection and support, and it will be very hard for him not to take it very personally if his brother or sister does not do well.

CHAPTER 15

. . . .

When You Get Home

MANAGING YOUR CHILD'S CARE

Once you get back home, you are in charge of monitoring your child's health. Being home is a big change, and though you may be happy to be back, it comes with its own emotional and practical challenges. Depending on what your child was in the hospital for, the challenges will be different. Some conditions require considerable ongoing medical care and adjustment of life at home; others will require going to many follow-up medical appointments and shifting the family's schedules.

If your child had an accident or surgery, managing mobility around the house may be difficult. If your child was newly diagnosed with a chronic illness, each condition will have its own particular follow-up treatment plan that will need to be understood and complied with. If your child was diagnosed with cancer and will continue to receive outpatient chemotherapy, you will need to ensure that she gets her medications and treatments as you manage side effects, take appropriate health precautions, and coordinate the rest of your family's schedules. If your child has just returned home from a stem cell transplant, the management of her care may take over a big portion of your life as she is likely to be weak, easily tired, taking many medications, and possibly having difficulty eating, all the while coping with a compromised immune system and attending frequent follow-up visits.

There are four primary goals of care that most outpatient medical teams will have for you and your child. First, that your child is being adequately cared for in terms of infection precautions, hygiene, nutrition, and general welfare. Second, that he is getting the medications he needs. Third, that you are taking him to all his medical appointments. Finally, that you are following instructions for his emergency medical care, including when to have the doctor on call paged to report any symptoms your child is having and when to bring him into the hospital.

You can be sure the doctors will let you know if they have any concerns about your child's medical care at home. They will discuss with you ways to manage the necessary care and will work with you to figure out what extra support they might be able to get for you at home in order for the goals of care to be met. For example, if you have a child just home from transplant, several young children at home, and no help, the hospital social worker might look into the possibility of getting you a home health aide.

INFECTION AND HEALTH PRECAUTIONS

Frequent handwashing and sensible infection precautions are a good idea when any child gets home from the hospital after an extended stay, but it is essential for children whose immune systems are compromised. The doctor will expect you to follow basic precautions upon returning home. Some of the most common practices follow.

If your child's blood count is being monitored

Most children getting outpatient chemotherapy will have periods during their treatment cycles when their blood counts are low and they will be particularly susceptible to infection, so special precautions are important during those times. Each institution has different recommendations on which activities are acceptable for patients based on blood count levels. For example, ask your doctor at what level they would recommend that your child not go to school.

By keeping track of your child's blood counts, you will get to know at what point in her treatment cycle she is particularly vulnerable. Common precautions for children with low blood counts are:

- Everyone coming into your home must wash their hands thoroughly and immediately, especially before touching your child or before touching food.
- Your child should wash her hands when she comes in and before eating.
- Your child should avoid people with infections, including siblings.
- Your child should put on sunscreen with at least SPF30 when going outside.

+ Your child should avoid crowds.
+ Report any exposure to chicken pox immediately.
+ Use recommended mouth care. Continue rinsing and careful cleaning.
+ Give your child stool softeners.
+ Do not use rectal thermometers.
+ Do not give your child routine immunizations (like flu shots).
+ Do not allow your child to swim in public pools or lakes.

....

AFTER A STEM CELL TRANSPLANT

All children coming home after a SCT will need themselves, caregivers, and family members to take consistent infection health precautions. Recommendations vary between institutions, so talk to your doctor about their specific suggestions. If your child has just returned from a stem cell transplant when her immune system is compromised, these additional precautions are typically advised even though the blood counts may appear normal.[1]

+ No children other than siblings should visit for three months after an autologous transplant and six months after an allogeneic transplant.
+ Carpets and curtains must be cleaned before your child returns home.
+ Your child should wear a mask when he is in any public space.
+ Your child should avoid anyone who has just been vaccinated with a live virus.
+ Your child should not receive a live virus inoculation until given the okay by his oncologist.
+ Talk with your doctor about your family's pets. For example, lizards carry the risk of salmonella and will need a temporary home elsewhere.
+ Move plants into a room in the house where your child does not go.

♦ Change air conditioning and/or heater filters and put away humidifiers for the season.

♦ Call your doctor or the person on call immediately if your child gets a fever or an infection. Prompt treatment is vital and sometimes is lifesaving.

. . . .

CALLING THE DOCTOR

After your child gets home, many parents struggle with deciding when it's appropriate to call the doctor. They don't want to be seen as oversensitive or a burden. But please remember it is far better to call when you don't need to than not to call when you do. A good rule of thumb is when in doubt, call the doctor. This is important because in any situation when the immune system is compromised, an infection, rather like a bush fire, can spread at lightning speed and the fire hoses need to start pumping at once.

Imagine your child with cancer has a low-grade fever. You have been talking daily to your doctor and following his instructions, which have been, so far, to stay at home unless his fever crosses the 101 threshold. On the third night your child's fever rises to 101.5. You worry you will bother the doctor on call unnecessarily by telephoning him, and want to see if the fever will go below 101 in the next few hours, but you decide to call anyway. Most likely the doctor will confirm how right you were to call and will tell you to take your child into the emergency room.

WHEN YOU GET HOME

Here are a few steps you can take to make your transition home go more smoothly:

■ Have the phone number of the doctor on call pinned up in a place where you or anyone else taking care of your child can access it easily.

■ In the same place, keep a list of the circumstances in which the medical staff want you to contact the clinic or the doctor on call (fever above 101 degrees, certain symptoms).

Remember, doctors far prefer you call too often than not often enough.

- Have your child's medication schedule written down and know your own comfort level dealing with the medications. If you are uncomfortable giving some of the medications, often you can request that a visiting nurse come to your home to give them. Sometimes the medical team will suggest this anyway.

- If the doctor suggests a visiting nurse, accept the help. Some parents like a visiting nurse to come, but others find it an unwelcome intrusion. If you are a parent who dislikes outsiders coming into your home, consider it as saving you additional visits to the clinic while ensuring your child gets the treatment and medications she needs to save her life.

- Ask the doctors to write down your child's future appointments at the outpatient clinic and the hospital. Pin them in a prominent place.

IT'S NATURAL TO BE ANXIOUS

When your child returns home from the hospital, it is hardly surprising if you are anxious about your child's health. Moreover, you have a new role. You are now the primary caregiver for your child without medical staff being there to help. It is one thing to be able to walk out of your child's room in a crisis to find a nurse, but another thing having to wait while the doctor on call returns your call. Other things may also cause you anxiety. If the original diagnosis was preceded by symptoms that were initially unrecognized, then a recurrence of any of the symptoms is likely to make you feel very anxious. Do not hesitate to call medical staff to tell them about the symptoms. They will understand your concerns and let you know if you need to bring your child to be examined. You can always explain to your child that your health worries may be excessive because of what happened before, but for your own peace of mind, it is necessary to consult with the doctor. If your child had a bad accident and is slowly recovering, expect that you will be concerned when he or she takes on new physical challenges. Perhaps you can be guided by his doctor about what is reasonable for him to do and what is not. Share with your child the reason for your worries and assure him that you are in consultation with the doctor and will be guided by her advice rather than by your fears.

....

NUTRITION AND WEIGHT

Most children have difficulty eating normally in the hospital. They are not feeling well. They are not exercising. The food is not appetizing. The available drinks are mainly sodas, and easily available unhealthy snacks may be more appealing to a child than regular meals.

If they are being treated for cancer, the problems are likely worse. Chemotherapy often makes a child feel nauseated. It wreaks havoc on appetite and taste, and can cause diarrhea, stomach upsets, and stomach pain. It can change taste and make food taste bland or even metallic. If your child is on steroids, his appetite may be voracious for a few days (but usually not for healthy food) and then disappear completely. Many children lose a lot of weight in the hospital. If your child had a stem cell transplant, the situation may be still worse. The mouth sores and intestinal inflammation that often go along with the transplant make it extremely painful to eat, on top of having no appetite. Your child may have had IV nutrition through his transplant. Your child's stomach will likely shrink during the hospitalization, and so it is easy for your child to feel full after a few mouthfuls.

If your child has lost more than 10 percent of his body weight, the doctors may have inserted a nasogastric (NG) tube, whereby liquid nutrition goes through a tube in the nose directly into the stomach. It is uncomfortable to insert, can get infected, and limits a child's mobility somewhat when it is in place. Sometimes doctors will prefer to surgically insert a gastrostomy tube (G-tube) directly into the stomach, particularly if the nutrition may be needed for several months. If a child has gotten used to feedings through a NG tube or a G-tube, transitioning back to normal eating can be challenging.

When you both come home from the hospital, eating is likely to be very low on your child's list of priorities and is probably very high on yours, as you are well aware that healthy eating is an important ingredient in her recovery. These different priorities can easily lead to a power struggle that you very much want to avoid if you can. So once your child gets home, how can you best address the issue of eating? Here are a few tips:

■ Acknowledge that a lot of kids going through what your child has gone through have a hard time eating.

■ Tell him it is quite possible his stomach shrank in the hospital, so it has gotten used to being less full and is sending incorrect messages to his brain that it is full when it is not. Tell your child that his challenge is to stretch it again.

■ Suggest when his counts come back up, after he is back home for a while and when his body begins to feel a little better, his appetite is likely to come back, which will make it much easier to eat more. Until then, the doctors still want him to eat as much as he can when he can and to eat whenever he feels like eating.

■ Remind him that the doctors have told you both how important it is for his body to be strong to help itself heal. And the more he is able to eat, the easier it will become for him to eat.

To help the process along you can:

■ Encourage him to eat little amounts often.

■ Make healthy high-calorie snacks easily available in between meals. Applesauce, granola bars, buttered popcorn, oatmeal, protein bars, cookies, cereal, cheese, and pizza slices are all good choices. Let him help himself if he can so you don't have to always put them in front of him.

■ Alternate these snacks with drinks like chocolate milk, milkshakes, or smoothies made with ice cream, or mixed with a supplement like Ensure. These drinks should be consumed between meals rather than at meals so the liquid does not fill his stomach before the food gets there, which would diminish your child's already small appetite.

■ Add protein to his diet. If he finds eating meat hard, substitute cheese, eggs, peanut butter, fish, or even crunchy roasted green peas. Add powdered milk to regular milk and use it to make milkshakes or pancakes. Grate cheese or slice hard-boiled eggs to put on top of other foods. Put melted cheese on top of hamburgers or hot dogs.

■ Offer your child plenty of peanut butter and jelly sandwiches if he likes them.

■ Add calories while minimizing sugar. Granola, pancakes (with milk), oatmeal, whole wheat bread, pasta, and potatoes are good options. You can add sour cream, full-fat yogurt, or cream to regular dishes or drinks.

■ If he needs more fat, you can offer him foods high in fat content like peanut butter, ice cream, avocados, olives, chocolate, and nuts. You can cook with butter, and spread butter on warm bread.

■ Get your child involved in choosing what to buy and perhaps even in cooking.

■ Try new recipes—after all, if your child's tastes have changed, it may be the moment that he will find something new more appealing than something old. Several parents found their children liked much spicier food than they used to—perhaps because it covered over an unpleasant taste change.

■ Make lists of what he likes in case someone other than you does the cooking at times.

■ Vary how you serve the meal. Some parents found their child ate more if the setting for the food changed. They suggested having a picnic in a different room (if that is not too difficult for you). The novelty may encourage your child to eat. Or serve a family dinner in front of the TV while watching a favorite movie (I'd suggest announcing the movie will be turned off if the dinner has not been eaten in fifteen minutes!).

■ Note what he likes and give it to him again.

If your child has had a transplant or has very low counts, he should not eat raw vegetables or fruit, but cooked vegetables and fruits that are peeled are encouraged.

Vitamin supplements should be used only in consultation with your child's doctor and a nutritionist. Some vitamins should not be used with particular chemotherapies.

Once your child begins to feel better, his appetite will likely follow. But it is awfully hard for a parent to sit waiting for that to happen. The ideas listed here will not necessarily bring your child's weight back up to where it was before, but they well may help reverse the downward trend in his weight and prevent him from having to be hospitalized and having IV nutrition or an NG tube or a G-tube inserted.

Sometimes staff would speculate that a child had developed anorexia, so adamant was her refusal and apparent incapacity to eat, but in all the time I worked at the hospital I never saw a child to whom I would give that diagnosis (and at another hospital I co-led a group for people with anorexia and bulimia, so I had plenty of experience working with people with eating disorders). When a child was refusing to eat, most often she had previously developed symptoms that had made it extremely painful or unpleasant to eat; she had lost a lot of weight and had become weak, fatigued, and in some instances, depressed; and could not work up the will or the energy to overcome the anxiety and fear she had developed over the experience of eating. Moreover, her stomach had shrunk, her appetite had disappeared, and she felt full the instant she did eat anything. Occasionally, she was angry at what was going on, and her eating was an area she could control and use to frustrate her parents and caregivers at the same time. In these instances, a power struggle was contributing to her difficulty eating. Should you get home and sense this is happening, there are several things you can do and ask your child's oncologist to do.

First, back off and stop trying to force your child to eat. Because you are at home and you are the person dealing with your child's meals, this may feel very difficult. You need to involve the doctors. Your child's weight and what he eats need to become an issue between the medical staff and your child—with you on the sidelines ready to help your child. The doctor must let your child know how seriously worried he or she is about your child's weight loss (the doctor will be very worried if your child is approaching the 10 percent weight loss mark), and tell her it threatens her health, her recovery, and her ability to be strong enough to fight her illness. Initially the doctor may want to weigh her weekly and note her progress or lack of it on a weight chart. A behavioral chart on which your child can earn points toward a selected prize whenever her weight goes up may be useful. Points are deducted if her weight goes down. If this does not stabilize your child's weight, the doctor may have to tell you and your child that if her weight falls further (perhaps below the 10 percent body weight loss mark), your child will need to be hospitalized and have an NG tube inserted. If she has previously had an NG tube, she most likely will strongly want to avoid this.

Brainstorm with your child how you can best help her avoid hospitalization and an NG tube. Review some of the ways listed earlier that have helped children with no appetite put on weight and see which of the snacks and foods listed appeal to her and what ways she would like you to help. Follow her suggestions. If she is not prepared to give you preferences, tell her you will put out some food options at different times during the day. You will leave them out for fifteen minutes and then remove them if they haven't been eaten. Tell her you will not be nagging her to eat, that will be up to her, although she may then have to be hospitalized and get an NG tube if her weight does not stabilize or increase. You can give her a five-minute warning that you will take the food away, and then do so with no comment whether she has eaten it or not. At the end of each day, ask your child if she would like you to do anything differently the next day.

For some children who dislike hospitalization and NG tubes this can be the necessary incentive.

TERESA

Teresa was a seventeen-year-old young woman who had lost a dangerous amount of weight. One attempt to insert an NG tube had failed in the hospital after she fought the nurse who tried to do it. She was later discharged and was at home but again eating and drinking almost nothing. Her weight was falling at each clinic visit. Several staff said they thought she had anorexia and I was consulted. I met with her and her mother and established that her mother was not prepared for her to have an NG tube inserted against her wishes, but was prepared for her to be hospitalized if her weight fell below a critical level. Her medical team encouraged her mother to stop begging Teresa to eat and cooking her special meals that Teresa would reject. It was clear that Teresa was furious at the way the staff and her parents were treating her. Her initial treatment had made her feel very nauseated and she would frequently throw up when she ate. She had minimum appetite and was choosing not to make the effort to eat or drink—an area she could control and use to torture her parents in the process. She did not want to go, however, to the hospital, which she also hated, and somehow, although her parents maintained she was still not eating or drinking, her weight held constant for two weeks. I then discovered she was drinking (and holding down) two cans of Ensure the evening before her clinic appointment, which guaranteed that her weight maintained itself just above the critical level when she was weighed the next day. I pointed out to her that this was an ingenious way to outsmart everyone, but interestingly, it showed she was able to hold food down, and we agreed it probably was not as good for her as eating regularly. We then made twice-a-week clinic appointments to monitor her weight more closely and enable her to see me more frequently. We talked about some of her future hopes and goals when treatment ended, and discussed other strategies she could use that would still give her control of what she ate but keep her out of the hospital. She gradually began to eat small amounts and feel better, and stayed out of the hospital. For her caregivers, including her parents, her weight gain was painfully slow, but for her, it was what she could manage.

SCHOOL

If your child has missed a certain amount of school and cannot immediately return to school after he gets home, federal law requires that the school provide a tutor. The criteria to get home tutoring may vary somewhat from state to state, but if your child meets the criteria, he should get a tutor at home three or four times a week. Using video programs like Skype can allow a child to follow what is going on in his classroom when he cannot be there in person. Ask if your child's school is equipped to set this up once your child gets home, or ask if they would be open to such a setup.

Ask if your hospital has a back-to-school program to help your child transition during his return. In our hospital, two staff members (nurses, psychosocial staff, or child life specialists) would visit the child's classroom—and sometimes the classrooms of their brothers and sisters—and in age-appropriate ways (via a puppet show for younger children, for example) would tell the children about the illness, treatment, and side effects that your child experienced and answer questions his peers might have. Usually, the child chose whether or not to be present. Those who did attend often answered some of the other children's questions. It was a very effective way to demystify what was happening, help the child transition back to school, and gain the support of his or her classmates.

Expect to feel anxious as your child returns to school for the first time since he was ill. You can take some steps that may somewhat alleviate your anxiety. You can start your child going back for part of the day first. You can tell the school about medications, physical limitations, or concerning symptoms. And your child needs to know he can visit the nurse's office if he feels tired or sick. You can tell your child,

"The school nurse is there to help children who feel sick and need to spend a little time away from the classroom. She will take you back to the classroom if you begin to feel better. And if you don't, she will call me and we will talk about what to do." But also remember that many children are quite skilled at using adult concerns to their own immediate advantage, so you may want to pay attention if there appear to be many visits to the nurse's office—particularly during your child's least favorite subjects!

If you plan for medical emergencies in advance, you will feel more peace of mind. Perhaps if you are working, you can assign someone who lives near your child's school to collect your child if he needs to leave school suddenly.

DISCIPLINE

Discipline and setting limits can be an issue for many parents when they get home. As we discussed in chapter 2, many parents find it hard to say no to a child or adolescent who is sick, and your rules and expectations about your child's behavior and other things may have changed somewhat while your child was in the hospital.

Moreover, however hard you may have tried to be consistent, your child will likely have gotten used to people waiting on him and paying him special attention in the hospital. He may well expect you to do everything his nurse did for him, and it will come as an unpleasant surprise that you cannot. Returning home, however, is an opportunity for you to go back to previous expectations. Children quickly notice if old rules of behavior have changed, and your other children will likely point out if he is being held to a different standard than they are. They probably will not hesitate to tell you if they think their brother or sister is getting special treatment. When your child gets back home, you can explain to all of them that a particular rule (the amount of video games played or TV watched) was relaxed only because he was in the hospital having a difficult time. It may be an opportunity to tell your child that for a while he was getting special treatment because he was sick, but now he is getting better and you are expecting he will gradually be able to do more for himself and help around the house like everyone else in the family.

ADJUSTING FAMILY LIFE

If you have a partner, perhaps you will need to consider readjustments of responsibilities divided while your child was in the hospital. If one person stopped working, can that person go back to work at least part-time, or should that decision be delayed for a while? My advice here is if you can possibly manage it, get used to being back home with your child for a while before taking on another large time commitment or responsibility. Parents are often surprised at the amount of time—for home care, regular clinic visits, and hospital appointments—that is still required on a day-to-day basis, let alone for unexpected emergencies. If your child is recovering from an accident, she may continue to need regular physical therapy appointments. For now, if extra time is available, divide it between the two of you so you can each get some time for yourselves and even take some time together.

If you are a single parent, the situation is more complicated, and you may have less flexibility. Whatever temporary emergency arrangements you made for your other children when you stayed in the hospital will likely now end. And you will be handling everything at home on your own with the added burden of overseeing your child's care as well as going with him to all medical appointments. Unless you have no alternative, this would be a very hard time to return to work. See if any of the people who helped when your child was in the hospital can continue to help in some way or if clinic staff can organize a visiting nurse to come to your home to do some of the medical care.

YOUR OTHER CHILDREN

Your other children will likely be very glad to have you home but may now expect that things will go completely back to normal and that you will have more time for them. We discussed in the last chapter how to warn your other children that your child who had the stem cell transplant may still need a lot of extra care.[2] But children coming home from the hospital for a variety of conditions may also require medical follow-up and extra home care, so warn your other children that, unfortunately, you will not at the moment have much additional time. Emphasize the positive—at least you are all back home together—but recognize that it is very common for there to be some resentment between siblings when your child who was in the hospital returns home.

So when your child is home and some of what you predicted is happening, here are some things you can do and say that are likely to make your other children feel better:

+ Give examples of ways in which your other children are helping and let them know you appreciate it.
+ Acknowledge any negative changes in your sick child's mood or behavior.
+ Ask your other children what they are thinking, noticing, wondering about.
+ Remind your other children they would be getting the special treatment and attention if they were sick.
+ Acknowledge the sacrifice that your other children are making (e.g., not being able to bring friends home, not seeing you as often, etc.).

If your child had a stem cell transplant:

+ Remind your other children that the recovery process is a long and slow one.
+ Reiterate that the transplant was successful even though your child may still feel ill.
+ If new symptoms—say, of chronic GVHD—occur, explain this may be a consequence of the transplant and does not mean the transplant did not work. The doctors will treat the new symptoms with medications that will hopefully improve the condition. Be understanding but not too sympathetic if your other children develop health symptoms—particularly if they resemble those of your child who has been ill. Obviously you do not want to miss a health problem, so first you need to check the symptoms out with your child's pediatrician. At the same time, you can also emphasize to your child the disadvantages of being sick and see your child has a boring time if he or she stays home from school! It is quite natural for your other children to try to gain your attention and time this way, and they may not have the slightest idea that this could be what they are doing, so a reassuring response is to pay attention to the symptoms but communicate and demonstrate at the same time how valuable and enjoyable being healthy is.

SCHOOL AND OTHER ACTIVITIES

After your child has returned home from the hospital, touch base with your other children's teachers to find out how they are doing in school. If other people have been helping out and doing special activities with your other children while you were at the hospital, try to ensure that they keep doing them for a while because you will likely have your hands full looking after your sick child without the nursing staff at hand. Maybe one parent, family member, or friend can do a few special activities with your other children, such as a trip to the zoo, a night out at the movies, or a nature walk. If your other siblings have gotten involved with SuperSibs, encourage them to keep that up.

Hopefully, your child who was ill will begin to feel better and stronger and will have to take fewer pills and visit doctors less frequently. Gradually your home will become less medically focused. Even if your child had a stem cell transplant, in six to twelve months your other children will almost certainly be able to ask healthy friends over and life should become a little more normal. The exact time may vary depending on your child's type of transplant and his or her particular situation. In some instances where ongoing medical care will be required, perhaps you and your other children will figure out ways to include their friends in home activities—maybe an extra adult could be on hand to help out or some spaces are kept medically free.

TAKING CARE OF YOURSELF

Similar to when your child was in the hospital, you may find it challenging to take care of yourself even when your child is at home.

Here are a few ideas to give yourself a break:

+ Ask a friend or relative (or your partner) to relieve you several times a week to allow you time for yourself—to exercise, or to do whatever gives your mind a break, be it reading, meditating, or praying. Or do this when your child is asleep or napping.
+ If your child is back in school and you are back at work, use the commuting time for activities you enjoy, such as listening to music, podcasts, or books on tape.

- ◆ Have healthy food and plenty of nourishing drinks in the house to encourage everyone, including you, to eat well.

- ◆ Encourage everyone, including yourself, to drink more water.

- ◆ Place a monitor in your child's room to reassure you and help you get a good night's sleep by relieving you from constantly feeling the need to check on your child.

··

SUMMARY

Your child's returning home may be a relief but also a challenge. You are likely to feel anxious at first. Get extra help at home if you can. Hospital staff as well as family, friends, and community groups may help you mobilize available local resources. And please remember to look after yourself as well as your child—just as in the hospital, the better you can take care of yourself at home, the more energy you are likely to have to take care of your formerly hospitalized child and your other children. Unless you absolutely have to, do not return to work or take on another major commitment right away. Give yourself time to get used to having your child home and see how much time and energy his ongoing care takes. Expect it will take everyone time to get used to the new situation and consider how to allocate responsibilities given the new demands.

PART II

. . . .

Survivorship

CHAPTER 16

. . . .

Transition to Survivorship

Various serious childhood health conditions have different trajectories and place different demands on you as the parent. Some serious childhood conditions do not have end points of treatment. Some do. Chronic conditions such as diabetes, sickle cell anemia, and some heart conditions require initial treatment that may stabilize the problem but require continuing, ongoing maintenance treatment for the stabilization to continue. There may be periodic exacerbations of the condition that are then hopefully controlled medically. In these situations, your child continues treatment, although the medical demands may lessen. You and your family face how to incorporate this ongoing reality into your family life. The treatment of childhood cancer, on the other hand, hopefully does have an end point and holds out the possibility of a complete cure along with the possibility of late effects requiring conscientious follow-up. A bad injury requires intense treatment initially and often only occasional follow-up later, which puts it into a similar category.

This chapter is most relevant to parents of children whose treatment has an end point or to parents of children where the medical demands have decreased significantly. Chapter 17 is about the follow-up care needed and possible late effects for children treated for cancer. There are important survivorship issues that are unique to this population that you need to know about if you have had a child with cancer. Chapter 18, "Emotional Effects of a Serious Childhood Illness," chapter 19, "Healthy Living," and chapter 20, "When Your Child Becomes an Adult" will be relevant to parents of children who have had any kind of serious medical condition, including those that require ongoing medical care.

....

ENDING TREATMENT

Your child has now finished his or her treatment. Perhaps your child has had the last hospitalization connected with his injury. Perhaps she has recovered from the rare viral infection that incapacitated her for some time. If your child had cancer, he may have had his last chemotherapy or his final necessary surgery. Now the visits to your child's oncologist or the specialist will be checkups and will hopefully occur with decreasing frequency. If your child had a central line such as a port-a-cath, it will likely be removed shortly. Your child should be able to attend school more regularly. Your family will assume a new normal where you will reestablish family life while recognizing and responding to new perspectives and attitudes in your family.

Don't be surprised if you feel a complicated mix of emotions. You may be enormously relieved and ready to get back to family life with fewer medical demands and as little contact with the medical staff as you can responsibly manage. Or you may find it very anxiety-provoking to see less of the medical staff. If your child had cancer, the treatment may have signified to you the disease was being held at bay. Once treatment stops, you may worry that the cancer could return. Sometimes parents miss the contact with the clinic and the familiar people there who have been a source of support and reassurance. For some parents and for parents dealing with different diagnoses, the change may not feel so dramatic because you may have already reduced the frequency of your clinic visits.

All of these reactions are normal and reasonable. Remind yourself that you will still have the continuing opportunity to ask questions of your child's doctor. Every large hospital has doctors on call in the emergency room. In most children's cancer treatment centers, there is an oncologist on call who will be available to answer your questions if something unexpected occurs outside normal clinic hours, even if your child has finished treatment. Depending on your child's condition, there are likely to be different resources and information available to you as you begin your child's survivorship journey.[1] Be sure the specialist has sent your child's pediatrician all the relevant information on his treatment and necessary follow-up care as you will hopefully gradually see more of the pediatrician and less of the specialist.

YOUR CHILD'S TREATMENT SUMMARY

It is enormously important that you obtain a treatment summary when your child's treatment ends, particularly if your child was treated for cancer. If your doctor does not volunteer the information, ask for a written treatment summary that precisely documents the treatment your child received. If your child had cancer, ask for the exact doses of chemotherapy agents and/or radiation amounts that your child received during the full course of the treatment. Everything is recorded in the hospital record, and your doctor knows what treatment your child received, so why should you bother? Here are a few reasons:

- It is not always easy to get precise information later from hospital charts, although the computerizing of many hospitals' medical records makes it easier.

- Treatment protocols change over the years as new research results emerge. Different chemotherapy regimens, for example, will have different possible late effects, and the information about what these could be will continue to come in as the years go by. Exact descriptions of the medications and precise radiation or medication doses for some chemotherapy agents your child received are vital information for the survivorship clinic or for any other medical provider who takes care of your child in later life.

- Doctors, particularly in a teaching hospital, often move elsewhere and may not be available for consultation or to help track down information about past treatments.

Each facility will have different ways to try to help during your child's transition to off-treatment. At our hospital, each child has a "transition visit." During this meeting, the child's providers review a treatment summary and follow-up care plan document. The document details medications, treatment, and/or surgery that a child received as well as the plan for follow-up moving forward. Also at this visit, the child's team gives every family a binder called "Transition to Survivorship." The binder includes possible late effects of a particular child's cancer treatment and emphasizes that children have a wide range of reactions even among those who received exactly the same treatment. Parents are asked not to assume that because a late effect is listed, a child will get it. It describes how researchers are trying to understand what leads to such different reactions among children who have gotten identical treatments and promises to keep parents updated about new information in follow-up meetings.

Our hospital has also offered group meetings for parents whose children are just ending treatment, to engage with providers and other parents who have been through the transition. You can ask whether your clinic or hospital has similar programs for the condition for which your child was treated.

THE TRANSITION TO OFF-TREATMENT

You may face many of the same issues after your child ends treatment as you did when your child came back from the hospital for the first time after getting treated initially:

+ Health concerns about your child.
+ Your child's adjustment back to school.
+ Family adjustment, including your other children.

YOUR HEALTH CONCERNS

Your health concerns are not surprising. Your child has survived a life-threatening illness or condition and you may be considerably more anxious than your child. Moreover, you will now have more time to worry, particularly since you are taking fewer actions involving her medical care (the clinic visits, the medical tests). Several studies have shown that many parents of childhood cancer survivors have post-traumatic stress symptoms.[2] Many parents of children who had other sudden severe health problems are likely to have similar reactions. So do not be surprised if you continue to find your heart beating rapidly when the clinic calls to make an appointment or when your child develops a symptom that vaguely resembles an earlier symptom he had when he was sick. You may feel incredibly worried when your child returns to school or stays away with a friend overnight for the first time. You may find yourself calling your child's doctor to get clearance for routine activities like sports. Of course you will feel protective. I'd love to tell you that most parents get over this as time goes on, but it seems to depend on your personality and how your child does. Many parents report worrying somewhat less if their child continues to do well, but even then, they can still find worries unexpectedly triggered. Some parents report that they become better at hiding their worries from their child. Later we will consider what to do if your worries are interfering with your life (see chapter 18, "Emotional Effects of a Serious Childhood Condition").

This parent speaks for many parents:

> John's treatment took a tremendous emotional toll on us all. This is the one chapter in our lives that I think we have ALL tried to erase. It isn't that we aren't grateful to everyone involved in John's care and treatment, because naturally we are indebted to everyone . . . but, honestly, the further behind us it gets the more our memories fade. Even time doesn't completely erase the fact that John suffered a life-threatening disease. It appeared from nowhere, but where is nowhere? Because it must be somewhere. In the back of my mind there will always be the concern that anytime John is sick we could be returning to nowhere/somewhere again, but it is not something to dwell on or even for me to ever speak aloud.

BACK TO SCHOOL: WHAT CAN YOU DO TO HELP?

■ If your child has been going to school regularly during his treatment, the transition off treatment may be relatively smooth from a school perspective. Perhaps he had a school reentry visit from his medical team when he first got out of the hospital and his friends and his teacher have supported him throughout his treatment. As school attendance improves and obvious signs of his illness (like hair loss or a physical limitation) decrease, you and your child may notice that he receives less special treatment. Commiserate with your child while giving the message that it is great that he is well enough again to be one of the group. When a new school year begins, his new teacher will not necessarily be aware of his medical history, so you will need to tell her.

■ If your child has been out of school for some time, the transition may be more challenging. For example, if your child has had an allogeneic stem cell transplant, he will have been out of school for nine months to a year with an individual tutor coming home or to the hospital several times a week. Schedule a meeting to speak with his classroom teacher about how challenging moving from having an individual tutor to returning to a classroom setting can be. You may wish to consider making suggestions such as having your child start school gradually (a few hours a day). Other suggestions might include asking the teacher to provide regular check-ins or asking that your child be seated close to the front of the classroom, making it easier for him not to be distracted by his classmates. Initially, your child may need you to help him at home to get organized for school the next day because he will not have done this for some time. If your child is suffering chronic physical effects from his condition, such as fatigue or weakness, you can advocate for reasonable accommodations to be made in his daily schedule. For example, a shortened schedule, rest breaks, use of the school elevator, or frequent access to the nurse's office may be appropriate accommodations. You may even want to consider an Individualized Education Plan (IEP) or 504 accommodations (described in more detail in the next chapter). Your challenge is to maintain a balance between encouraging your child to return to as normal a life as possible and keeping reasonable expectations.

Hopefully with or without these accommodations your child will gradually adjust back to the classroom setting. Some children who had a treatment or condition that affected the central nervous system may be vulnerable to neurocognitive late effects that can result in learning challenges. Ways to identify ongoing learning needs and address neurocognitive deficits in school are discussed in the next chapter. Most children treated for cancer or other serious childhood health conditions do not have this vulnerability. Your doctor will tell you whether your child could be vulnerable or not.

FAMILY ADJUSTMENT

In time, hopefully, your family life will become a little more predictable. You may have more time and energy to do things with your partner. If you shifted responsibilities around to accommodate your child's treatment schedule and hospitalizations, maybe this will be the time to reassess the changes you want to keep and those you don't. If you left a job or changed work schedules to be with your child, you may be able to reevaluate those changes, too. If your family finances suffered during your child's treatment, you may now have a chance to recoup some financial losses.

Brothers and sisters may take up activities that they could not do while their sibling was getting treatment. It is not unusual if a brother or sister who has been accommodating throughout treatment suddenly starts being more demanding. Brothers and sisters may have had to put their interests, needs, and wishes on the back burner, and some may have not wanted to make any fuss while you were obviously upset and worried. Now it feels safer to voice complaints and make demands. If you are able to respond with patience and understanding while making clear what is and is not possible given your family's financial situation, logistical difficulties, and other constraints, your other children may become more reasonable. If they do not, you can always consult a family therapist.

NEED FOR ONGOING FOLLOW-UP

The follow-up care required by childhood cancer survivors and the reasons for it are described in the next chapter. Other conditions will need varying amounts of follow-up. Your child's doctor will tell you what is needed, and your task will be to see your child gets the needed follow-up care regardless of any protests from your child about it being unnecessary! Children have a great capacity to think that if something does not hurt, nothing is wrong, so why should they have medical tests and go for doctor's visits when they feel just fine? You will need to explain simply and clearly why the follow-up is necessary and ask the doctor to do the same:

- You need to see the doctor today so he can check that :
  - your bone is growing in the right way after your surgery.
  - the medicine did the job and no lumps are growing anywhere in your body.
  - the white blood cells, the red blood cells, and your platelets are working together the way they should.

CHAPTER 17

· · · · · · · · · · · · · ·

Childhood Cancer Survivors

· ·

CHRONIC AND LATE EFFECTS

This chapter describes the development of and modifications to treatments given to children with cancer. It stresses the vital importance of follow-up care and where that care can be obtained. It lists possible chronic and long-term effects of the treatment and suggests concrete steps you can take as a parent if you and your child are faced with some of these chronic or late effects (academic, physical, vocational). The chapter may be tough to read. But please remember two things:

1. Specific treatments are associated with specific late effects and not others, so check with your doctor which, if any, late effects can be associated with the specific treatment your child received.

2. Children have a wide range of reactions even among those who received exactly the same treatment, so you should not assume that because a late effect is listed in connection with a particular treatment that your child will get it.

As of 2011, almost 400,000 pediatric cancer survivors were living in the United States.[1] The intensive treatments used since the 1960s saved the lives of these children. The treatments included high levels of chemotherapies and sometimes radiation treatments and/or surgery. Because of the relative rarity of a diagnosis of childhood cancer, different cancer centers have cooperated in research projects about survivors.[2] And pediatric cancer centers in the United States, Canada, and Europe have collaborated to come up with comprehensive guidelines for long-term care of childhood cancer survivors.[3]

Findings over the years have unfortunately shown considerable adverse health and neurological effects for subsets of pediatric cancer survivors. The good news is that in response to these findings, major modifications were made and continue to be made to the treatments (for example, radiation doses have been reduced or eliminated for some diagnoses,[4] some chemotherapy doses have been reduced or capped, and special treatments have been given to protect a particular organ from damage from a particular chemotherapy). This has substantially reduced the severity of some late effects for children currently receiving treatments. However, early follow-up research showed two complications. First, many patients treated years ago (in the 1970s and '80s) could not be tracked down, and some in their peer group were showing serious late effects. Second, adverse health effects increase over time, but the likelihood that vulnerable groups will receive appropriate survivorship care decreases over time,[5] which suggests that many early patients with possible severe late effects were likely to be approaching a point at which they would need help but were not being followed by medical professionals knowledgeable about the care they would likely need.

To address these problems, pediatric cancer survivor clinics have been established across the United States (and in many other countries) to provide ongoing care and follow up information to childhood cancer survivors and their parents as well as to keep better track of survivors.[6] The survivor clinic will monitor your child regularly and appropriately given her particular diagnosis and treatment. Staff are knowledgeable about recent research on late effects. If your child has any ongoing effects from the treatment, the medical staff can also help you manage them. The benefit to you as a parent for your child to be seen regularly at a childhood cancer survivor follow-up clinic is that the staff are experts on the subject. You and your child will have professionals from different disciplines (doctors with relevant specialties, nurses, psychologists and/or social workers) on your child's medical team who will consider your child's situation from various perspectives and will make recommendations to you and your child incorporating their different viewpoints. You can reasonably expect the following services from a cancer survivorship clinic:

- Clinic staff will keep you abreast of your child's appropriate medical follow-up plan based on the latest research given his diagnosis and the type and amount of treatment he received.[7]
- They will tell you about possible late effects given your child's particular disease and treatment.

+ They will recommend appropriate monitoring to detect any problems as early as possible in order to lessen the severity of possible late complications.

+ They will help manage any chronic ongoing effects.

+ They will offer support or make relevant medical or psychosocial referrals to help deal with physical or emotional complications from the disease or treatment chronic or late effects.

+ They will offer relevant information on healthy living for childhood cancer survivors.

+ They will keep you up-to-date on research on late effects relevant to your child.

+ They will work with you and your child as your child gets older to help her transition to appropriate adult medical care.

At our hospital, sometimes a survivor continued to be followed by his oncologist in conjunction with the survivorship clinic and sometimes his or her follow-up care would be transferred entirely to the clinic. The decision was based on the family's choice and the doctor's availability.

If your child's hospital or clinic does not have a follow-up clinic, check the follow-up recommendations for your child match those indicated by the Children's Oncology Group (COG) guidelines for your child's diagnosis and make use of the Health Links for parents on the website.[8] Discuss any differences with your child's doctor. And see that the oncologist communicates test results to your child's pediatrician or primary care doctor.

....

CHRONIC AND LATE EFFECTS

There is a formidable list of chronic and late effects that can be broken down into six main categories. But please remember it is a comprehensive list, not a list for each individual. Any one child might have none, one, or several effects but is extremely unlikely to have all of them. I will describe the broad categories of effects and then suggest some things you, the parent, can do if your child has any of them.

Possible Immediate and/or Chronic Physical Effects

Some treatments are much more likely to cause immediate physical effects than others. Some immediate effects may be temporary. Several types of chemotherapy cause temporary hair loss. Others can cause muscle weakness or walking difficulties that usually pass after treatment ends, but sometimes continue. Steroids can dramatically alter your child's appearance and mood temporarily. Other physical effects may be longer lasting. For example, some types of chemotherapy can cause some hearing loss. Surgeries for sarcomas or a brain tumor may cause long-term physical effects. Some surgeries may alter a child's appearance. Some chemotherapy may cause chronic tiredness or make a child more susceptible to infections. Some of these effects can impact a child's energy, motivation, and mood over time. On balance, evidence suggests that many survivors do have some functional impairments, reduced energy, activity limitations, or some negative health symptoms over time, although a majority of survivors still report their general health as good.[9]

Your doctor will be able to tell you if an effect is likely to be temporary or could be longer lasting. If temporary, you can reassure your child that it will pass. If it could be longer lasting, you can always say "We hope it will pass." If you notice your child tires easily, you may need to prioritize and limit activities for her so she gets to do what is most important and less of what is not. If your child seems less enthusiastic about an activity, it may be hard to figure out whether this is more attributable to his mood or to a reduced energy level. Your child, his teachers, or school counselors may be useful partners in trying to understand what is contributing to his attitude or behavior.

Possible Physical Late Effects

Particular therapies can affect different parts of the body in various ways over time.[10] This is one very important reason why your child needs regular, ongoing medical follow-up.[11] Different chemotherapies can impact particular organs, so depending on the chemotherapies and the doses your child received the doctors may want to regularly check the current functioning of a potentially vulnerable organ.

Your role here is to check with your child's oncologist whether your child's particular chemotherapy regimen might have affected particular organ(s) and, if so, to follow their specific recommendations for follow-up care in which the functioning of these organs is appropriately monitored.

Effects on Fertility and Sexuality After Total Body Irradiation and Chemotherapy

Total body irradiation (TBI), radiation near the ovaries or the testicles, and certain alkylating chemotherapies may adversely affect a child's sexual development. The testicles or ovaries may have been damaged and therefore are less able to produce testosterone or estrogen. Some surgeries or radiation on particular sites like the pituitary gland may impact growth and regular pubertal development. In some cases, treatment can cause infertility or place someone at risk for delayed puberty and early menopause—leaving a smaller window of time for an adult to have children biologically compared with the general population. You should have been told by the doctors at the time of his treatment if your child could be affected in this way.

As your child gets close to adolescence, you may want to review with your child's doctor what he or she understands is the actual situation for your child. You may want to encourage him or her to tell your child at this time what the likely facts are. Your child may well have misapprehensions about whether he or she can have children. He or she may have a range of emotions about the situation depending on his priorities, his values, and his stage of life.[12] For some survivors, different health concerns may take priority; for others, possible infertility may have a major impact and affect their view of themselves and their confidence in forming lasting relationships. Others may hold on to hopes that they will have children. Your child's views may change as he or she gets older. Practically, your child may need to be educated about using contraceptives. Some adolescents or young adults who came into our clinic were having sexual relationships but were not using contraceptives because they assumed they were infertile—perhaps they had only infrequent menses or assumed because of a low sperm count that they could not father a child. This was not necessarily the case. It is important for survivors to have accurate and relevant information from their medical providers. You will be the best judge of whether you, your child's pediatrician, or his or her caregiver at the survivors' clinic is the right person to discuss these issues with your child. Recent research looking at sexual functioning suggests that though a majority of young adult survivors are satisfied with their sexual functioning, more women than men are not. However, sexual dissatisfaction had a greater impact on life satisfaction for men than for women.[13] Survivors may become sexually active somewhat later than their peers. If you think your child may be having sexual concerns, you can suggest she meet with the endocrinologist or psychologist on her team. Information and resources about fertility issues are included in Appendix A (see page 332). If you feel fertility is a worry for your child, suggest he talk with his doctor or see if his doctor would make a referral to a therapist experienced in dealing with reproductive concerns. Some doctors may not be comfortable bringing it up without prompting, but avoiding the subject may adversely impact your young survivor.

If your son, as an adolescent, used sperm banking and is now in a serious adult relationship, you may want to ask him if he wants to find out what his options are at this point and whether he would like to talk to a medical professional.

Growth After Radiation or Chemotherapy

Some treatments such as surgery, radiation, or particular chemotherapy can affect growth. Your child's oncologist will tell you if your child could be affected this way.

You have an important role here. You will observe how your child is reacting to her height and whether she seems bothered if she is shorter than her peers. If you are concerned, you can always request an evaluation by an endocrinologist at the survivors' clinic. You may be asked to consider with your child and the medical team whether growth hormone stimulation injections might be desirable for your child. This is an individual and complex decision. A family's genetic makeup is important. If both parents are tall, an adolescent who grows a few inches less than he would otherwise will likely be of average height, whereas if both parents are short, a couple fewer inches may make a child feel conspicuously shorter than his peers. Your child's oncologist will review your child's medical picture thoroughly before recommending the injections.

Body Development After Surgery or Radiation

Surgery or radiation to a particular part of the body at a young age may affect how that part of the body develops later. If the treatment was around your child's face, her appearance may change, sometimes significantly, as she gets older. If she received treatment elsewhere on her body, the effect may be less obvious to others but still evident to her as she grows.

Your role here is to observe her reactions to her appearance as she gets older as well as to check with her doctors whether other surgeries are available or desirable that could, for example, correct a facial imbalance or hide an obtrusive scar. When your child is younger, you may be the one who has to decide if the benefits potentially outweigh the downsides of another surgery. As your child approaches adolescence, she may have more decided views on the subject that will be important for you to understand and consider. You may need to think twice about strongly advocating for a cosmetic surgery that your child is resisting. Sometimes it will be a decision that your child can revisit in a few years, but in other cases, the doctors may recommend surgery be done while your child is still growing.

SECOND CANCERS

Some treatments can increase the risk of a second cancer. For example, a new tumor may form in the field of a prior radiation site.

As scary as this is, your first job here is to check with your child's doctor whether any of the treatments your child received could increase the risk of a second cancer. If there is a risk, you can help your child by understanding what the risks are by seeing that he is followed by providers with an understanding of those risks, by adhering to the recommended screenings and follow-up, and by knowing symptoms of concern so you can report them promptly if they occur.

Possible Learning Effects After Brain Surgery, Chemotherapy, and Radiation

Some brain surgery and its associated postoperative trauma can cause immediate learning effects. Cranial radiation, some brain surgery, and chemotherapy administered into the spinal fluid (intrathecal)—chemotherapies usually given to treat leukemia and brain tumors—can cause delayed learning effects. The higher the doses of radiation and chemotherapy and the younger the child, the greater the risk of later learning effects, although there is considerable variability in effects even among similarly aged children who received the same treatments. If there are effects, they can surface anytime from months to years after treatment ends. Sometimes they are noticed when a child faces more challenging tasks during key transition points (such as moving from elementary to middle school or middle school to high school). No one knows exactly what leads to this unhappy consequence, but researchers are slowly identifying contributing factors. Chemotherapy may adversely affect the sequence and the flow of brain development and the development of white matter, particularly in younger children. Some treatments may affect the networks of the brain that develop rapidly during adolescence (including executive and organizing functions that allow adolescents to think creatively, flexibly, and abstractly).

Children (excluding brain tumor patients) who get a stem cell transplant, if they are at least six years old—even if they receive doses of total body irradiation (TBI) in the 12 to 14 Gy (Gray) dose range before the transplant—appear to be at minimum risk for adverse neurocognitive effects later.[14] (Gy is the unit of absorbed radiation dose, and radiation levels given are now expressed in these units.) Younger children and those children who had learning difficulties previously may be at greater risk, although by five years posttransplant, socioeconomic level was a greater determinant of both cognitive and academic outcomes than any other factor. The authors speculate that the 12 to 14 Gy TBI dose may not cause the neurotoxicity associated with higher levels of TBI dose. The TBI dose now commonly given to children with high risk acute lymphoblastic leukemia (ALL) is 18 Gy—reduced considerably from the 22 Gy dose given initially to children with ALL, which was associated with a range of neurocognitive and other negative late effects.

Steps to Help Your Child If He or She Is at Risk for Later Learning Effects

If your child could develop later learning effects from treatment, inform yourself what they could be. Even though the information may worry you, you will be more prepared to notice issues should they arise and you will certainly be better informed in talking with your child's teachers. Nancy Keene's book *Educating the Child with Cancer* describes many of the possible types of later learning effects, suggests steps you can take to identify them, and gives concrete recommendations for teaching methods and services that may help your child.[15] If you fear the information would be too upsetting or that you will become hypervigilant with your child, then perhaps you could simply follow recommendations about the frequency and type of testing your child needs and get further information only if your child starts to show learning problems.

Alert the teacher to the possibility that your child could develop some of these difficulties. You can give her information about types of learning effects that your child might have later and continue to do that at the beginning of each school year when your child gets new teachers. When your child seems physically fine, a new teacher may have difficulty understanding that a learning difficulty may be a delayed consequence of a treatment received several years earlier and should not be attributed to laziness or lack of effort, particularly when the learning effects may be quite subtle and difficult to pinpoint initially.

The following story illustrates how a child and parent can work together to contend with the challenges that these subtle types of learning difficulties can produce.

A SURVIVOR'S STORY—MOLLY

TREATMENT

In 1997, Molly was diagnosed with ALL at five years of age. She was treated for two years with chemotherapy. In 1999, shortly after her treatment ended, Molly relapsed. She received a stem cell transplant and was given chemotherapy, some specific radiation, and total body irradiation (TBI) in preparation for the transplant.

I met Molly, her parents, and her older brother shortly after her diagnosis and worked periodically with them during her initial treatment, later stem cell transplant, and follow-up. I continued to see Molly and her family on some medical follow-up visits and then, many years later began to meet with Molly annually in the Perini Quality of Life Clinic for childhood cancer survivors.

SCHOOL

After a year of individual tutoring at home and in the hospital after her transplant, Molly started school on schedule. Initially Molly's parents focused on her social reintegration.

Molly's mother: "Molly's first three or four years of school were during the time of her initial treatment and subsequent relapse and healing. Our focus was more on her healing and social reintegration. I really did not want to be too involved because I felt it was important for Molly to feel as normal as possible and start to learn to advocate for herself."

Molly did well in school but had to put in increasing effort to do so. A family friend provided some tutoring at home.

AWARENESS OF CHALLENGES

Molly's mother: "As she got older and the demands to keep up grew, I needed to take a more active role in getting support for her. Molly always put a great deal of expectation on herself to keep up and, until just recently, did not feel it was appropriate to ask for help. The biggest challenge for me was to stay in communication with her teachers behind the scenes to keep them aware when Molly's challenges became overwhelming for her. Starting in middle school, Molly spent an inordinate amount of time on her homework and her tests. Being granted extra time to complete her tasks was not the best solution, because that meant Molly just had to work longer to get everything done, and that took a toll on her. I met with Molly's individual teachers at the beginning of each school year to give an overview of her processing difficulties."

When Molly was fourteen, the school organized a neuropsychological assessment.

Molly's mother: "Having neuropsychological testing performed by the school and then having a follow-up consultation with the school by someone from Dana-Farber (School Liaison program) to explain the testing, in relation to the effects of Molly's treatment, was invaluable. It not only helped the teachers understand her disability, it helped me to understand how Molly was being affected by her disability. Molly had an unusually large gap between her comprehension and her processing time. Her frustration at feeling she should be able to do the work and the amount of time it took to actually complete it was often very overwhelming and she started having recurring headaches and depression."

Molly, her parents, and the school worked out a 504 plan (see p. 217). The plan included the following items, among others:

♦ Molly would have some extra study time in school.
♦ She could have extra time for tests, for some assignments, and for class transitions.
♦ She could handwrite lengthy assignments.
♦ She needed to complete fewer math or science problems if the standard number was too much.
♦ Teachers could use alternative testing options (oral, not written) if that would not alter the test's standard.

By the time Molly was fifteen, she had an impressive insight into her own learning style. She told me:

"I'm an auditory and visual learner, but I can't listen for long. I do best if the teacher is interactive. I'm a perfectionist—I want to show what I know. I know I can do the work and can do it well, it just takes me forever."

She was also noticing that trying so hard was affecting her emotional and social life.

"Too much material makes me feel overwhelmed. Then I can feel anxious and sad because I have to work so hard and I have no time for a social life."

High school, with its multiple teachers and large size, was a challenge and was not meeting Molly's needs. Her mother advocated forcefully for practical and uniform ways in which Molly could use the accommodations made in the 504 plan. A family friend who was also a math tutor worked with Molly at home to allow her to spend more time on other subjects in school.

A few months later Molly started taking Lexapro, an antidepressant. "I went to different therapists and none of them could figure out why I wasn't happy. I had good grades, friends, was good at sports, and had a great home life. They suggested antidepressants. We figured treatment might have created a chemical imbalance."

At sixteen, Molly reported finding schoolwork a little easier. She thought Lexapro helped her feel less stressed, less anxious, less irritable, and better able to focus, but most of all, it made her headaches go away. She did notice she felt tired much of the time. "But my therapist kept telling me it was normal for someone my age to be tired and want lots of sleep."

COLLEGE

Molly entered a local college.

Molly's mother: "Molly wanted a fresh start in college without using her diagnosis as a crutch, so finding potential advocates for Molly early on was key. I went to a meeting for newly enrolled students and their parents. I then followed up with an e-mail to a potential support person, so it gave me a contact. Finding real support in college was very difficult. She was given extra time to complete tests, but the staff was stretched thin with their own workloads."

Molly did find the new environment challenging. She took on a hard course load, and found the social life exciting but stressful.

"It was not easy—there was too much work, and it was a completely new environment. I thought I could handle the same course load as my peers, but it was way too much. I also wanted to have a social life. This was the first time for me not being known as the girl who had cancer—it is generally a very public ordeal in the community when a child is diagnosed with cancer."

At the end of her freshman year, Molly was put on academic probation. This was revoked, but by the end of her first semester of sophomore year, she decided to take a semester off. She lived at home, but stayed busy with a job and some nonprofit activities. She returned to college, taking a lighter course load and classes during winter and summer breaks, but she noticed a pattern.

"Sometimes I didn't ask for help or know who to ask. Then I'd fall further behind. I was also chronically tired to the point where I could not muster up the energy to do even fun things because I was so exhausted."

And she did encounter various challenges in getting the help to which she was supposedly entitled to in college that would have helped with her learning needs.

Molly then developed different kinds of severe headaches that were caused by a benign brain tumor—a likely consequence of her prior treatment—which necessitated taking further time off while it was surgically removed. After the surgery she returned to college part-time.

Molly was greatly supported by her parents during her college years. "In college my mom helped me prioritize and my dad helped me organize my work. The more orderly, the less overwhelming it felt. But sometimes their needed involvement led to difficulties in our relationships. It took a lot of time to figure out how to work together cohesively and peacefully."

Molly's chronic tiredness made it doubly difficult to keep up with course assignments and exams. After consulting with a new psychiatrist and with her mother's encouragement, Molly decided to discontinue taking her antidepressant, Lexapro, and began taking a nonstimulant medication, Strattera, used with some people with ADD, instead.

"It has made a huge difference. My friends and doctors and even my parents tell me I'm like a different person. I just wish I had done something sooner and not just accepted it. I feel so much less tired."

Molly has just graduated and is now considering what professional area to pursue.

MOLLY'S ADVICE TO PARENTS

"Ask your child's social worker or doctor for information about a Serious Fun network camp (info@seriousfunnetwork.org; 1-203-562-1203). Your child will probably have many positive experiences that come out of having had their illness, but being in the spotlight and being called a hero is a lot of responsibility and will make them feel different. This does not mean that these experiences are not great ones for your child to have, but it is important for your child to have a place to be just a regular kid where they don't feel different, and Serious Fun camps can be just that place. For me, the Hole in the Wall Gang Camp was the only positive experience I had relating to my cancer where I wasn't pointed out as, or didn't feel, different. Even Make-A-Wish made me wear a big pin with a bald child on it.

"Be prepared to advocate for your child when he or she is young.

"Advocate with the school to get the right supports in place. If you are worried, see that your child has a neuropsychological evaluation sooner rather than later so the school can concretely understand the areas in which your child may have learning difficulties and can plan how to address them promptly.

"You can also notice and bring to your child's and the school's attention what is happening at home—if, for example, your child is taking a very long time to complete homework.

"Find out exactly which accommodations could be made available in the school and speak up if you think they are not meeting your child's needs.

"Do the same when your child gets to college—though not as much. Encourage your child to advocate for herself, but be a safety net. Remember that though other kids the same age may be able to handle their own affairs at school, they do not have as much to advocate for and will not need to ask for as much from their school. Do not be too afraid to ask for what they need. Ask questions and make suggestions if your child asks you."

MOLLY'S MOTHER'S ADVICE TO OTHER PARENTS

"Follow your gut instincts and do not be afraid to question authority when it comes to your child's health. Continue to share your child's story to anyone willing to listen. Through networking, you may find the solution to your child's problem.

"Be open to really listening to your child and following his lead. Take an active role behind the scenes, but allow your child to grow and experience life on his own terms at his own pace."

· ·

MOLLY'S ADVICE TO OTHER CHILDREN, ADOLESCENTS, OR YOUNG ADULTS WITH TREATMENT-INDUCED LEARNING DIFFICULTIES

In school: "Recognize you are perfectly smart but you may have challenges in writing down or explaining what you know. You may have some difficulty keeping focused and organized. It may take you longer than your classmates to do a problem or assignment. But getting help and using accommodations can make things easier. Don't be afraid to use the 'cancer card'; in fact, don't even consider it that. Effects of treatment are not black and white. If something is hard for you, it's probably not your fault, and school should be a level playing field for everyone. It's not always clear what equipment you will need, but you can't be expected to play ball with your classmates without the proper equipment, so don't feel bad about asking for a glove when you realize that you aren't catching the ball as well as your peers.

"Notice if a particular accommodation is actually helping with the problem or if it is just being counterproductive. Ask for help if you are having difficulties. Do not delay, because the problem will get worse.

"If you were diagnosed at a young age, you don't necessarily remember what it felt like to be 'normal,' and finding your normal can be challenging. Be attuned to your own body and if you ever suspect that something is different or not normal, don't be afraid to ask your doctor. This doesn't mean you need to be afraid of every headache, blemish, or stomachache, but make sure you pay attention to what your body's patterns are.

"Don't be afraid to say something about an abnormality, even if it's just a small discomfort. It may be fixable with a change of medication, a change of dose, the elimination or addition of a medication, or an adjustment to your diet."

In college: "Look into each college's disability services before making your decision. I did, but not well enough. I ended up needing a lot more help than I thought I would.

"Consider the size of the school. Because my school was so big, nobody noticed if I didn't show up for the extra time testing, or if I wasn't in class. A smaller school would have been better for me in that respect. I would have gotten a lot more attention.

"Go talk with the resource center staff. Find someone you like and work with that person right from the beginning. But be aware that the person you work with is not guaranteed to be there all four years you are there, so find out what the disability services program(s) do and don't do for you, and what your responsibilities will be in terms of advocating for yourself. Find out what accommodations are available.

"It is easy to take on too much at the beginning, and planning a reasonable course load in the first semester is important. Recognize there will be lots going on. Getting used to the college environment, the social events, new demands, and completing assignments is quite challenging.

"That being said, a good social life is important and don't let anyone tell you it isn't. You need to be happy in order to be healthy, and you need to be healthy to do well in school. When you take a tour of a college, ask yourself if you could see yourself being friends with the kind of people that go there.

"Remember that your body has already taken quite the beating, and keeping this in mind is important. So when I say 'good social life,' I also mean a healthy one. . . . I knew that my body was very different from other kids my age.

"Also look into extracurricular activities that are available. I found that I did best in school and was able to get the most work done when I had balance between schoolwork and other things. Not just relaxation time, though that is important too, but balance with a sport or an activity, or even a job you like."

As Molly and her mother show, a parent's role is vital, particularly when your child is young. You can be an advocate, a proactive supporter as well as a cheerleader. And remember the first thing to do is inform yourself. If your child is vulnerable to later learning effects, organize that he gets a **baseline neuropsychological testing** when his treatment ends to show his baseline intellectual functioning.

Neuropsychological testing:

+ Assesses intellectual functioning and learning style.
+ Looks at strengths and weaknesses.
+ Recommends ways to improve your child's academic performance.
+ Gives baseline information with which to compare future scores.

The Children's Oncology Group (COG) guidelines for follow-up care recommend a complete neuropsychological battery for a child susceptible to neurological late effects every three years (sooner if you have particular concerns) and regular school testing every year. The thorough neuropsychological assessment of a childhood cancer survivor will look at your child's general intellectual functioning (more routinely covered in a school psychological assessment) but also at particular areas of functioning sometimes adversely affected by particular cancer treatments, not usually covered in the school evaluation. Possible areas affected include:

+ Intellectual functioning (verbal knowledge and fluency, nonverbal reasoning)
+ Academic achievement (math, reading, and spelling)
+ Attention (focus, flexibility, and sustained attention)
+ Memory (visual, verbal, and working memory)
+ Executive functioning (initiating, planning, organizing, and solving problems)
+ Speed at processing information
+ Nonverbal reasoning and tasks (visual and spatial motor skills)

Regular testing will allow your child's current results to be compared with his past performance and his performance relative to his peers.

A full neuropsychological and behavior battery for vulnerable survivors should be given by a neuropsychologist who has specialized knowledge about neurological late effects for childhood cancer. The review should include tests that zero in on the presenting problems of a particular child. Parents' and teachers' evaluations are likely included in the assessment. Sometimes a neuropsychologist will add information to an ongoing evaluation (see the following box). The Children's Oncology Group (COG) have developed a brief standardized neuropsychological and behavior assessment primarily used for research across pediatric cancer centers.

Neuropsychological testing is expensive, and insurance companies may be reluctant to pay for it. The following box suggests how to get and pay for appropriate neuropsychological testing.

HOW TO GET APPROPRIATE NEUROPSYCHOLOGICAL TESTING AND HOW TO GET IT PAID FOR

- Ask your child's oncologist whether your child should get a thorough neuropsychological assessment, and if so, whom the oncologist would recommend. Your hospital may have neuropsychologists who are specialized providers of these services. The neuropsychologists may have a list of other local qualified providers if they cannot do it themselves.

- Check your insurance company's coverage and see whether they will pay the specialized provider whom you are considering.

- Understand that rules vary from state to state (only Connecticut requires insurance companies to pay for neuropsychological testing for vulnerable childhood cancer survivors). There are also big differences between insurance companies within states regarding what they will cover. These differences include:
  - Whether the neuropsychological testing is a covered benefit.
  - Extent of prior evaluation that needs to occur before neuropsychological testing is approved.
  - The criteria for a "medical necessity" (often the grounds on which payment for a neuropsychological evaluation is approved).
  - Number of hours of evaluation allowed and covered.

> ▸ The proportion of the service the insured person has to pay (deductibles, co-payments).

- If your child's oncologist and/or a neuropsychologist document a medical necessity for the testing, it will increase the chance that an insurance company will pay.

- Medicaid will usually pay for testing if your child's care is taking place in that state. Mass Health will pay for it in Massachusetts. However, if most of your child's care is occurring in a different state, they will not. You will need to investigate what the rules are in the state where your child is receiving the most treatment.

- If your child's school is getting a psychological evaluation done by a school provider, ask if that person has specialized knowledge about late effects of cancer treatments. If not, ask that the provider consult with someone with the appropriate knowledge or that the school contract with a specialized provider. An experienced neuropsychologist can use prior testing, do an abbreviated assessment and integrate the findings to come up with an overall formulation and plan for your child.

- If you can support or participate in any effort to have legislation passed that makes it easier for parents to get testing paid for, you would be doing a great service to future parents and for children in similar situations as your own. In Massachusetts, effective advocacy has produced three improvements: "medical necessity criteria" needs to be clear, any denial must include a specific description of why the request did not meet the criteria, and there is now a uniform request-for-authorization form.

WORKING WITH YOUR CHILD'S SCHOOL

Some childhood cancer centers have staff who can continue to work with you and your child's school to see that an appropriate educational plan is in place to meet your child's needs. Dana-Farber's School Liaison

program organizes appropriate neuropsychological testing, consults
(by phone or in person) with the family and the school, does on-site visits, provides information on neurological late effects to the school, and
tells you how to access relevant services from federal, state, and community resources. If such a service is not available to you, the following
list summarizes the steps that may be helpful for you to take if your
child could be vulnerable to developing learning difficulties:

■ Inform yourself and your child's current and future teachers about
potential late learning effects that can occur given your child's particular treatment. Useful references are Nancy Keene's book[16] and the
Association of Pediatric Hematology Oncology Educational Specialists
(APHOES) practice recommendations for managing the educational
needs of pediatric hematology and oncology patients.[17]

■ Get an appropriate neuropsychological test battery done within a few
months of your child finishing treatment so you have baseline information on your child's intellectual functioning. (See the box on page 214.)

■ See that your child gets annual screening in school and follow-up
neuropsychological testing every three years—or sooner if you have
concerns.

■ Check if there is a parent special education advocate with whom you
could consider working.[18] The person's training, relevant experience,
fees, references, understanding of your child's needs, fitness of match,
and role he or she would play with the school are all factors to consider
in your search.[19]

■ If you or your child's teachers suspect your child is developing some
of the possible late learning effects, *request a school assessment*. The
school needs to get its own evaluation done, although you can request
that the neuropsychological testing that may have been done already
be part of the evaluation. A school is required to consider (though not
necessarily to accept) an outside evaluation. All children are entitled to
a free and appropriate public education (FAPE), regardless of disability.
The classification "Other Health Impaired" is the eligibility criterion
usually used for children with cancer or other serious health conditions
if they are to qualify to receive special education services. Some schools
may ask your child's oncologist or another specialist to document the
condition. You and school staff will meet after the initial evaluation has
been done.

■ If it is determined your child has a disability that is affecting his or her ability to make effective progress in school, he or she may qualify to receive specialized instruction and related services through an individualized educational program (IEP) In this case, a formal IEP team would be assembled in which you and any other expert you invite will be important participants.

■ Consider if a Section 504 plan, which provides reasonable accommodations or modifications for a child with a disability that substantially affects a major life function (i.e., walking, seeing, learning), may cover services that would be helpful in supporting your child in school. Accommodations can be included in a formal IEP or can be outlined in a separate 504 plan.

■ The IEP and 504 accommodations can include a range of specific services with designated goals: concrete services (a classroom aide); supplementary services (resource room help, specific skill development); accommodations (longer time for tests, hearing aids, wheelchair accommodation, class seating). An IEP is a legally binding document, but a 504 plan is not, which may make it less enforceable in a complicated high school setting.

■ You have ten days to sign the proposed IEP once it is complete. If you are not satisfied, you can reject it and request additional meetings. You may want to consult http://www.wrightslaw.com, which is the leading website about special education law and advocacy.

■ Check how the school will ensure that all your child's teachers are aware of the educational plan and will implement the plan. This is especially challenging in a large high school where a child has different teachers with different styles and practices.

■ If you do sign the plan, continue to communicate and collaborate with your child's teacher and other school support staff to ensure that the services and accommodations in place are addressing your child's needs and are resulting in some academic progress. If you think they are not, communicate this in writing to your child's team and request that changes be made. An additional meeting may need to be convened.

■ An IEP must be reassessed at least once per school year and more frequently if necessary. Rules for reviewing a 504 plan vary from state to state.

■ Check if any of the existing programs in the list below designed to help children with these kinds of learning effects might be available near you or online.

■ As your child gets older, be sure that you are comfortable with the required transition plans in the IEP that will move your child toward the next stage after high school, be it vocational training, a job, college, or a community-supported program. The IEP transition plans are intended to anticipate needs and see that sufficient supports will be available in these settings to allow your child to succeed. Be sure they are realistic, and double-check whether the support services still exist.

■ If your child is considering college, discuss with him and school staff what kind of college would suit him best and find out if appropriate learning and emotional support services exist there. Colleges want their students to succeed, but some have better resource and support programs than others and are better at detecting when students need these services. (See Molly's advice to patients on page 211.) If you and your child can find out about such services or even visit the resource center prior to your child enrolling (the admissions office will readily volunteer the information if asked), your child may find it easier to use the services should he need them. He could even work with staff in the resource center to plan an initial reasonable course load.

REMEDIAL PROGRAMS OR MEDICATION TO IMPROVE SKILLS

Special needs staff in school will often teach study skills and organizational and learning strategies as part of your child's IEP. In addition, various approaches have been specially designed or adapted to address the particular learning difficulties sometimes experienced by childhood cancer survivors. These include:

+ Cognitive remediation program
+ Other learning approaches
+ Computer-based cognitive training
+ Psychopharmacological treatments

One cognitive remediation program was especially designed for childhood cancer survivors and consisted of twenty two-hour individual sessions. It combined approaches from brain rehabilitation, educational psychology, and cognitive behavioral strategies. It has shown some slight but positive academic effects.[20] Other programs have been designed to give feedback on learning styles, to teach problem-solving skills, to teach visual motor skills, and/or to improve memory and attention. More general computerized learning programs focus on improving attention and memory by repetitive practice and are already used widely in schools.[21] Some learning programs use Internet games or brain exercises to help a child gain new learning strategies and to increase cognitive flexibility or processing speed. In some programs, an individual therapist works with the child; in others, intensive group sessions are held over several weeks. The programs may be offered as summer courses, sometimes by private educational groups and sometimes by a university or cancer center, or perhaps as part of a research study. These programs have shown some positive but limited results.[22]

Some medications, mainly stimulants (similar to those used to treat children with ADHD), have helped some pediatric survivors improve their focus and attention over time, according to the children, parents, and teachers.[23]

So what are you supposed to do given this smorgasbord of offerings, which have shown some promising results but are definitely in the still-being-investigated stage and may not be generally or easily available near you? Is it worth pursuing them? Probably so, but most important, be sure you are satisfied with your child's educational plan, which hopefully includes the recommendations of the neuropsychologist and is designed to meet your child's particular needs. The annually assessed plan will likely have the greatest influence on the quality of the daily learning experience your child has. Some schools will have more skilled professionals and more resources than other schools even though any school is required by law to meet your child's needs or to contract with outside people or agencies to provide them. In some instances, a learning program may supplement what a school is offering and may meet a particular need your child has. The neuropsychologist who tested your child would be a good person to ask about local or online remedial programs. If your child seems to be developing short-term memory or attention difficulties, look for computer remedial programs that address those areas. I would suggest you inform yourself about the content and the demands of any program your child is considering. If your child already had learning difficulties before the cancer treatment, be cautious about enrolling him in a program where he might feel frustrated or inadequate. He would likely do better in an individualized program that adjusts to his skill level. For the same reasons, you should monitor how your child is responding to an online course.

If you are noticing your child is experiencing increased academic difficulties, perhaps accompanied by increasing difficulty with attention, organization, motivation, and initiating tasks, talk with the neuropsychologist about the pros and cons of medication, most likely a stimulant. You and your child would also need to consult with your child's pediatrician or a psychiatrist before it could be prescribed.

Just as the extent of learning effects can vary considerably even among children receiving the same treatment, so the consequences of a particular learning difficulty can vary considerably. The effects can be lessened if your child is offered and learns ways to compensate for the difficulty. The effects can be alleviated for some children with appropriate support in school. For others, an outside program may provide your child with the strategies and skills he or she would not be taught in school.

HOW TO WORK WITH YOUR CHILD AT HOME

You are not alone if you struggle with how much or how little to do to help your child keep track of or do his schoolwork—how to keep a balance between being supportive while also encouraging independent study skills. Working with your child who has developed late learning effects from her treatment may be even more challenging because you may find it hard to believe that she is struggling with tasks that used to come easily. Read the "Recommendations" section of the neuropsychologist's report carefully and ask the neuropsychologist for concrete suggestions about how you can implement them at home.

For example, let's say one recommendation was to keep assignments simple, concrete, and specific (i.e. avoid the open-ended and complicated tasks). How can you help your child do this when she seems to be getting nowhere with a complicated assignment and it is already suppertime? Perhaps you can encourage her to brainstorm about the process, to outline the assignment, to ask herself questions like "What does the teacher want to know?" You may also need to send a note to the teacher asking her to make the assignment more specific.

Let's imagine another of the neuropsychologist's recommendations was to allow more time to complete tasks and transition activities. How can that be implemented at home? Can you allocate specific times for certain tasks, including a few minutes of advance warning when it is close to the time to switch tasks?

Some programs encourage parents to work with their child at home to support the "metacognitive strategies" that the child may learn relating to preparing for a task, doing the task, completing the task, and generalizing from it.[24] So if your child is receiving some study skills training, be sure to request that any information sheets are sent home to you so you can review and reinforce the strategies at home.

Once your child is in high school, you can usefully monitor how much time he or she is spending on homework assignments at home and inform the teacher. A child like Molly may feel compelled to finish an assignment no matter how long it takes. Remember, it may be more difficult for your child to organize and produce the knowledge in a timely manner than it is for her peers, and she may be feeling overwhelmed. The demands of your child's workload should match her production and processing capacity, and if you see the two are seriously imbalanced, you can request an accommodation be made to the type and amount of homework she is given.

....

EFFECTS ON SOCIAL SKILLS AND PEER RELATIONSHIPS

You may have concerns about your child returning to school and being amongst his healthy peers. You may worry he could be teased, feel ill, or feel left out. The evidence in general is encouraging. Childhood cancer survivors who have not had treatment involving the central nervous system seem to do well with their peers. Classmates rated children who had had or were being treated for cancer, as, on average, more likeable than other classmates.[25] However, children with brain tumors were, on average, seen as more vulnerable.[26]

Specific interventions have been developed to address the complex needs experienced by brain tumor survivors and their caregivers including various group programs. The most helpful programs often include separately facilitated groups for the children and parents. The parents group may combine discussion with more formal presentations on topics like educational advocacy or sibling needs. The Family Pediatric Neuro-oncology Outcomes Clinic at Dana-Farber/Boston Children's Cancer and Blood Disorders Center has run these concurrent monthly gatherings for many years. These parents and survivors describe spending time with others who "get it" as helpful and informative. If you want to find such a group, you can contact your local hospital, clinic, or other agencies in the community that may run programs for individuals with complex needs. Ideally the children's group will have a professional facilitator and other children in the appropriate developmental age range as your child to ensure your child's needs are met. If such a group does not exist at your institution or locally, you could see if other parents might be enthusiastic about collaborating with an interested nurse or psychosocial staff member to start one. If you cannot find a facilitator for a children's group, you could always start with a group for parents. You could experiment with different formats, for example, inviting outside speakers versus having informal discussions on topics of interest. You may also want to explore camp options for children with chronic illnesses including brain tumors. Some camps include the whole family. Appendix A includes some camp listings, and your hospital staff may know of local resources. Children with chronic illnesses and their parents have described greatly benefiting from connecting with others with similar medical experiences and challenges at these camps.

VOCATIONAL EFFECTS

Although many childhood cancer survivors have excellent jobs with which they are very satisfied, there is some evidence that a lower percentage of childhood cancer survivors get and hold jobs than the general population.[27] Risk factors for survivors being unemployed were being in poor physical health; having had a brain tumor, leukemia, or some sarcomas; or receiving high levels of cranial radiation.

Several studies found that childhood cancer survivors had difficulty obtaining health insurance and sometimes were reluctant to change jobs because of difficulty obtaining new health insurance.

Some survivors choose to avoid the risk of rejection by not including their cancer histories when filling out employment application forms. A fair number of survivors reported health problems that had caused them to miss work sometimes. Employers showed different degrees of understanding about missed time.

There are several ways that you can help your child negotiate the workplace. Whatever your child's condition, be aware of the legal statutes that exist to protect workers, including:

◆ The Americans with Disabilities Act (ADA) 1997. Employers are required to make "reasonable accommodations" for those with disabilities who "can perform essential job functions."

◆ Family Medical Leave Act (FMLA). In a company with more than fifty employees, the employer is required to allow up to 12 weeks of unpaid medical leave per year.

◆ Consolidation Omnibus Reconciliation Act (COBRA). Larger companies must continue to provide insurance coverage for eighteen or thirty-six months depending on the "qualifying condition" that led to an employee being laid off or fired.

◆ Affordable Care Act 2010. It forbids insurers to exclude or significantly increase costs of coverage based on most pre-existing conditions including cancer. It allows children to be covered by parents' insurance till age twenty-seven. It forbids absolute lifetime limits on medical expenses. It requires all adults to have health insurance and states to facilitate people procuring insurance at affordable rates.[28] This bill is currently under attack and efforts to repeal it with or without a replacement bill that might leave some of the provisions intact are ongoing.

Whatever your child's condition, encourage him to take whatever actions are necessary to manage his symptoms and allow him to work regularly. (See chapter 19, "Healthy Living.")

Finally, think with your child about his career choices. If he is likely to have health problems that will regularly interfere with his ability to travel daily to a particular workplace, consider if some jobs have greater flexibility in this regard than others. For example, telemarketing likely requires less regular attendance than working in most factories. A disadvantage could be that it may have fewer or limited benefits. Some white-collar jobs can be more easily done from home than others.

A FINAL WORD ON CHRONIC AND LATE EFFECTS

There can, unfortunately, be a range of chronic and late effects that are associated with childhood cancer treatments. Your child's oncologist can prepare you for what these could be (and what they are likely NOT to be). Even the possible effects may not occur. But if they do, there are many ways that you can help your child alleviate, compensate for, and live with the effects. Remember, there are other professionals and other parents who are available to be with you and your child to answer questions and give suggestions along the way.

CHAPTER 18

. . . .

Emotional Effects of a Serious Childhood Illness

The experience of having had and survived a serious childhood illness can influence your child's emotional makeup. For some survivors, having endured and survived is a major part of their identity which can leave room for little else. For other survivors, it has little impact. This latter group likely includes children who were babies or toddlers when they were first diagnosed. In this case, your child likely has little conscious memory of the experience of treatment, although he may have some body and unconscious memories that may cause him to have reactions that surprise him or you at different moments. The impact for your very young child may be influenced by the presence or absence of chronic or late effects and on how you treat your child later. A child who remembers little and has few effects is not so likely to view his illness as a major part of his or her identity—unless it makes you extremely protective.

For your child who gets sick once conscious memories are forming, the experience can be powerful. It can take over your child's life and perhaps your family's life, too. One or two years of your child or adolescent's life may be focused on hospitals, doctors, feeling sick, getting treatment, and enduring medical procedures and appointments. Your child may miss friends, peer activities, and the developmental milestones children of his age are going through. How a young adult integrates these medical experiences with the other priorities in life can be an important task over many years before the illness is placed in a balanced perspective. Talking with a therapist who is able to listen and help your child understand his reactions in light of those experiences can be very useful.

In general, a majority of pediatric cancer survivors rate themselves as similarly or more positively psychologically adjusted compared with siblings and the general population.[1] This is true even if they report some adverse health effects. Other challenging childhood conditions can produce similar reactions. The next two sections describe some of the more obvious positive and negative emotional effects that can occur for a child who has survived a major health problem.

POSITIVE EMOTIONAL EFFECTS

"I've learned not to sweat the small stuff."

"It gives you a sense of perspective."

"I felt more mature than my peers after what I went through."

"I sometimes think of the paths I might have taken, but the illness also teaches you how to survive."

A child may experience several types of positive emotional effects:

- ◆ He may have developed useful ways to cope.
- ◆ He may become very motivated and determined to succeed.
- ◆ He may even know the area in which he wants to make his mark (often related to health or the health care field).
- ◆ He may appreciate his own personal strengths.
- ◆ He may be more mature and have a wider perspective on life than his peers.
- ◆ He may be able to find meaning in negative events and to see the positive side of challenges.
- ◆ He may have better relationships and be more aware of the value of turning to others for help.

Your child has survived a challenging and life-threatening illness. He or she has probably had to endure unpleasant and uncomfortable treatments and hospitalizations in the process. He or she may have learned special skills to help cope with pain or anxiety that can be used in difficult situations in later life. A marvelous video titled *No Fears, No Tears: 13 Years Later* showed how some children continued to use the coping skills they learned during cancer treatment in useful ways afterward.[2] Your child may have received much positive attention for what she had to go through, not only from her family but also from society in general. She has been treated in special ways. She may have attended popular baseball events, gone on trips especially for children with her condition, or been visited by athletic stars. She may have observed how other people got together to help her and her family. She may have been able to choose a wish for herself and her family. The outside world may regard her as a hero for overcoming her condition; even her friends may regard her as rather special. She may have come to believe she went through what she did for a purpose. (You may wonder the same thing.) She may be more mature than her peers and have a wider perspective on problems. She may have come to appreciate the value of life and good health and may be determined to make the most of the opportunities she now has, even if the opportunities have been limited by the illness, the treatment, and its consequences. If another adverse event happens she may be able to tell herself, "I got through my illness, I can certainly get through this."

NEGATIVE EMOTIONAL EFFECTS

There are also potentially negative emotional effects that can be associated with having been very ill as a child. First, some of the positive emotional effects can be double-edged swords. The increased maturity and changed priorities a survivor may experience may also lead to her feeling somewhat different and isolated from her peers. A survivor may justifiably feel her peers' concerns are trivial in comparison to what she has faced, and this can affect the quality of the relationships she forms. Second, there also may be mixtures of attitudes, abilities, and styles that can interact in problematic ways with being a childhood survivor. Imagine a child who has gone through a difficult treatment and is now a survivor. She has become used to others taking care of her, looking out for her, paying close attention to how she is feeling. She has been given special treatment—rules at home and in the hospital may have been relaxed for her. She has been the center of attention in her family. She may have had a tutor at home. She has experienced some of those unique privileges as well as the hardships that often go along with a challenging treatment. Maybe she already had a difficult time making friends. Maybe she is a child who found it harder than most to give up being treated specially. (And maybe her parents found it harder than most to worry less and to return to normal expectations about her behavior.) Indeed, she may have somewhat resented returning to normal life. Now let's imagine she has been back in school for a while and is finding it increasingly difficult to do the schoolwork. She finds it hard to take initiative, to organize her homework, to concentrate, or to focus on academic strategies that could help. Part of her feels it is not fair that she had been sick and does not think she should have to make any special effort to succeed academically. She may blame her difficulties on her illness. If other people find it easier to do things than she does, why should they not do them for her?

In other words, her learning difficulties are interacting with her feelings of specialness. She is noticing that others are doing better than she is, but she has a hard time taking any action that could help. She becomes a little bitter. She may begin to experience some continuing health effects that may leave her easily tired with less energy than her peers. She begins to worry about her future health. These worries reinforce her sense of hopelessness and helplessness. She could easily become depressed, particularly should new stressors occur.

There are some ways you can interrupt this cycle. While you are reinstituting prior expectations of behavior, you can tell your sick child that you will have higher expectations for her behavior now. But you can also tell her you are so glad that she is well enough to be able to meet these expectations and you are looking forward to doing some of the things you could not do with her while she was sick. In other words, you will be emphasizing the positive side of wellness as well as the challenges that come with getting better. If she seems less motivated in school, consider whether she could have learning effects from treatment. If so, arrange a neuropsychological assessment. If she is highly unlikely to have these effects, consider what else could be going on. You can talk with her teacher and discuss ways to increase her motivation, such as focusing on a special interest at home and in school. If she has continuing health issues and seems worried about her health, warn her doctor so these concerns can be discussed when you next meet. If your child's daily functioning seems to be suffering, consider meeting with a therapist who is experienced in survivorship issues.

OTHER EMOTIONAL EFFECTS

There do seem to be some survivors who are at risk both in childhood and adulthood for emotional difficulties, particularly when positive or negative stressors occur in their lives, like a new job, a new relationship, or a new health difficulty. Your child may exhibit:

+ Anxiety symptoms
+ Behavioral issues
+ Depression and sadness

I discuss these symptoms and ways to address them in more detail in the following pages. Your child may be more vulnerable to developing some of these difficulties if:

+ Your child received cranial radiation or intrathecal chemotherapy.
+ Your child suffered learning effects or has had other major medical issues.
+ Your child was diagnosed with an illness requiring multiple surgeries that negatively affected his or her appearance.
+ Your child has negative perceptions of his or her experience and of his or her health and future health risks.
+ Your child has a prior psychiatric history.
+ Your child, upon reaching adulthood, has had limited education, is unmarried, unemployed, or has few economic resources.

Some of these factors are associated with greater likelihood of negative psychological health quite apart from being a survivor. And please remember that many children who fall into these categories (even into several of them) do not develop emotional difficulties.

Anxiety Symptoms, Including Post-Traumatic Stress Disorder (PTSD) Symptoms

It is not uncommon for childhood survivors and/or their parents to experience serious anxiety, particularly related to health issues. There are some situations for you and your child where some anxiety is

completely normal. For example, if your child is being screened for second cancers, you are both likely to feel very anxious. If you or your child
encounters something that has associations with a particularly hard
experience during treatment, do not be surprised if you feel a sudden
rush of anxiety. If you and your child hear about survivors you know
who have developed serious complications or other problems, your anxieties are likely to be triggered. In some instances, it may help to think
about the differences (based on different diagnoses or treatments)
between your child and the other survivor to remind yourself that
everyone's experience is different.

Parents are as likely to develop post-traumatic stress disorder
(PTSD) as their children—so if you are noticing that you become acutely
anxious, consider whether you could be one of these parents.[3] Perhaps
you understood the seriousness of the medical situation much more
fully than your child. Perhaps you were in the extremely difficult situation of seeing your child having very painful but necessary procedures.
The order and structure in your life could have been upset dramatically,
and the outcome, although hopefully positive, may have pitfalls and setbacks and you may be faced with constant reminders of the uncertainty.

You or your child could be vulnerable to severe anxiety or PTSD if:

 ♦ Your child's diagnosis and treatment has been particularly
   stressful and hard to witness.

 ♦ You or your child are genetically predisposed to be
   anxious.

 ♦ You have few outside supports and resources.

 ♦ Other stressful events are going on in your life.

So the signs of severe anxiety or PTSD you should look out for in
yourself or your child are if your child or you:

 ♦ Are significantly anxious and avoid certain activities.

 ♦ Become acutely anxious before regular medical
   appointments.

 ♦ Have flashbacks or nightmares about past medical
   experiences.

 ♦ Have panic symptoms (heart races, you experience sudden
   shaking).

If you or your child is experiencing some of these symptoms, reach
out to a psychosocial clinician experienced in dealing with anxiety and/
or PTSD for help. There are excellent treatments for these symptoms.

POST-TRAUMATIC STRESS DISORDER (PTSD)
A SURVIVOR'S STORY—SUSAN

Susan was thirty-one years old when she reached out to me. She had been diagnosed with cancer when she was twelve, and I had worked with her during her extremely difficult treatment. She had experienced dramatic mood swings as a side effect of prednisone, had several medical complications, and endured very painful procedures. When she was thirty, she was diagnosed with a second cancer, likely caused by a complication from her first treatment. She received six weeks of treatment that required her to be immobilized. Several months later she began having panic attacks and her family persuaded her to get in touch with me again. Susan told me that for a decade she had canceled or avoided medical appointments many times. "When medical issues confronted me, my anxiety level was uncontrollable. I would be in a constant state or worry, obsessing about worst-case scenarios until I made myself physically sick." She avoided thinking about and had minimal conscious memories of her first cancer treatment. She avoided taking risks. "I thought that if I maintained control over what I experienced and was exposed to, I would be able to control my future. I would be able to limit any future fear, pain, or unpleasantness of the sort I experienced during treatment." She had limited her social contacts and the activities in her life and felt most comfortable with her close family.

Susan said she wanted to feel better and to feel less trapped and controlled by her fears. She wanted to be able to have necessary medical appointments without feeling utter terror. She wanted to expand the activities, interests, and people in her life. If possible, she wanted to avoid medication. We agreed to meet weekly with the specific goal of preparing for follow-up medical appointments in our survivor clinic. Over the next three months, Susan practiced and used slow breathing every day as a way to calm herself. She faced her fears about remembering her treatment. We used her hospital chart and my notes to prompt her memory. She wrote down and retold her experiences. She remembered that she had an extreme reaction to prednisone, experiencing major mood swings: "I had rage outbursts. I felt different, out of control." She remembered multiple painful bone marrow aspirations and spinal taps without anesthesia. She remembered severe leg pain and weakness. She remembered that at one point the doctors feared she had relapsed. She remembered several unexpected hospitalizations. "I hated surprises like the unexpected bone marrow at the end of treatment. I remember anger, helplessness, a visceral wish to refuse and escape but knowing I could not. I felt trapped because I knew my family would make me do it." I was able to corroborate many of her painful memories.

Susan gradually noticed that her anxiety about remembering and the anxiety she felt waiting in the pediatric clinic to see me were both decreasing. She identified some of the negative things she was saying to herself (about her appearance, about her employment skills, about her illness, about the role her illness had played in her family), and we brainstormed what she might say to herself that would be truthful but more encouraging and accurate.

Susan made a hierarchy of challenging tasks in the medical area and in the rest of her life that she had simply avoided acting on till then. She selected one task each week in the nonmedical area to try. We prepared for the medical appointments (what she could expect and what to do, questions she could ask the doctors, what to do if she felt anxious).

During her medical appointments, Susan used her breathing to calm herself. She did not feel extreme anxiety during the medical interviews and asked the questions she had prepared. She did have a flashback feeling of anxiety when the hospital bracelet was put on her wrist. She told herself there was no need to be anxious now and reminded herself that it was good that she was there having the medical appointments. She was encouraged by the feedback she was given by the doctor—that she was doing well and did not appear to have many late effects other than the second cancer, which had been successfully treated. She noted that feedback allowed her to shift her perspective on her illness and its consequences. She now felt "that I was one of the lucky ones, not one of the unlucky ones."

Susan decided she wanted to expand her goals further socially and professionally and over time has been able to do this in an impressive way. She has married, has a satisfying job. She notes:

"Reaching out for help was the best thing I have ever done. It was in these sessions that I realized why I was doing what I was doing. I also learned of tools and techniques that I could use to help me navigate those inevitable uncomfortable situations. The techniques aided me in changing both my mind-set and physical reaction in circumstances that would typically be stress triggers.

To this day, I still use some of the relaxation techniques to calm myself for both medical AND professional appointments. I am so very grateful that I no longer have the exaggerated reactions to medical appointments, as I know am able to address my health and wellness in a functional and healthy manner."

To work with Susan felt like a gift. What she had gone through during her treatment had been extremely upsetting to witness even though the treatment had saved her life. Susan's remarkable qualities—determination, intelligence, conscientiousness, and a strong motivation to feel better—helped her use the tools provided to her effectively and opened new windows in her life.

If you suspect your child or young adult is experiencing high levels of anxiety associated with medical follow-up, you will help her enormously by seeing she gets the treatment that can alleviate her distress and allows her to function effectively again.

BEHAVIORAL PROBLEMS

You'll be relieved to hear that there is not good evidence that children who have had major health difficulties are more at risk for behavior problems than the general population. If your child is showing behavior difficulties, consider that the illness may not be to blame. Perhaps it is your child's developmental stage or outside stressors.

Certainly act if your child is:

+ Being destructive to self or others.
+ Doing risky things (driving dangerously or using drugs or alcohol).
+ Breaking rules at home and school.
+ Having serious difficulties with peers.
+ Increasingly getting into family fights.
+ Cheating.
+ Lying.
+ Withdrawing or isolating himself.
+ Being preoccupied.

- Having obsessive thoughts or showing compulsive behavior.
- Having serious insomnia.
- Spending irrational amounts of money.
- Having bizarre thoughts or hearing voices that are not there.

You have every right to be concerned and should consider consulting with a psychosocial clinician or therapist. The behavior may or may not have anything to do with your child's illness experience and may need a thorough evaluation to understand. There are several ways to find an appropriate therapist. You can talk with counselors at your child's school and see if they can recommend someone. You can make an appointment for your child at the local mental health clinic. Staff there will likely apply to your insurance company for coverage. You can find out from your insurance company whether they have a list of approved providers, then go through the list and see if there is a professional who seems suitable for you and your child to consult. If there is no appropriate professional, you can request an out-of-network provider, which may or may not be approved if the insurance company feels one of their providers can offer the service. If you are worried about your child's or anybody else's safety, take your child to the local emergency room, where he will be evaluated and some follow-up recommendations will be made.

DEPRESSION AND SADNESS

Some children are more prone to becoming depressed than others. A chronic or serious illness can be an added precipitant for depression. Some childhood illness survivors are at a somewhat increased risk to experience depression than others based on various factors:

- If your child's illness and its treatment have affected either his learning skills or a particularly valued area of your child's life that is key to his sense of himself—for example, if your child was a star athlete and can no longer play sports.
- If your child has other major life or family stressors.
- If your child continues to suffer major health effects from the illness or its treatment.

♦ If your child has negative ideas or feelings about the treatment and its outcome (past, present, or future) and/ or views himself negatively.

Again, please remember that many children who might fall into one or even several of these categories do not become depressed. Moreover, some children who happen to be childhood illness survivors may become depressed for other reasons (genetic, personal, or environmental) that have little or nothing to do with having been ill.

Signs of depression in any child include:

♦ Negative mood (sadness, low tolerance for frustration)

♦ Suicidal or self-destructive ideas or actions

♦ Low motivation (lack of interest in usual favorite activities)

♦ Difficulty concentrating

♦ Difficulty sleeping

♦ Changes in appetite

♦ Fatigue

♦ Dropping contact with friends

♦ Increasing disagreements with family members

There are easily available and effective treatments for depression, primarily cognitive behavior therapy and antidepressant medication. However, identifying depression particularly in a survivor of a childhood illness can be complicated because some of the symptoms of depression—for example, lack of motivation—may have other causes. Difficulty initiating tasks or concentrating, associated with learning difficulties developed by some pediatric cancer survivors, may easily be confused with lack of motivation. Similarly, fatigue can be a late effect of treatment or accompany depression. Indeed, posttreatment fatigue can have multiple medical causes. If you see some of these signs in your child, consult with a mental health professional experienced working with childhood illness survivors.

Distinct from a clinical depression, your child may feel considerable sadness at moments in his life when the reality of something he may already have known hits home. Knowledge of likely infertility or limited fertility can have a strong emotional impact, for example, when your child begins a serious relationship.

Some children may have marks or scars or changes in appearance because of an accident, radiation, or surgery that as a young child they hardly noticed but that begins to affect their view of themselves when they reach adolescence.

A young adult will naturally feel sad if new negative consequences of his or her illness and treatment appear—for example, if he develops another major health complication or has difficulty getting new health insurance.

In any of the above instances, if your child has trusted friends, family members, or a therapist with whom he can share his sadness and talk about his discomfort or his regrets, he will be less likely to get stuck in a morass of negative thoughts and feelings that can lead to depression than if he is facing them alone. And in observing his reactions, sharing his sadness, and supporting him, you may help him and yourself endure it.

HOW COPING STYLES AND ATTITUDES CAN AFFECT MOOD

Differences in attitudes and response styles both in your child and yourself may influence how you react to the same adverse event. Let's imagine your child has finished his treatment and has returned to school, but finds he is exhausted after half the day.

Your child could think:

1. This is really unfair. First cancer, now this. I'll never be able to do what I did.

2. This is hard, but I guess I'll just have to get used to it.

3. This is hard, but I'm lucky to be alive and maybe I can figure out how to do what I want to do most.

You could think:

1. This is just too much. He has had cancer and then he has to face this. He won't be able to handle it. I wonder what will hit us next.

2. This is hard, but he has adjusted to a lot already and maybe we can help him figure out how to pace himself.

3. This is a small price to pay for his survival. We can help him deal with it.

You and your child could go through several of the reactions at different moments. But which reactions predominate in each of you is likely to influence how you both feel, how you act, and how you integrate the new reality emotionally into both your lives. Your child may need to feel your empathy and may even feel comforted by your anger and sadness, particularly if he shares those emotions. If you combine that reaction with the underlying message that you have faith that together you will be able to deal with the situation, you are more likely to transmit confidence and hope to your child. Reactions and feelings you express are powerful models for your child, and sometimes children take on the response styles—positive or negative—of their parents. Children are also predisposed to have pessimistic or optimistic attitudes, so in some cases your child's attitudes may have little to do with you. Regardless, try to understand his reaction before you share your own, particularly if your reaction is a negative one.

....

WHAT HELPS?

If you could wave a wand and summon certain qualities to act as buffers for you and your child against the often uncertain, anxiety-provoking, and extended survivorship path, here is a starting list:

+ Flexibility if faced with bad news.
+ Being hopeful and positive but realistic.
+ Having a problem-solving bent.
+ Having ways to manage anxiety.
+ Accepting the reality—but not being overcome by it.
+ Being able to ask for help if you need it and to use whatever resources may be around you.
+ Being able to communicate clearly about what you or your child needs.

If you or your child already have many of these qualities, they will be invaluable. If these reactions do not come naturally to you or your child, are there ways you could add these skills to your own or your child's repertoire of responses?

It appears adults and children can learn some of these skills—not necessarily transforming a pessimist into an optimist (as we will see in the next chapter, an excess of either attitude can cause problems depending on the situation), but moderating thoughts and behavior in a positive direction and learning new skills that increase flexibility and expand perspective.

There are several types of therapy that help to develop these skills, and determining which will suit you and your child best will likely depend on your particular styles and the needs of the moment. During the time your child was having treatment, you or your child may not have had the time, interest, or energy to pursue therapy outside the hospital or clinic where your child was treated. Your focus then was on getting through the treatment, and any therapy you may have received was likely primarily directed to that end.

Now you and your child may have more time and distance to reflect on the experience, as well as to have an increasing understanding of the uncertainty of the path that lies ahead. At this point or at other difficult moments along your family's journey, a range of therapies could be helpful depending on your or your child's particular style and what you see as the main issues currently facing all of you.

You might consider three broad categories of therapy. The first is insight-oriented therapy, sometimes called psychodynamic therapy. This therapy aims to increase self-understanding, objectivity, and perspective and to allow someone greater freedom of choice in thought and action by removing self-imposed roadblocks to personal progress. This therapy can help people to understand feelings and thoughts that they may not even be aware of or that they may push away because they find them unacceptable. These feelings and thoughts may lead someone to act in ways that are harmful, repetitively negative, or self-destructive. The relationship with the therapist and his or her ability to listen and reflect back may be one of the routes through which insight about these matters is gained and previously unavailable choices become available.

The second category includes cognitive behavior therapies. These therapies are more structured and usually time-limited. They help someone recognize negative thought patterns that are leading to more depression, worry, or anxiety than necessary. In addition, they provide structured tools to counter these thought patterns and to generate more positive thoughts and behaviors. Cognitive behavior therapy seems particularly effective in treating depression but may not be sufficient to help someone with a complicated clinical picture. It has been adapted and used with children individually or in group settings. It has also been adapted to use proactively with vulnerable children to bolster their resistance to future adverse events. (See Martin Seligman's work at the Center for Positive Psychology in Philadelphia https://ppc.sas.upenn.edu.)

The third category includes therapies extending the tools and skills offered by cognitive behavior therapies. These therapies often emphasize mindfulness and acceptance of painful emotions, and teach skills that help regulate and tolerate negative emotions. They are often time-limited and structured, and may be taught individually or in groups. Examples are 1) Mindfulness Based Stress Reduction (MBSR), an eight-week group program (www.mindful.org; Kabat-Zinn) that teaches mindfulness meditation, body awareness, and yoga to people with chronic illnesses. 2) Acceptance and Commitment Therapy (ACT), a relatively new structured therapeutic approach that incorporates mindfulness into its world view. This approach cultivates awareness, acceptance, distancing, figuring out values, and taking actions that would support those values. It may increase psychological flexibility. 3) Dialectical Behavior Therapy (DBT) teaches mindfulness, tolerance of powerful negative emotions, effective interpersonal skills, and emotional regulation to people with severe difficulties within a highly structured framework that incudes group and individual work and telephone consultation. Mindfulness meditation is also being taught in other settings including in some hospitals and clinics, in individual therapy, and in schools.

Skilled therapists may combine elements of different approaches as therapy progresses, depending on your or your child's needs. Interestingly, your choice of therapist may be as important as the methods she uses. If your child has a good relationship with a skilled therapist, that may be as important as the approach she takes, so do take time in selecting someone who feels a good match for you or your child.

HOW YOUR OTHER FAMILY MEMBERS MAY BE AFFECTED BY YOUR CHILD'S ILLNESS

There may also be emotional effects on your other family members over time. The severe illness of a child changes your family and has an emotional impact. You may become a different parent. Your relationship with your partner and your children may change. Your expectations for each of your children may change somewhat. You may give up some hopes and develop other hopes. You may find your own attitude toward health and your family somewhat changed by the experience of your child having been so ill. You may find that your priorities change. You may take on new causes and encourage others to work with you for particular goals that may or may not relate to your child's experience.

We have talked already about some of the immediate effects on brothers and sisters. Longer-term effects on brothers and sisters vary considerably and depend on many of the same factors that make predictions for the survivors themselves so difficult. Relevant factors for brothers and sisters include their personal characteristics, temperaments, their place and role in the family, environmental factors including family functioning, and how the survivor does, amongst many others.[4] Survivors may feel more the positive impact their illness had than their brothers and sisters do. Their brothers and sisters may have felt more of the negative effects on the family (less parental attention, more disruption, more worries) and fewer of the special benefits.

There can be a myriad of ways in which serious illness affects the family. Maybe it caused a financial impact that was hard to recover from and led to sacrifices among family members. Maybe it brought out irreconcilable differences within the family. Maybe it gave a new direction and purpose to the family. Maybe it affected a brother or sister's worldview or even influenced the choices he or she made about a future career. Maybe it increased the empathy that family members felt for others with health problems.

Your family's story will be a unique one. There may be some things you have lost or not been able to do, some priorities that have shifted. There may be other things you have learned or ways that you have grown as a family. Whatever the changes are, it is very likely that your family's story will be changed by your family experience of your child's illness.

· ·

A FINAL WORD ON EMOTIONAL EFFECTS

There is enormous variability in positive and negative emotional effects shown by survivors of childhood illnesses, both individually and over time, which is likely influenced by who they are and what is currently happening in their lives, some of which may be related to effects of their treatment and some of which is likely not to be. Surviving their illness may have given some survivors unique strengths and resilience. For others, it may have supported prior negative expectations about the unfairness of life (providing ammunition to construct a negative view of the world and the future). For some, there will be serious late physical effects; for others, no physical late effects.

Your role will change in the coming years, but it will be no less important. For you, overseeing your child's follow-up until she can take over, tolerating any ups and downs, empathizing with setbacks if they happen, remaining positive with your child, cultivating resilience in yourself and your child, seeking expert help if you or your child needs it, encouraging independence in your child, and, if possible, gradually helping your child take on responsibility for his own health care follow-up (the subject of chapter 20) are just some of your vital and challenging tasks.

CHAPTER 19

. . . .

Healthy Living

In this chapter I discuss ways in which you can help your child be as healthy as possible by the time she reaches adulthood. You want your child to treat her body with respect as well as to give her body the best chance to counteract whatever health difficulties could come her way.

. . . .

HEALTHY HABITS

Healthy living habits may be even more important for survivors of childhood illnesses because many of their organ systems may be more vulnerable to challenges of various kinds. Crucial ingredients of healthy living are:

- ◆ Eating well.
- ◆ Exercising regularly.
- ◆ Not smoking or abusing substances including alcohol.
- ◆ Using sensible precautions against cancer, such as sunscreen.
- ◆ Using protective measures such as good dental care against potential late effects.

Unfortunately, there is little evidence childhood illness survivors do any better than the rest of us in these areas. In fact, in some areas, like getting enough exercise, they may do worse. You have a window of opportunity to model and educate your child about healthy lifestyles. If you can introduce your child early to healthy habits, you will do yourself and the rest of your family a service. As a young adult, your child may be away from home and health habits may be more ingrained. Should you wish to make a few changes and to maximize family impact while minimizing conflict, here are a few general suggestions:

- ◆ Whatever changes you introduce, make them for the whole family and not just for the child who was ill. First, the changes will likely be good for everyone—including you—even though they may be most important for your survivor. Second, it will prevent your child from feeling singled out.

- ◆ Make sure your partner is on board and agrees with the changes.

- ◆ Begin to discuss the importance of healthy lifestyles with your child's specialist and pediatrician before your child reaches adolescence. The doctors will be pleased to take the lead in making specific suggestions to you and your child. You can report the progress or lack of it on these fronts annually. This will give the doctor a chance to reinforce the importance of healthy life habits in front of your child and for you and your child to ask questions. If your doctor brings these subjects up, your child is less likely to perceive you as nagging and more likely to see you both as following the doctor's instructions.

- ◆ Take advantage of any programs and information offered as early as possible.

Eating Well

We all benefit from eating well, particularly a child who has been very sick. If you can offer your child a diet of grains, fresh vegetables and fruits, healthy snacks, and foods with low sugar content while managing to keep very little junk food around, hopefully he will get used to eating healthy food. Your child's doctor most likely would also be happy to discuss healthy eating with your child. If you have particular concerns, many medical centers have a nutritionist on staff who can discuss with you both in more detail the benefits of fresh foods, reading labels, balancing different food groups, and eating reasonable portions. These foods may be somewhat more expensive, so bulk buying or being in a co-op can help with the expense. It can be difficult to break eating habits, and the surest way to prevent returning to junk food is not to have it in the house.

Exercise

We all benefit from getting regular exercise, particularly if we have been sick. Your advocacy may be needed to make this happen. At school, some survivors of serious childhood conditions may have difficulty keeping up with the school's athletic program because they tire easily or because of other physical challenges. The school athletic staff may worry about overtaxing your child, and so rather than designing an appropriate athletic schedule, they may allow your child to sit out gym completely. If this is the case, advocate for a modified exercise program rather than no program. You can also discuss which accommodations to request with your doctor or your child's physical therapist. If your child's school has few exercise opportunities, you have a different challenge. Are there physical activities you can organize during the week for your child—soccer, activities at the Y, swimming? At home, can you make sure your child gets some regular exercise during the week, even if it is only walking or climbing up the stairs to an apartment? Could you introduce a weekend family activity that involves exercise, walking, hiking, jogging, biking, or even a family soccer game? Can this involve the whole family and not just your child who was sick? Bracelet pedometers register the number of steps each day someone takes, and simple ones are not expensive. As insurance companies focus more on prevention of health problems, perhaps your child's health insurance would cover the cost? Or could you afford to get pedometers for all family members and make it a family competition?

No Smoking

Childhood cancer survivors and young adults with serious medical challenges as children are likely to be strongly advised not to smoke by their doctors. In fact, a surprising number of pediatric cancer survivors do smoke. One study found that 28 percent of pediatric cancer survivors had smoked, and 17 percent currently smoked despite the increased risks.[1] If you smoked before your child's diagnosis, giving it up will send a powerful message. During his childhood, you can share your concern about any other family members who smoke and involve your child in trying to persuade a family member to quit. (Your relative may not thank you, but your child could be a powerful advocate!) Ensure that the doctor tells him annually about his own particular vulnerability to smoking—as well as the general dangers of smoking.

If, despite your best efforts, your child begins to smoke, you can find out about smoking cessation programs and encourage your child to call one of them. A few suggestions for getting started with quitting smoking are listed here.

- ◆ Call the Help Line 1-800-QUIT-NOW (1-800-784-8669). They can tell you about local resources and programs. They also talk to your teenager and help individualize his own plan to quit smoking. Depending on the state, they may be able to send nicotine replacement products (gum, patches, or lozenges) to your teenager.

- ◆ Smokefree.gov is a website with great information that takes someone through the process of quitting. This site offers two free apps: 1. QuitGuide: "Helps you understand your smoking patterns and build the skills needed to become and stay smoke free." 2. quitSTART: made for teenagers, though adults can also use it. The app uses information from your teenager's smoking history "to give individualized tips, inspirations and challenges." It suggests things to do to get ready to try to quit. It suggests how to get back on track after slips. It suggests how to manage low moods, offers distractions to deal with cravings, stores helpful information, and makes it easy to use social media to describe progress.

- ◆ Each state health department is likely to have a list online of smoking cessation programs that may include programs run by local hospitals and clinics.

- ◆ There are also several smoking cessation programs that have been designed especially for adolescents and young adults who had cancer as children—one program used a telephone intervention done by trained cancer survivors and resulted in twice as many survivors quitting as in a comparison group.

- ◆ Your child's doctor can stress the risks of smoking as well as tell your child of the multiple resources out there to help quit smoking. The doctor may have a particular local smoking cessation program to recommend.

- ◆ Many insurance companies as well as Medicaid and Medicare will cover most of the cost—if there is one—of a smoking cessation program, including a certain number of individual sessions.

Staff in these programs are skilled at increasing a client's motivation to quit, so if you get your child to make the first call, you may have set her on the right path. Don't get discouraged if it takes several attempts for your child to quit. Quitting is difficult, and all you can do is to encourage your child to keep trying.

Alcohol and Drug Use

Encouraging responsible behavior related to drugs and alcohol is a challenge. Nearly half of college students overuse drugs or alcohol, and one study found that the rate is only slightly lower for pediatric cancer survivors than their peers despite the added risks.[2] There is no reason to suppose the statistics are any better for survivors of other serious childhood conditions. Of course, you want to encourage your child to be part of the responsible group. You can remind your child of the added risks for him and get his doctors to talk with him about the risks. You will know if your child's specialist, pediatrician, or someone else is the best person to deliver this message and to give the reasons behind it. If you think your child has a serious problem with alcohol or drug use, your child's primary care doctor should be informed and will certainly be able to give you and your child referrals to get help.

Sun Protection

Sunscreen with high protection levels is desirable for everyone but essential for many formerly sick children who may be particularly vulnerable because of the treatments they received. Make it a family practice to use sunscreen liberally when you're leaving the house each day, no matter what the weather is like. If you all use the high protection cream, perhaps the habit will become ingrained even when your child is away from home, especially if you put a tube of sunscreen in his bag.

Dental Care

Chemotherapy and radiation to the head and neck often affect the salivary glands and mouth tissue. Young children who have not developed their permanent teeth are particularly vulnerable. So pediatric cancer survivors may be more prone than most to getting tooth decay, mouth sores, and infections. Therefore, good dental care is likely to be even more important for your survivor (regular brushing and flossing and regular biannual cleanings) than for your other children. If you have encouraged these habits from an early age, hopefully your child will continue to have good dental habits even if he is away from home as a young adult. Your child's dentist will likely be happy to reinforce the message regularly.

A FINAL WORD ON HEALTHY LIVING

We all benefit if we can live healthy lives, exercising regularly, drinking and eating in moderation, and generally taking care of ourselves. There are resources out there that can help. If your child has had a serious childhood illness or condition, healthy living habits are likely to be particularly important for his future health. If you can help him incorporate these habits into his lifestyle as he grows up, making use of whatever resources you can find, you will be setting him up for a longer, healthier life.

CHAPTER 20

. . . .

When Your Child Becomes an Adult

The Transition to Adult Medical Care

A child becoming an adult is a transition that every parent has to negotiate. It is often a time of mixed emotions. Feelings of pride and accomplishment are mixed with other feelings of fear and sadness. It can be challenging. The situation at home, the number of children you have, what your child is going to do, and how resilient or vulnerable you think she is can influence your reactions. It may be harder for you if you are a single parent, if you are not working, if you do not have other consuming interests, or if you do not have fulfilling relationships with other people. It could be more stressful if your child has decided to work in a dangerous place in the world or if you see your child as especially vulnerable. Because your child has experienced a serious childhood illness or condition, you could easily feel she is vulnerable. Moreover, depending on her condition, a good portion of your time may have been devoted to taking care of her, so you may have had less time to work or to develop other interests. A parent's natural fears about a child's ability to negotiate life in the real world may be increased by your worries about your child's health and thoughts about what she needs to do to maintain and protect it. You may also find you have more time on your hands to worry. Do not be surprised if you find yourself quite anxious when your child is moving out or moving on.

This chapter talks about how you might work with your adolescent and his doctor to see he gets the follow-up medical care he needs as an adult. Adult survivors may no longer be eligible for or comfortable with follow-up care in a pediatric clinic, and a pediatric specialist may not be comfortable having overall responsibility for the care of an adult patient, so the survivor will need to seek adult medical care. Unfortunately, many adult survivors of serious childhood conditions currently do not get appropriate medical follow-up care.[1] This is true of a majority of childhood cancer survivors.[2] I describe some of the reasons your young adult may be reluctant to take over his own follow-up medical care, and I offer some ideas for you to consider.

There are three separate but related practical challenges about medical care you will likely encounter when your child gets ready to leave home and is becoming more independent—all of which will affect the quality of medical care your child gets and will influence how you can best help your child take over her own care. The first is determining the most appropriate long-term follow-up care that will meet your child's needs and preferences throughout adulthood. Your child's pediatric specialist will be the caregiver who can give you the relevant advice about your child's follow-up guidelines. The second challenge is managing the difficulties you and your adult child will encounter as your child transitions to the adult medical world. The third challenge is getting your child to take responsibility for his or her medical care. You have an important role to play in negotiating all three challenges.

· ·

FINDING THE RIGHT LONG-TERM FOLLOW-UP CARE

Many chronic childhood conditions will require specialized follow-up care during adulthood. This follow-up care will be of varying types and frequency depending on your child's condition, and again your child's specialist doctor will be the person from whom to gain this information. Different medical organizations and subspecialty groups are coming up with their own condition-specific recommendations for adult follow-up care.[3] Almost all childhood cancer survivors will need life-long follow-up medical care of some kind. The frequency and intensity of that care will depend on the specifics of the diagnosis and treatment (which will determine your child's level of risk), your child's age, and how long ago your child completed treatment.

The models of adult medical follow-up care for pediatric cancer survivors include:

♦ Intense cancer-center-based specialized long-term follow-up care with a backup primary care provider.

♦ Primary care provider with periodic specialized cancer follow-up care visits.

♦ Primary care provider only.

In an ideal world, the following would occur:

1. Higher risk pediatric cancer survivors who received radiation, a bone marrow transplant, and/or multiple surgeries as well as chemotherapy would be followed closely by a specialist cancer survivor follow-up clinic, perhaps several times a year, with backup care from a primary care provider.

2. Medium risk survivors (who received multiple-agent chemotherapies) would be followed by a primary care provider, initially a pediatrician, later a primary care physician who communicates regularly with a cancer survivor clinic. Your child is checked in the survivor follow-up clinic every two or three years and the results are communicated to the primary doctor. The primary care doctor reports any major health changes in your child to the clinic.

3. Lower risk survivors (who had simple surgery or limited chemotherapy agents) would be followed by a primary care provider who communicates if necessary with a cancer survivor clinic. The provider has all information about your child's cancer treatment, possible late effects, and follow-up guidelines for your child's particular treatment and diagnosis and follows them.

Your child's oncologist should be able to tell you which risk category your child falls into and how that has factored into your child's current follow-up care plan. Check that there are no complicating factors in your child's medical picture that would require more frequent specialized follow-up. You can compare your child's follow-up plan against the Children's Oncology Group (COG) clinical practice guidelines.[4]

ROADBLOCKS TO NECESSARY ADULT MEDICAL CARE

The second challenge relates to systems difficulties for adult survivors of serious childhood conditions as they transition to adult medical care. Some roadblocks he or she may encounter include the following:

1. Adult providers may lack expertise in issues specific to the childhood condition the child had. For example, primary care providers can lack relevant knowledge about potential late effects for childhood cancer survivors and will not necessarily be aware of the recommended follow-up guidelines.[5] There may also be a shortage of specialized adult providers for some conditions.

2. Communication between the pediatric specialists and the adult primary care provider may be intermittent or inadequate, as may be the communication between different adult care providers.

3. Adult medical care is often more fragmented and less easy to access than pediatric medical care, so it is much more difficult to make appointments and follow through with all the follow-up care recommended.

4. The close personal relationship between you, your child, and the pediatric specialist may be difficult to replicate in the adult medical world.

These obstacles have made it difficult for many young adult survivors with chronic childhood conditions to get appropriate and well-coordinated adult medical care. Moreover, if a young adult survivor has not kept in touch with his pediatric providers, he may not learn about new research that could have important implications for his follow-up care. Adult and pediatric medical professionals have recognized there is a problem across chronic childhood conditions and are trying hard to identify ways to improve the transition of care with feedback from patients and parents.[6] Electronic medical records, continuing medical education programs, earlier and more complete educational preparation, patient navigators, transition readiness questionnaires, young adult clinics, joint visits, and a formal transition program in which an older adolescent is taken to the appropriate adult care facility and introduced to the adult providers are some of the newer initiatives. But progress is slow and uneven across states, institutions, and childhood conditions.

Some roadblocks may be easier for you, the parent, or your young adult to navigate than others. Your child needs to get an adult primary care provider. You can ask your child's pediatric caregivers to recommend an adult medical practice or a medical professional with whom they are used to working. If they have no recommendations, you can check with your insurance company and see which practices and individuals they have listed as providers and whether any seem appropriate for your child. If a desirable individual or group practice is full, ask for your child to be added to the waiting list. This can be a frustrating and difficult experience, so starting sooner rather than later is wise because it can take a while to get care with which you and your child are satisfied.

If your child is being followed by a specialist clinic and a primary care provider, advocate for appropriate communication. If your child is a pediatric cancer survivor, you have probably already requested that the clinic sends the treatment summary, a list of possible late effects, and follow-up guidelines to your child's primary care provider. If your adolescent changes providers as he nears adulthood, remind your adolescent and the clinic that the information should be sent to his new providers.

Encourage your young adult to check that any test results and diagnostic findings are sent regularly to the primary care provider and that the primary care provider is informing the specialist clinic of any significant health changes—so there is ongoing and two-way communication between caregivers.

Perhaps, at least initially, you can also help your young adult negotiate the challenges of managing the adult medical world—in which patients usually have to make their own follow-up appointments across different medical specialties and departments that are located in different places and have different appointment times available. This is very different from the pediatric world, where you or a medical staff facilitator may have coordinated the follow-up appointments that occurred close together with familiar medical staff involved. Do not be surprised if you receive mixed messages from your child, who may both want greater independence in managing his care but may also want your help.[7] This ambivalence is common.

In addition to checking that appropriate and ongoing communication occurs between caregivers, useful questions to ask about the adult care that is being suggested for your child includes:

- ♦ Is the adult medical caregiver or facility equipped to do the specialized follow-up care themselves?

♦ If they are not, how will your child continue to receive the specialized follow-up care he needs? Will your young adult continue to have periodic appointments with his current pediatric provider or in a separate adult facility, like an adult cancer survivor clinic?

♦ How will the several health care providers continue to communicate with each other?

♦ How will the new providers stay abreast of new research coming in about late effects of your child's particular treatment?

You may also influence when and how your young adult transitions to adult care providers. Parents in our facility had a range of viewpoints on this. Some parents did not want their child transferred to an adult care provider during college. These parents pointed out that needed follow-up care would be more likely to continue if they made the appointments during their child's vacations. Some parents wanted their young adult to continue follow-up with us even if he or she moved elsewhere to start a new job, arguing that he would be more likely to come to follow-up appointments with familiar people. The children usually concurred with their parents' wishes.

In contrast, some parents preferred that their adult child transition care to an adult provider earlier. Perhaps their young adult was no longer covered by parents' insurance, perhaps a new job offered a different type of insurance, or a planned move was seen as a good opportunity to switch caregivers. Sometimes a parent encouraged a gradual transition— a survivor might come in to meet with us first annually and then every two or even three years, which helped us establish regular contact with the adult health care providers. Your provider will likely follow your lead about when to make the transition to adult medical care because in the United States, unlike in many other countries, there is no automatic transition of care when your child reaches a certain age.

There may be circumstances in which you might reasonably worry whether a complete transition of medical and psychological care to an adult care provider would be a good idea for your child. What might be such a circumstance?

■ Has your child had neurocognitive effects from a brain tumor or some leukemia treatments and has a hard time functioning on his own? Do you see continuity of care for your child as a high priority? Even if some of his care needs to be with adult providers, is your child functioning at such a developmental level that he might be more comfortable in the pediatric clinic world? Does he want to continue seeing familiar people who knew him and you over the years? If the answer to these questions is a resounding yes, you can advocate that some of his care remain in the pediatric clinic with input from adult providers. Different clinics may have different policies about this, but there is no harm in trying.

■ If your child has a complicated psychiatric or social history, she might benefit from some continuity of physical and/or psychological care and you can advocate for this. You can ask if the same staff can see patients in the adult setting as well as the pediatric setting. You can make the same request for psychological support. For a while, our adult nurse practitioner shifted from seeing some older patients in the pediatric survivor clinic one year to seeing them the following year in the adult survivor clinic—their transition involved shifting offices, not caregivers. Occasionally, I would continue to see a patient in the adult survivor clinic so we could offer continuity of psychological as well as physical care. Usually, psychological care would be transferred to the psychosocial staff in the adult clinic. But make it a priority to work out with your child and his caregivers the mixture of pediatric and adult medical care that would match his needs best and strategize about the timing of the transitions.

Occasionally we saw a much older person in the pediatric clinic who had received treatment in the 1950s or 1960s. They might have been referred to the clinic by their primary care physician or have made the call on their own because they wanted to talk about their early experiences. Often the topic they wanted to talk about was the dramatic and lasting effect the treatment had on them and on their relationship with their parents. In those days, a child could be brought in and left at the hospital. Parents were not allowed to stay overnight. Parents could visit during the day, but only if they could stay nearby. There was minimum explanation about what was happening. A child could easily feel isolated and abandoned. Another child might feel guilty at the hardship and expense she thought she was causing her parents. Yet another child might feel angry and resentful toward her parents. These older survivors often had in common that they had not talked with outsiders or even with their parents about their feelings. Sometimes they had put off coming to specialized follow-up appointments for years. These older survivors said talking about their experience was an enormous relief. It also helped them understand their parents' likely perspectives. For us, the clinicians, talking with them showed us the enormous benefits of a more open communication and the considerable toll the secrecy had on the ongoing development of the child and his relationship with his parents.

AN OLDER SURVIVOR'S STORY—SIMON

Several years ago, Simon, a man in his fifties, came to our clinic. Simon wanted to tell his story to people he felt would understand what he had been through. He had been diagnosed with cancer as a young child. His parents had brought him to the hospital and left him there to get his treatment. He had felt horribly ill. He did not see his parents again for several months. They had little money, lived far away, and had other children at home. He did not know what was happening. He blamed himself and thought he had been left to die. Many years later he married, had children and noticed he felt extremely anxious whenever his wife left home. He never talked about his early experience with his parents until his mother became ill a few years ago. Then he learned from her how helpless and sad they had felt leaving him, how they had debated not taking him to the hospital for the treatment but had been told it was the only chance to save his life. Back then there was no thought of explaining to him what was happening. We were the first people other than his mother to whom he had described his experience. He was referred to a group of older cancer survivors with whom he could share experiences. Simon said talking to his mother and talking to us made him feel as if a massive weight had been lifted from his shoulders and helped him understand the extreme anxiety he had felt whenever his wife went away.

EMPOWERING YOUR CHILD TO BE RESPONSIBLE FOR HIS CARE

The third challenge, how to encourage your young adult to become responsible for his own follow-up medical care, is a facet of the general challenge of how to start trusting your child to make his own decisions. When your child's health is involved, how can a conscientious parent not feel extremely anxious about this transition? If your adolescent is reluctant to pursue follow-up care recommendations and take responsibility for his own medical care, he is not alone. Not only do many young adult survivors of chronic childhood conditions share the same reluctance, but young adults in general are notoriously casual in keeping medical or therapy appointments or looking after their health in general. For example, a health clinic at Yale has recently changed from scheduling medical appointments to a drop-in model. Unfortunately, many chronic childhood conditions do require lifelong medical follow-up care, so strategies to ensure this happens are necessary.

Many parents in our clinic worked hard with their child's oncologist to get their child ready to take more responsibility for their own medical care. The following lists positive steps parents took, often over several years, to encourage their children to be involved in and responsible for their own medical care. These strategies have been documented as being effective for children with other chronic childhood conditions besides cancer:[8]

■ Some parents encouraged the doctors to meet alone with their child and gradually educate their child beginning in early adolescence about the importance of regular follow-ups. The doctor meeting with your child alone gives your child the message you and his doctor see him as an important, independent player in his own care. In addition, if you let your child meet first and then come in for the second part of the meeting, you can ask that any key information be repeated so your child hears the information twice.

■ Some parents encouraged their older adolescent to make his or her own follow-up appointments.

■ Some parents encouraged the doctor to describe to their adolescent what sometimes makes it hard for young survivors to keep to medical follow-up recommendations despite the importance of doing so, and to find out what might help their particular adolescent follow up appropriately (prompts from parents, from the clinic, help in getting insurance, help looking into appropriate follow-up clinics, help in scheduling?).

■ Some parents gradually turned over the responsibility completely. They would slowly pass along different components of care to their child. For example, they might progress along these lines:

  ▶ Having your child spend some time alone with the doctor— gradually increasing the time your child spends with the doctor alone, though you may want to still be part of complicated debriefings where a lot of information is conveyed.

▸ Looking at your child as the doctor speaks will help the doctor start to talk to your child instead of you when explaining medical things.

▸ Going over with your child in advance the questions to ask the doctor.

▸ Encouraging your child to ask the questions.

▸ Going over with your child when she needs medical appointments.

▸ Encouraging your child to make the appointments.

▸ Having your child take the lead in getting to the appointment (driving, getting a ride).

▸ Encouraging your child to come into the clinic with a different family member, friend, or on his own.

Becoming responsible for her own care is likely to be a big change for your child. You have probably managed all medical follow-up since your child's diagnosis. You may have conscientiously followed the doctor's recommendations, made the necessary appointments, and brought your child to them. Undoubtedly, the doctors told you how important it was you do so. If your child's condition began when he was young, you will have done this for many years and your child's is probably accustomed to you doing so. If your child was diagnosed in adolescence, you are probably still coordinating all the appointments with the clinic and your adolescent is probably also used to that. Your child's or adolescent's role has been to come to the appointments. Now she is expected to remember when her follow-up tests are due, make the appointments for tests she may dislike, and juggle appointments with an increasingly complicated schedule. Is it surprising she "forgets" quite often?

Moreover, it is likely to be much more complicated making appointments in adult facilities than in pediatrics. You may be tempted to take it on again. Some young adults are not above giving the subtle but clear message: "If you want me to go to my follow-up appointments, you can make the appointments for me." You will be the best judge of whether this is a reasonable request because of the many competing demands on your child or whether your child could do it himself. Both statements may be true! And deciding when and if to say "Now it needs to be you to make your own appointments" is an individual decision. I urge you to discuss the matter frankly with your child. Offer support, but encourage your child to realize that the day will eventually come when he will have to handle his own medical care. And you want to be sure that he is adequately informed about why the follow-up is so necessary. For example, if your older adolescent is a pediatric cancer survivor, you may want to encourage his pediatric oncologist to review specifically with him at this point his treatment, late effect risks and follow-up guidelines. And see that he has it in written form. If you were given a transition to survivorship workbook at the end of his treatment, giving the book to your child is an explicit message that you are handing over primary responsibility for his medical care. (You would only be human if you had made a copy of some of the key pages before you did so!) Many childhood cancer survivors are not aware of important facts about their treatment and late effect risks even if their parents have received treatment summaries, so his own review with his oncologist is important.[9] The same is true of childhood survivors of other chronic conditions where significant knowledge deficits have been found.[10] As your child approaches adulthood, perhaps you can go over with him the current follow-up plan for the next five years and decide together how to allocate responsibility for making the follow-up appointments—as well as what to do if the appointments are not made.

Occasionally, other psychological and practical factors may make your young adult reluctant or unable to be a responsible partner in his or her own follow-up medical care despite your and everybody else's best efforts.

+ Your adolescent may not understand that he needs medical
  follow-up or not be able to keep track of a complicated
  follow-up schedule. His learning and organizational
  difficulties could have always been present or been caused
  by treatment.

+ Your adolescent may not be able to get to medical
  appointments or know how to make the appointments.

+ Your young adult may face financial barriers—for
  example, limited medical insurance.

In such instances, your young adult may need you to remain in charge of overseeing his medical care. He may need you as a second ear in his meetings with the doctors. He will certainly need your help as he transitions to adult facilities. You will perhaps be able to hand over some of the medical responsibilities but maybe not all. If there are insurance questions, maybe your provider can help you. And your child may well need your help when it comes time for him to get his own insurance.

In other instances, your young adult may resist follow-up care for a mixture of developmental and personal characteristics or situational stressors—and you may well have some idea about what the reasons are. You know your child best and will probably be able to guess which of the following examples might apply to him.

- Your adolescent may assume he or she is cured or invulnerable, so follow-up care is not really required. This kind of magical thinking is not uncommon in adolescents and young adults.

- Your adolescent may assume you made all those follow-up medical appointments because you were overly concerned and that many of them were and are unnecessary.

- Your adolescent may wish to be independent, to live normally, and not to be burdened by his or her medical history, at least for a while.

- Your adolescent may wish not to be bothered and may have other priorities on his or her mind at this moment.

- Your adolescent may be very busy trying to make his or her mark in college or in a new job and be very reluctant to take time off for medical meetings thus showing vulnerability in this new competitive adult world.

You may want to calibrate your response based on what you think is causing your child's resistance. If, for example, his resistance appears to be because of the unique pressures of the moment, you can acknowledge this but tell him you will be reminding him again when he is under less pressure. If, however, his resistance appears to be rooted in denial or avoidance, you may want to bring in others like his doctor to challenge his viewpoint.

....

MATCHING YOUR ADVICE WITH YOUR CHILD'S ATTITUDE

The way you phrase the advice you give is likely to work better if you match your words with your child's style. I will give an example. We have talked a lot so far in this book about the benefits of optimism. As a well-known psychologist named Lazarus pointed out, some self-deceptions and illusions may be necessary for our positive mental health.[11] However, some illusions may not be of benefit. Compare these three optimistic statements:

> "I'm sure I won't get serious late effects; therefore, I never need to go for medical follow-up."

> "I'm sure I won't get serious late effects, so I'm not going to go to my checkup this year (but probably will next year)."

> "I'm sure I won't get serious late effects, but I will go to my checkup anyway (just to be sure)."

Optimism was followed by avoidance in the first case, procrastination in the second case, and compliance with recommended follow-up in the third case.

And let's compare these three pessimistic statements:

> "I'm bound to get late effects and the doctors won't be able to help, so there is no point going for medical checkups."

> "I'm bound to get late effects, so I might as well enjoy whatever time I have and not go to my checkup this year (but probably will next year)."

> "I'm bound to get late effects, so I'd better go for my regular checkups so they can be found as soon as possible."

The three pessimistic views are followed by a similar behavioral outcome as the optimistic views: avoidance, procrastination, and compliance with recommended follow-up. So an optimistic or pessimistic attitude, in and of itself does not guarantee compliance with follow-up recommendations, though it is likely that the people with the more optimistic attitudes will feel less burdened and more hopeful.

The arguments that you use to persuade your child to go for follow-up might be different based on how your child is looking at the situation. If your child has an overoptimistic attitude, can you stress the positive? Can you emphasize that your hope too is that the checkup will confirm your child's belief? This approach could be more likely to persuade him than if you talk about the percentage of people with his condition that get late effects.

If your child has an overpessimistic attitude, can you stress the importance of catching anything early and resist the temptation to tell him that many people with his diagnosis do not get serious late effects? The more closely you are able to align your arguments with his attitudes, the more likely you may be to influence him.

Let's remember that by this time you may have a primarily advisory role, and your pleas may fall on deaf ears for the moment. However, perhaps your young adult is the procrastinator, at the stage in her life when she simply wants a break in her medical regime and wants to forget that her life has a shadow over it. You may find this very hard when you start worrying about what could be brewing while not being attended to. You can be forgiven if you start thinking about the sacrifices you and your family made for your child to get successful treatment and be angry and sad that she is not taking proper care of herself, running the risk that something preventable will be missed because of her negligence. You will likely try again the following year to remind her to go for a follow-up appointment. Some parents extracted a promise from their child that if he or she missed the appointments one year, he or she would go the following year—and did not hesitate to remind their child of the promise a year later. Maybe your child will take your advice or maybe he needs a longer break away. Do not despair if your child initially resists your pleas to keep up with his medical follow-up care. Sooner or later, hopefully, he will be back. He may be prompted by you, maybe by a new girlfriend or boyfriend, maybe by worries about children, maybe by reading a random article, maybe by seeing a TV program, maybe by a minor symptom that worried him. Many survivors came to us having missed follow-up appointments for many years, and gave any one of the reasons above as what led them to finally come for the follow-up appointment.

MAKING A SUCCESSFUL TRANSITION TO ADULT CARE

You can influence your child's successful transition to adult medical care and how he views his responsibility for his own medical care in various ways. Ideally, your efforts begin well before your child becomes a young adult and can take many forms:

- Giving your child a sense from early on in his medical journey that he is a partner in a joint enterprise.

- Understanding from your child's pediatric doctors what long-term follow-up care your child will need and why.

■ Gradually handing over to your child in early adolescence some responsibilities for his medical care and encouraging his doctor to do the same.

■ Deliberately playing a less active role in meetings with the doctor and seeing they meet alone for some of the time.

■ Seeing that his doctor gives him the information he needs about his diagnosis, treatment, possible late effects, and follow-up needs.

■ Talking over with your child and his doctor what to expect in the adult medical care world

■ Getting specific recommendations for adult medical care referrals from your child's doctor.

■ Making the transition of care as gradual as possible and actively supporting your child during the transition, including advocating for and taking advantage of any transitional services available like a patient navigator or transition program.

■ Helping your child, at least initially, navigate the adult medical world so that his medical needs are met and his caregivers develop the practice of communicating appropriately with one another.

■ Communicating to your child that you do, despite some natural anxiety, have confidence that he will be able to take care of himself.

■ Understanding and managing your anxiety so it does not communicate itself to your child.

■ Matching your guidance to your child's style.

■ Understanding that your child may go through a period of avoiding his responsibilities while recognizing this may be a temporary phase. It is likely extremely anxiety-provoking for you, but may well pass.

■ Accepting that the most you can do during this phase may be to offer reminders, incentives, bargains, and prayers while containing your anxiety and your temper.

. . . .

A FINAL WORD ON THE TRANSITION TO ADULT MEDICAL CARE

The transition to the world of adult medical care can be difficult to navigate for you and your child. Advance preparation, patience and careful listening can make the switch easier. Efforts that seem to help the transition go smoothly include:[12]

- ♦ communicating the idea to your child that this transition is a positive and normal development

- ♦ checking your child has realistic expectations (neither too rosy nor too gloomy!) about adult medical care

- ♦ seeing your child knows the details about his diagnosis, treatment, and future health risks, and feels competent to manage his illness

- ♦ ensuring the timing and the details of the transfer have been carefully planned with input from you, your child, and his doctor, who has hopefully recommended where and with whom the adult follow-up care should happen

- ♦ making use of any resources available to support the transition process (joint visits, using a liaison coordinator)

Making these efforts over time and tolerating your child's ambivalence during and after the transition of care has occurred while remaining in the background ready to help when your child is faced with particular medical roadblocks mean you are doing all you can to ensure your child gets the adult medical care she needs and in the long run sees herself as responsible for her own long-term health.

PART III

When Your Child's Treatment Does Not Work

CHAPTER 21

. . . .

Challenges for Parents

Sadly, some children do not get better. A child may lose his battle very shortly after a diagnosis or many years later after a long series of treatments when doctors finally tell you that they have no more options for cure. Doctors may speak to you about continuing to treat your child's symptoms in order to keep him as comfortable as possible, and perhaps will tell you they may be able to help him live a little longer. But, if you are reading this section, the heartbreaking truth is that your child is one of those unlucky ones for whom a cure cannot be found.

These were the words you hoped, above all else, that you would never hear, and they may feel like a physical blow to your stomach that leaves you stunned, immobilized, and terrified. Your challenge will be how to absorb this terrible news in a way that still allows you to be there for your child and continue to function in a suddenly bleak world. Be understanding with yourself. Your thoughts are likely to spin in every direction. You may well be struggling hard to manage your emotions. Your immediate reactions may be instinctive and protective and not immediately under your conscious control. As time goes on, you may find that your method of dealing with the news slowly changes or you may not. You may experience any of a range of possible reactions immediately and over time.

. . . .

A RANGE OF REACTIONS

Nothing challenges the mind and heart quite like having to absorb such painful information about your child and then trying to continue to live your life as normally as you can for the sake of your child. People have very different styles of dealing with terrible news and living with the reality afterward.

So do not be surprised if initially:

■ You do not believe the news. Your mind may search desperately for alternative ideas, views, options, and scenarios. Perhaps you demand a second opinion or spend hours on the Internet researching experimental treatments for your child's condition. Your efforts to explore these alternatives may give you energy, hope, and comfort. You will also be doing everything you can to try to save your child—and taking every possible action may bring you comfort later. Or you may turn to other sources of comfort and hope such as your faith in God and the belief that God will not let your child die. You may want to talk with your priest or minister or the hospital chaplain and share your reactions with that person.

■ You hear the news and acknowledge its likely accuracy given the present state of medical knowledge, but immediately hope that some other cure will appear or that your child somehow or other will beat the odds. Hope buffers you against the blow. And you can remind yourself, accurately, that occasionally a child does recover contrary to the doctor's predictions.

■ You start preparing yourself immediately. You want a great deal of information about why this has happened, what will happen next and how. You question your child's medical team intensely and look up information on the Internet. You want to know the details of what you and your child will be facing in order to get ready.

■ You and your partner become angry with each other for having different ways of reacting. For example, you may believe the news right away and want more information while your partner does not believe the news and wants to hear no details. Understand that you are each trying to cope with the news in your own way and may need other family members or friends to talk to as well as having separate meetings with the doctors for some time.

■ You or your partner becomes angry with the doctor, especially if he or she was initially quite positive about the outcome of treatment. The messenger who gives bad news has a long history of being reviled. The doctor will understand, but remember that he or she 1) has a responsibility toward both you and your child, 2) knows parents want to make decisions in their child's best interest, 3) wants you to be in a position to make informed decisions about your child's care, and 4) wants to give you the option of having a treatment plan that is more focused on comfort than on intensive measures, which could have long-term benefits for your child and for you. There is some evidence that parents who have earlier discussions with their doctor about their child's likely death are more satisfied with the end-of-life care their child receives.[1] If you do continue to feel angry over several months with your doctor and this is impacting your communications, consider whether you would be more comfortable working with someone else who you could trust more to walk with you through this agonizing time.

■ You are irritated with your other children for behaviors and actions that you would normally tolerate. You are under great stress and may need to explain that to your child's siblings.

■ You find yourself resenting other children who are healthy and are not having to endure what your own child is enduring. Indeed, they are not.

■ You feel enormous rage that comes on unexpectedly, even toward people who are unconnected to your child. Anger and sadness are closely related emotions, and some people feel easily enraged when they are very sad.

YOUR CHANGING REACTION OVER TIME

You may notice over time that your thoughts and feelings change a lot, a little, or hardly at all. You will likely have been absorbing the news in your own way—and there can be many different ways—as you continue the extraordinarily difficult task of supporting your child as he gets sicker.

You may notice any or several of the following reactions as time goes by:

■ You begin to acknowledge to yourself that your child is likely to die. Perhaps you needed time to absorb the news and needed the evidence of your child becoming weaker and sicker before you could recognize this. But do not be surprised if the focus of your attention still goes back and forth. You may notice the focus of your thoughts and your emotions fluctuate between acknowledgment, sadness, new or changing hopes, other family concerns and activities, and reassessing what is happening. These fluctuations in focus might last all the way up until the time your child dies; in fact having ever-changing feelings may be what help you keep going. Few people can bear a relentless truth without some reprieves.

■ *"You need to be told only once your child is going to die. It's not something you forget."* You may have immediately acknowledged that your child's death is likely once the doctor told you it was a probable outcome. Some parents take in the bad news right away, but they compartmentalize it to allow other things to occupy their mind and heart. You might find that you focus on something besides your child's impending death, such as a short-term objective like getting your child home for Thanksgiving or a new potentially curative treatment you read about on the Internet. Sometimes you may still find yourself hoping for a different outcome or praying for a miracle. As I said earlier, it is true that some children do defy the odds and their doctors' expectations. The human spirit can use that knowledge to endure the darkest times. This division between your rational mind and your hopes may sustain you and allow you to enjoy the time with your child. As another parent said, *"I cannot think of him dying right now, I want to be fully present and available to him right now."*

■ You may want as much information as possible about what is happening and what will happen. You want to know about the way your child is likely to die in order to prepare yourself.

■ *"I can't believe I've planned his funeral already, but I know I won't be able to do it when the time comes."* You may notice you have done some advance planning for your child's death You may have thought about the funeral home you want to use (hospital staff can help here), who you want in the hospital with you and how to reach them, how you will get home afterward, and even whether or not you want your child to have any kind of postmortem—often a doctor is obliged to ask you about this if your child has been on an experimental protocol after your child has died. Some parents say no immediately but might have said yes if the reasons were explained beforehand and they were told then that the results could benefit others. If you are a planner, these are all decisions that can be made in advance that may spare you pain and effort later.

■ *"I don't want to be so sad that I cannot enjoy whatever time I have left with him." "I'm not going to grieve for one second longer than I have to or before I have to."* You may understand that your child is likely to die but want to protect yourself from experiencing emotionally what that means because you want to be sure you can be emotionally available to your child.

■ *"Once I start crying, I'm afraid I won't be able to stop."* You may be afraid to cry because you fear that you will be overwhelmed by grief and will not be able to support your child.

■ On the other hand, you may be a parent who deliberately makes a space in your life where you can feel some anticipatory grief and you find that releasing some of the emotional sadness and tension you are carrying inside you helps you continue to function. *"When I'm driving home from work, that's when I let myself cry. Then I'm ready to face my family again."* Or you may select a time or place where you can express your feelings. *"I need to talk to you today. I've got to have a safe place where I can cry."*

■ *"The doctors kept telling me he was going to die. I just did not believe them. I don't know why."* You may continue to deny the information entirely over time, perhaps because you fear at some level that if you allow the knowledge in, you will not be able to protect yourself from the incapacitating emotions that could follow.

■ *"How can I be there for Jane when I feel so devastated that I cannot look at her without crying?"* Or you may be so grief stricken that it becomes very hard to visit or be with your child. Sometimes strong emotions can be overwhelming and negative thoughts can take over. I will talk below about the importance of getting help immediately in this situation.

■ You may have moments of thinking you will not be able to go on living if your child dies. Many parents have fleeting thoughts or questions about this and wonder how they will continue to live without their child. I will also say more about this later.

ARE YOU RECOGNIZING REALITY?

It is often a process. You may be taking some conscious steps to prepare yourself for your child's likely death. But you also may be taking unconscious steps that you don't even realize you're taking that help you prepare yourself. You may notice any of the following:

■ You have acknowledged to yourself that your child is likely to die even if you find the strength of that acknowledgment waxes and wanes. You may notice that you still go back and forth in what you are thinking about and focusing on between your child's likely death and other hopes, preoccupations, and activities. One week you may want to talk with the doctors about your child's imminent death and the next week about the possibility of his returning to school. This is perfectly normal, and indeed this back-and-forth process may be exactly what helps sustain you and allows you to be with your child in the way you want.

■ You are gradually adjusting your hopes for your child—from hopes for a cure to hopes that your child will be able to be part of a particular family event to hopes that his death will be peaceful and pain free.

■ You have done some advance planning for your child's death. You have taken positive steps to help yourself when the time comes and when you fear you will feel incapacitated, yet you are still able to be with your child and be a source of strength for her.

■ Even if you may still not consciously believe what the doctors are telling you, you may hear it at some level but not want to acknowledge it consciously to yourself or to the doctors while you are unconsciously preparing yourself, as Frankie's mother appears to have been doing.

FRANKIE AND IRIS

Frankie was a six-year-old boy who had relapsed after a stem cell transplant and a series of aggressive treatments. His mother, Iris, had been continuously upbeat throughout his difficult treatment. His tumor was growing again, although he was still managing to go to school. His doctor told Iris no more curative treatments were available and that tragically Frankie would soon die. Iris showed little reaction and continued to maintain that new symptoms and the growth of the tumor were related to conditions other than his cancer. The doctor repeated his opinion during future visits, and Iris did not acknowledge it. On their last visit to the clinic Iris talked to me about different families she had been thinking about whose children had died. She said she had reached out to their parents in the last several months and knew how they were doing. She continued to attribute Frankie's condition to benign causes other than cancer. Frankie did get worse but continued to go to school until about a week before he died. He became weaker at home and his mother was helped by a visiting nurse. He died at home peacefully. The doctor was very worried about Iris, since she had seemed so unprepared. Although Iris was immensely sad, she did not seem surprised that Frankie had died. It appeared that she had been unconsciously preparing for his death even though it was not obvious to his doctor nor to me. Her conversations with the bereaved parents may have allowed her to see that parents could survive the death of their child. Several months after Frankie's death, Iris told me that she had hoped above all else that Frankie would not be afraid. She believed he had not been afraid when he was dying and that her positive attitude had allowed that to happen.

So what hints suggest you may be unconsciously preparing yourself? Be aware of dreams you have about friends or relatives who have died. Or notice if you suddenly think about other families who have lost a child and you feel an urge to contact them. Follow that urge. These experiences may be preparing you at some level for your child's death and may buffer you somewhat against the shock when it happens.

Also know that if you do not appear to be taking in the seriousness of the news, the doctors will likely become worried about you and continue to repeat the bad news. If this repetition is very hard for you to hear, you can always tell the doctors you have heard what they said but that you believe there will be a miracle and will deal with a contrary outcome if or when it happens. You can add that until then, the hope for a miracle is what is sustaining you and allowing you to support your child in the way you want.

But if you really have not recognized that your child's death will occur, you could feel completely blindsided and your grief path will be affected by how you react afterward. If you can, like Iris, say, "I helped him die without fear," that will be a comfort. If you accept your child's death as "God's will" and manage not to be angry with God because of that but still find your faith a comfort, you will ease your grief path. But the next section mentions other factors that can make this attitude more complicated and may require you to get help before or after your child dies.

....

WHEN HELP IS NECESSARY

There are three situations in which it is vital to get help for yourself or for others to get help for you before your child dies.

■ If your denial that your child is dying is combined with several of the following factors:
  ▶ feeling uniquely responsible for saving your child
  ▶ actively using alternative treatments
  ▶ consulting less rather than more with your child's medical team as your child gets sicker
  ▶ being physically and mentally exhausted from taking care of your child

Under such circumstances you will be particularly vulnerable to a massive and destabilizing shock when your child dies. If you are unable to ask for help for yourself, your family members need to take matters into their own hands and to communicate their concerns with your child's team—and try not to be angry with them if they do and understand they have your best interests at heart. You *do* need help, and before your child dies.

■ If you are seriously considering whether you can go on living if your child dies. We discussed earlier that many parents have fleeting moments of wondering whether they will be able to go on living if their child dies. This is not uncommon. However, if you find these moments are becoming more frequent or are preoccupying you, or if you are thinking of how you would act to accomplish this goal, it is essential you talk with the medical or psychosocial staff and let them know what you are thinking and feeling. Or family members need to tell the medical staff about their concerns for you. And try to understand they are trying to help you. You are under extreme stress and carrying such a heavy burden that you may not be thinking clearly. You may not recognize the enormous loss you would be creating for those who love and depend on you. If the medical staff think you are at emotional or physical risk, they will probably make a plan with you for your own safety, which may include finding you a therapist and speaking with family and community members to ensure your safety. To start with, a psychiatrist would likely consider if any medication might provide a buffer for you against the pain and stress you are feeling or, at minimum, allow you to sleep. Medical staff may also suggest that as your child gets sicker, he or she is taken care of in the hospital, both for his or her own comfort and so that you will have the support of a medical team around you. Lastly, the team will also talk to other family members and people in the community to ensure that they will be available to be with you when the time comes.

■ If you are feeling so completely overwhelmed by the news that you are unable to get it out of your mind and are having a very hard time functioning or being with your child because you feel so sad, you need help immediately. You may have become seriously depressed and you need to meet with a therapist and consider a trial of antidepressants. Both options could help you feel better. Therapy, talking to an experienced professional about what you are going through; some behavioral interventions like meditation or relaxation strategies; cognitive therapy, which offers ways you can interrupt your negative thoughts; and antidepressant medication that could help you sleep and eat better—all are interventions that can help you feel better. These interventions can allow you to mobilize your internal strength and energy and be there for your child. If you do recognize that you are feeling this way, please agree to try some of these recommendations. They can make an enormous positive difference to both you and your child, immediately and when you look back and remember this time.

CARA AND IRENE

Cara, an adolescent, went through a long and difficult series of medication trials. No treatment had worked, and she was now receiving palliative care only. Her mother, Irene, had been her main support throughout her long hospital stay and had taken care of Cara's father and their other children at home as well.

Cara, though still terminally ill, briefly stabilized and was able go home and to return to school. Irene developed difficulty sleeping and eating, felt overwhelmed by sadness, and lacked energy and interest in her normal activities. This continued for several weeks. It was obvious to her and to the medical team that she was having great difficulty functioning on a daily basis and had developed a major depression. She agreed to meet with a therapist and to start taking an antidepressant. She had been so busy and active when Cara was in the hospital, moving from handling medical crisis to medical crisis and being the mainstay of the family, that she had not allowed herself any time or space to grieve about what was happening. Now that Cara had returned to school temporarily, Irene had time and space on her hands and was flooded by the emotions she had held at bay before. Her insight into the situation helped her understand what was happening and the antidepressants improved her eating and sleeping. Her depression gradually lifted. Although she remained very sad, she was able to be support her daughter and her family again. She continued to meet with the therapist in order to have a place where she could express her own feelings. She was enormously glad to feel sufficiently better that she could function and be present for her daughter again.

WHEN TO SIGN A DO NOT RESUSCITATE (DNR) ORDER

As your child gets sicker, the medical team will at some point want to discuss a Do Not Resuscitate (DNR) order with you. A DNR order is a medical order that instructs medical caregivers *not* to perform some actions like cardiopulmonary resuscitation (CPR) if a patient's breathing stops or advanced cardiac life support (ACLS) if a patient's heart stops. If the patient is a child, the form must be signed by his parent or legal guardian. In the United States, different states have different versions of a DNR order, but every state now has some version of it.[2] Depending on which state you live in, this order will have one of the following names:

- DNR (Do Not Resuscitate) order
- DNAR (Do Not Attempt Resuscitation) order

- ◆ DNAR verification form
- ◆ MOLST (Medical Orders for Life-Sustaining Treatment)
- ◆ POLST (Physician Orders for Life-Sustaining Treatment)
- ◆ AND (Allow Natural Death) order

The naming of the form "Do Not Resuscitate" is unfortunate, misleading, and often very upsetting to parents. Naming the form "Allow Natural Death" would be more accurate and would better explain what you, the parent, are actually being asked to decide.

The important fact for you as a parent to know is that if the relevant order has not been signed by the parent and your child has a medical crisis at home, the responding medical team is legally required to take aggressive and invasive measures to preserve life, including performing chest compressions and intubation. This may or may not be in your child's best interest, or what you as a parent wish for her.

Parents and medical staff frequently delay discussions about resuscitation status until a time of crisis because of the shared reluctance by caregivers and parents to have such conversations. Such a discussion requires acknowledging that your child could die and prompts you to think about the ways that are in your child's best interest for this to happen, which are extremely difficult tasks. Some parents do not yet believe that their child could die, so any discussion about it feels intolerable. Many parents feel they are being asked to sign their child's death warrant. This does not need to be your experience. Hopefully you have a doctor who has described to you the legal constraints on medical emergency staff as well as the medical condition of your child and the likely progression of his illness, including whether or not his condition is reversible. This is important information because it puts you in a better position to make an informed choice about what you want for your child before a medical crisis forces you to choose under enormous stress. Considering the following questions and your answers to them might help you decide whether signing such an order is in your child's best interest:

- ◆ Is maximizing comfort a valued treatment goal for you in your child's end-of-life care?
- ◆ Do you know that a MOLST form or DNR order need *only* exclude extraordinary measures likely to cause suffering (like chest compressions and intubation), while measures that can increase comfort temporarily (like oxygen support) can still be provided—and you can decide which measures to exclude or include?

◆ Has your child indicated directly or indirectly what his or her wishes are as death approaches? For example, "not to be in pain" or "to be at home," and, if so, how might these wishes influence your decisions about DNR and comfort care?

◆ Is your child's disease process reversible or irreversible?

◆ If your child's condition is not reversible, have you considered that aggressive emergency measures like intubation might not only inflict suffering but might also lead to maintaining your child's life artificially, probably in the hospital, with minimal quality and no hope of recovery?

◆ Could careful advance planning now minimize your child's suffering later and avoid your having to make major decisions during the stress of a medical crisis?

◆ Did you know if you have a MOLST form at home you can choose whether or not to show it to medical personnel in an emergency?

◆ Did you know you can revoke or change DNR orders at any point should you change your mind or should your child's condition change?

If the doctors have told you that your child's condition is not reversible and your goal for her end-of-life care is maximum comfort, you may decide you are furthering that goal if you verify the order excluding emergency measures that inflict suffering while allowing those measures that provide comfort.

If your child's condition could improve for some time at least, you may be more reluctant to exclude any measures being used in an emergency and you might decide not to sign the form.

If you cannot bear to think about your child dying or signing any order that would limit measures that could temporarily save her life, you may not be able to sign a DNR form under any circumstances. But, unfortunately, you could have to endure your child's dying after being on life support in the hospital, which can be heartbreaking to witness—your child could be intubated, on a ventilator, appearing agitated or sedated for comfort, and in either case unable to communicate. On the other hand, it will allow you to know that you did everything you could to preserve your child's life for as long as you could and may slowly bring you to understand the sad inevitability of your child's death.

··

HELPING YOUR OTHER CHILDREN UNDERSTAND YOUR SICK CHILD'S WORSENING CONDITION

Your other children will be greatly affected by your child's worsening condition. Depending on their ages, personalities, and relationship with their sick brother or sister, their reactions may be very different. Some children, particularly younger ones, may become more demanding and clingy. Some may withdraw or become angry. Others may try to be helpful and mask their own reactions to protect you. Some siblings, particularly older ones, may protect themselves by spending a great deal of time out of the house. Many children may feel helpless and not know how to help.

So how can you help them when you already likely feel overwhelmed, sad and, drained yourself? Three words are key:

+ Explain
+ Involve
+ Understand

Can you—or someone to whom you entrust the task—*explain* what is happening medically? You do not want your other children to be blindsided by their brother or sister's death or to feel misled by you. The more you can gradually prepare them for what is going to happen, the more they can begin to absorb the news and the less devastating the shock of your child's death may be. If there is time, younger children can be told that their brother or sister is getting sicker and that the doctors are very worried. As the time gets closer, you can use simple words to tell your other children it is possible that their sibling will die and you can even prepare them for how it may happen. *"He will probably get more and more tired. He will sleep more and more. His breathing will get slower and slower, and finally he will stop breathing."* But be prepared that some younger and older siblings, like some adults, will not believe the news and will not want to listen however much you try to prepare them. For them, the death of their sibling is likely to be very hard, and we will talk about that in chapter 23. If you feel you are unable to prepare your other children, you can consider letting them meet with psychosocial staff or a doctor in your hospital or clinic who could prepare them.

You may also need to explain, particularly to younger siblings, that as their brother or sister gets more sick, he or she may become more irritable or withdrawn and less able to play or talk, and that these

changes are because of the illness and have nothing to do with anything the sibling has done.

Siblings will form important memories of their brother or sister during his or her last sickness. Try to think of simple ways to involve your
other children in their brother's or sister's care as he or she gets sicker.
Case studies from way back suggest that siblings are helped by feeling
included in their brother's or sister's care, and this is more likely to occur
if your child is at home.[3] Involvement can take many forms, including,
for example, if their sick sibling is in the hospital, visiting him there. Our
inpatient staff often facilitated joint activities, such as taking photographs of the children together or making handprints or footprints
together. These activities create positive memories during a difficult time,
and what the children create together may have significant meaning for
siblings later on.[4]

Depending on the age of the sibling, he or she may react differently
to becoming involved in the world of their brother's or sister's treatment.
A younger sibling may tolerate spending only a short time with his
brother or sister before going to the playroom with another adult. If a sibling cannot or does not want to visit her brother or sister in the hospital,
can she call, text, Skype, or email, send pictures or a handmade present?
You can act as the go-between and can tell your daughter that her brother
was asking after her or was talking about something they did together.

The decision whether to bring your other children in to see their
brother or sister when he or she is close to death is hard. At any age it is
painful for a child to see his sibling very ill. You will need to make the
decision for your younger children. If you decide not to bring them in
because you think it would be too traumatic, they can communicate in
one of the ways mentioned above—sending in a drawing or even a
favorite toy as something special for him. If your sick child looks very
different, is sedated, unconscious, or uncomfortable, your older children should know this before they decide to visit. You may also need to
tell them that their sibling is unlikely to respond to them.

If you are bringing in your other children perhaps for the last time
to see their brother or sister, consider if it would help to have them
meet with a psychosocial clinician before and after the visit. It may be
easier for someone other than you to help prepare them and talk about
it afterward.

If you are taking care of your child at home, encourage your other
children to do simple things that might help them to feel involved, such
as sitting with him while he watches a favorite video, bringing him
drinks or snacks, or helping run errands. Older siblings may even be
able to help with some simple medical care.

At home, siblings may benefit from your update on how your sick child is doing during the day when they return from school. "He's had a rough day, so he is not in a good mood," will make it less likely they will take it personally if their brother appears withdrawn and silent.

Make sure your children know that you understand how hard this is for them too and you appreciate the sacrifices they have made. Thank them for their help. Tell your younger children that you understand how hard it must be for them that their brother or sister is no longer able to play with them as he or she used to. Tell older siblings that you understand their wish to spend time out of the house. Ensuring that all members of the household feel heard and understood is very important for the emotional health of your family during this hardest of times.

••

SCHOOL AND FRIENDS

In addition to family members, teachers and friends are important people in your child's world who will need some information about what is happening. Even when the picture is bleak, many parents prefer at first to give general information—for example, that their child is back in the hospital—for teachers to pass on to students. Keep in mind that school-age children and adolescents in particular may well be in touch with their classmates themselves. No one wants a teacher to give more negative news to the class than your child or adolescent has been giving to her friends. So although classmates do benefit from preparation about your child's condition, it can be done in an age-appropriate way that allows the possibility of your child returning to school without exposing her to thoughtless comments from young classmates. The teacher can say something like "Jane is getting some more treatment in the hospital. We can be in touch with her and let her know we miss her and hope she will be back in school as soon as she feels better." If your adolescent chooses to tell her good friends what is happening, that is her choice. For many adolescents, peers can be a tremendous source of support. I will discuss this further in the next chapter.

Some children choose to go to school for as long as they can, sometimes up until a very short time before they die. In this situation, it may be necessary for the teacher to inform younger classmates that your child's illness could affect his strength, mood, or behavior. Furthermore, emergency medical plans will need to be put in place if he continues to go to school as his condition worsens. Once he can no longer go to school, teachers will have to prepare younger classmates that their friend will not be returning to school and why. If a teacher would like guidance, and you are willing for him or her to contact a psychosocial clinician at the hospital, that person could likely help the teacher plan what to say to the class and how best for the teacher and the class to communicate with your child. If no guidance is available, ask the teacher to prepare the other children as gently as possible. You can suggest the teacher say something like "The doctors are worried about Janet—they are keeping her comfortable at home right now, but she will not be able to come to school. I will let you know how she is doing and we can figure out ways to let her know we are thinking about her." The next week the teacher could say, "Janet is still very sick and the doctors are helping her be comfortable. What can we send her that will let her know how much we miss her and care about her?" If a student asks, "Will Janet die?" you can give the teacher permission to say something like "the doctors are worried that she will die—and her mommy and daddy are very sad but are taking the best care of her that they can."

A HEARTBREAKING JOURNEY

You are facing an unbearable possibility and are likely to go through a series of different emotions throughout your child's journey. Respect your reactions and understand that your manner of dealing with things may be protecting you and allowing you to spend time with your child in the way you want. The human mind sometimes modulates the information it takes in, depending on its ability to tolerate it. If you are a parent who cannot acknowledge your child's likely death and cannot imagine agreeing to a DNR order, you may be preserving your strength in order to be with your child now, but you may suffer more later. If you are a parent who acknowledges, either immediately or over time, your child's likely death, it may allow helpful advance planning and important conversations with your child to take place. You may also get respite from this knowledge in various essential ways that allow your focus to go back and forth. If you are a parent who is so devastated by the news that you get no relief or feel that you cannot go on living without your child, you can and should get help from a psychosocial clinician on the medical team or in the community.

If you are able to discuss in advance the interventions that would or would not be in your child's best interests when his disease becomes irreversible, you may be able to spare your child suffering. If you cannot discuss the desirability of these interventions in advance, your child may be with you a little longer, but he may not be in a condition in which he can communicate or respond. Remember that you can always seek assistance from medical professionals to help you make these heartrending decisions.

Dealing with your other children adds another layer of complexity. If possible—and I recognize sometimes it is not—prepare them in advance for your child's death. They will likely experience less of a shock when it happens and may find it easier to deal with as time goes on. If you are emotionally unable to prepare them, you can delegate that task to someone you trust to deliver the news in a clear but supportive way. Furthermore, including your children in their sibling's treatment can make a world of difference to them, as well as to your sick child. The memories they make in the hospital or at home while their sibling is very ill will be important to them down the road. Letting them know you understand how difficult this is for them, too, allows them to feel included, rather than separate from events that have a massive impact on their family.

CHAPTER 22

Giving Your Child Bad News

In this chapter, I will try to show the myriad ways that parents, young children, and adolescents can approach death. I will tell stories that illustrate the courage and resilience of many children, adolescents, and parents and will consider, depending on your child's age and your respective styles, how to talk and listen to each other in ways that feel right to you at the time and may be of some comfort to you later.

There is no right or wrong way to walk this heartbreaking path. You and your child will be the ones who figure out what path is for you. You may meet medical staff who urge you to speak openly with your child. For some parents and children speaking openly may comfort children, may allow parents to say good-bye, and may help parents afterward feel they have traveled with their child as far as they could.

But outside circumstances sometimes allow no acknowledgment— if your child dies suddenly or unexpectedly. Or you may not have acknowledged to yourself that your child will die, or even if you have, you may not want to talk with your child about it.

Some parents and some children prefer indirect acknowledgment. If you are one of these parents, indirect acknowledgment may allow you to express your love and appreciation to your child and allow your child to express his or her love for you effectively and perhaps less painfully than a more explicit verbal acknowledgment would do. You are doing what feels right to you under excruciatingly difficult circumstances.

On top of coping with the difficult news of your child's illness yourself, you also have to decide how and when to talk with your sick child and your other children about what is happening. The next two chapters discuss several factors that may influence how and whether you choose to do this, such as:

◆ The age of your child and what he understands about death

◆ What you think about open communication and including your child in medical decisions

◆ Whether your child is signaling directly or indirectly that he could be worried about dying

◆ Whether you can find bearable ways to talk to your child about his condition

◆ Whether you prefer more indirect ways that you and your child can say good-bye

AN OPEN DISCUSSION

As discussed in chapter 3, there is a growing trend in America's medical culture to believe doctors have an ethical obligation to keep a patient, even a child, appropriately informed about his condition.[1] Many ethicists in America and Europe also think that the voice of the child should be included as much as his age allows in decisions relating to his end-of-life care, so it is likely your child's team will recommend that your child be told about the progression of his illness in an understandable way that allows him the chance to ask questions while respecting his hopes and fears as much as possible.[2] An older child may often want to be included in planning end-of-life medical care.[3] However, some medical professionals now recognize that fully open communication may not suit all families and are adjusting how they speak with families accordingly.[4] Many parents are comfortable letting their child know that he has to get shots and take medicine to get better, but may be more reluctant to tell him the medicine has not worked the way everyone hoped it would, or, particularly, to tell him he cannot be cured. You are certainly not alone if, at least initially, you are reluctant to communicate with your child about the severity of his or her condition.

You could have various reasons for your reservations:

■ You may not have acknowledged the news yourself and are still in a state of shock and disbelief. If so, ask the doctors to delay saying something to your child till you feel more prepared. Many parents find that once they have acknowledged the prognosis to themselves, they can find the right moment and the right way to talk with their child. If you continue not to acknowledge the news, you may need to discuss with the doctors what you are willing for them to say to your child and how you wish them to answer questions your child has. The doctors will probably not agree to lie to your child.

■ You may wonder whether you are giving up by acknowledging your child's prognosis. But acknowledging is very different from giving up. Acknowledgment can allow open conversations and valuable advance planning.

■ You may feel you do not want to burden your child with bad news. But your child may have picked up that something bad has happened and it may be a comfort to him to know for certain rather than imagine what is going on. He is likely to feel less alone and more supported.

■ You may fear that speaking about relapse and the possibility of death will make it happen. But speaking about it makes things more manageable, not more likely—and can allow you to answer your child's questions, help him feel less alone, and speak with him openly as well as making plans in advance.

■ You may believe deeply that God will not let your child die. This belief may indeed be helping you function, but can you listen to the medical information and follow the team's recommendations for appropriate care anyway? You can also consult with others in your religious community.

■ You may fear you could not speak about it without crying, and this would upset your child. But you can explain to your child you are very sad that he has to go through all this because you love him so much. Your feelings are natural and your child may feel less upset if you can cry with him rather than coming into the room with red eyes obviously having been crying somewhere else.

■ You may fear you will not know what to say. But you can discuss with a psychosocial clinician or trusted friends what you might want to say. You can start by asking your child what he thinks happens after death and follow his lead. You can tell your child what you think about how people are remembered or, if you are a believer, your views about an afterlife.

....

AGE-APPROPRIATE DISCUSSIONS OF DEATH

Children understand death in different ways depending on their age and on how much they have been exposed to death in their lives. The way a child understands death changes in striking ways as he gets older and conversations need to change accordingly.[5]

Babies and Toddlers (Infants to Two Years Old)

A baby gradually recognizes familiar faces, sounds, places, and experiences separation anxiety when a familiar person leaves him. He has little understanding of permanence, and cannot grasp that a person continues to exist even after he can no longer see them. He also has little concept of time, so for him there is no distinction between separation and death, and no concept of what could cause death. His understanding about death and fear of death is likely to be minimal, but his reaction to separation from loved ones may be considerable. He is able to register his emotional reactions to situations, places, and people in nonverbal ways.

Preschool (Three to Five Years Old)

A preschool child may have seen a dead animal or even have known someone who died. He understands that sadness is the usual reaction when someone dies, but he thinks of death as temporary, reversible, and avoidable. When I tried to explain to my three-year-old son that the doctors had told us that his grandfather was going to die, his first response was "I don't believe the doctors." Once his grandfather did die and I delivered the news, he said, "The doctors will make him come alive again." When I said that, sadly, they could not, his next statement was "Well, the magicians will," and he was not happy when I did not accept that idea either.

Children of this age have their own unique logic that may work through association rather than reason. This is the age when a child may ask, "Why is the moon following me?" so it is very easy for them to assume that something they did or saw caused their condition or the condition of their brother or sister. For example, I knew of a three-year-old who after seeing his father eat peanut butter the morning before he died of a sudden heart attack developed a phobia of peanut butter. His thinking became: "If I eat peanut butter, it will kill me too." Young children around this age are very literal and egocentric.

For children of this age group the description of death needs to be simple and clear in order to avoid confusion.[6] Try to communicate the points below over the course of several conversations about death with your child:

+ The body stops working.
+ The body does not breathe, talk, move, or feel things anymore.
+ The spirit may live on in different ways (depending what your own beliefs are).
+ Usually people's bodies are buried in the earth and the body gradually becomes part of the earth.
+ If you have chosen cremation, explain that the body is exposed to very high heat and turns to ashes. The ashes can be buried.
+ Dying itself does not hurt.
+ Everyone dies sometime—usually when they are very old.
+ Death is part of the cycle of life.
+ Each person has made a special contribution that will be remembered.
+ People often feel sad and sometimes angry when someone they love dies because they will miss them and are so sorry they will not see them every day.

You should AVOID telling a young child:

+ Death is like going to sleep (then they may become afraid of going to sleep).
+ Beliefs you might find comforting, but which may be frightening, such as "God and his angels will take you away." Your child will always be keeping an eye out for God and the angels!

The content of the conversation may be less important to your child than the fact that you appear comfortable and open having the conversation and that you listen to him.[7]

School-Age Child (Six to Eight Years Old)

Children at this stage gradually understand that death is permanent, that someone cannot be brought back to life, and that everyone dies—although they may think that there may be a personal exception if they are smart and can figure out how to avoid death (death may be understood as a figure with a scythe or looking like Darth Vader). At this age, a child may fear that the death of someone they know is just the beginning of many deaths and loss—that if death can happen once, it can happen again. A child may become afraid that other people he or she loves may also die. After her paternal grandmother died, my six-year-old granddaughter asked not to hear stories where people were killed. She said she woke up at night and felt scared. She also began asking me about my health.

A school-age child is developing some idea about time—two nights away is more than one night away—and can recognize the difference between separation and death. Children this age may still be quite confused about what causes death. They may still imagine death is catching and want to avoid the people and places associated with death. It remains important with this age group also to stress that nothing they did caused their brother's or sister's condition.

A young school-age child is often interested in facts about how the body works or stops working, so in addition to the simple description of death given for younger children, she may also need more details about how the body stops working (for example, "the lungs that help us breathe do not work anymore"). She can begin to understand the idea that the soul or spirit may be different from the body and can live on in some way after someone's body stops working. She can begin to understand that someone can "live on" in another person's memories.

School-Age Child (Nine to Twelve Years Old)

An older school-age child is aware of the finality and permanence of death and that everyone dies. He is by now more aware of the possibility (but low probability) of his own death. He can also better anticipate the effect of his own death on his parents and worry whether his parents will be all right. He is also more likely to worry about the way someone dies. Children of this age are better able to understand the distinction between being sick and being so sick that you are likely to die. Many children this age will also want more explanation about the physical process of dying.

It is important to tell a child this age that she may feel sad, angry, and hurt if she or someone she loves is going to die and that it is okay to talk about it. If she sees you are sad, you can tell her the reason is because you love her very much and will miss her being with you every day, not because death itself is painful or awful in itself.

Adolescents Twelve to Seventeen Years Old

An adolescent has an intellectual understanding of the finality and permanence of death. He knows everyone dies at some time. However, he combines this knowledge with a strong emotional sense of his own invulnerability and therefore often has considerable difficulty believing that he is going to die. He may acknowledge it one moment and not the next. An adolescent is keenly aware of his parents' feelings and may worry greatly about how his parents will manage should he die. If this is obvious, it may be important to tell your adolescent that even though you will be heartbroken without him, you will be all right.

....

IS YOUR CHILD SIGNALING THAT HE COULD BE WORRIED ABOUT DYING?

In a study in Sweden—a country where openness of communication about medical conditions is stressed as much as in the United States—only about one third of several hundred parents had discussed death directly with their children compared with two thirds who had not. None of the parents who had such discussions regretted it after their child died, whereas over a quarter of those who did not discuss it regretted not having such a discussion.[8] A more recent study in Holland found somewhat similar numbers, with most parents being satisfied with the particular route they had taken but some parents in each category being dissatisfied.[9]

So try to stay attuned to your adolescent's mood, behavior, and statements and be on the lookout for signs that suggest your child of any age could be worried about dying, such as:

♦ A direct question from a child of any age: "Am I going to die?" You want to let him know that it is all right for him to ask such a question. You also want to know what is behind his question before you answer it. If you ask him what is making him wonder, you will then be better able to direct your answer to the particular issue that led to the question. Hopefully his answer will help you gauge the strength of his belief and his readiness or lack of it to hear bad news. You may discover your child has noticed how upset his family is. Or he may have overheard a conversation you were having with the doctors. Or he may have remembered that another family member died of cancer. Or he may feel so ill that he thinks he will not get better.

♦ Talking about other people who have died (grandparents, friends, other patients, famous people, even pets).

♦ Doing schoolwork, writing, or drawings that reflect concerns about death. A younger child may bring death into her play. Stuffed animals die or are killed, dinosaurs fall down and don't get up. Toys representing family members get put in different parts of a doll's house and some "family members" have covers put over them or are deliberately left outside the doll's house.

♦ Showing a greater interest in books, stories, or films about death.

♦ Showing increased anxiety. A younger child might experience increased separation anxiety from you. An older child might be unwilling to leave you and go to school. He could have difficulty sleeping or wake up with nightmares. He could be afraid to leave the house.

♦ Becoming depressed, withdrawn, and increasingly isolated from friends. This is different from the quiet withdrawal that people of any age can show as they approach death.

♦ Showing uncharacteristically aggressive behavior.

♦ Having difficulty sleeping or having nightmares.

WAYS TO ADDRESS YOUR CHILD'S FEARS

If your four-year-old child is showing feelings or behavior that could suggest fears about dying, you or a psychosocial clinician can use animal toys, a puppet, or dollhouse figures to explore worries that you think your child may have and see how your child reacts. Based on your child's responses, the puppet or animal toys can become the vehicle through which these conversations continue. You can ask, "How come Ducksie [your child's glove puppet] is looking sad today?" or "What might Ducksie be mad about?" You could wonder with your child if Ducksie is upset about what the doctors told him yesterday about his relapse—maybe he has to stay in the hospital for a while to get more treatment? And comment "I guess Ducksie is not feeling too great today—I guess he is pretty unhappy having to stay longer in the hospital and get more medicine? Do you think he could be wondering if he is ever going home? Anything else he could be worrying about? Let's think what we should say to him."

If your child is six or seven years old, he may respond if he is told a story about a child in a similar situation to his own and asked what the child might worry about or hope for.

JOSÉ

An emotionally expressive seven-year-old boy, José, who had a progressive and incurable illness, was showing increasingly aggressive behavior, getting into fights at school and at home, and kicking parked cars in his neighborhood. His mother and I met with him and I told him a story about a boy called Peter who had become very ill. We told José that Peter had started getting angry very easily and was suddenly getting into fights with his friends at school. Peter just wanted to kick things even if it hurt his foot. We thought he could be worrying about something. Did José have any idea what Peter might be worrying about? José said that Peter might be worrying about dying. We asked what in particular might Peter worry about dying. He said Peter might worry that dying would hurt and that he would be alone when he died. He added it was the big monster inside him that got so angry. It was not him. We told José that getting angry was a natural way to feel if you got very sick and worried if you were going to die—that big monster had a point, but perhaps Peter did not want the monster to be in charge. José agreed. We also said that Peter perhaps needed to know that dying itself did not hurt, and if there was hurting on the way to dying, there were medicines to help. Also Peter needed to know that his mother and father would do their very best to be with him when he was dying. Perhaps we needed to tell Peter all this and then maybe he would feel less angry? This information seemed to comfort José. In later meetings we talked a lot more about angry monsters and how not to let them be in charge as well as other ways to deal with worries about dying. José did show less aggressive behavior and seemed more at peace. He asked his classmates to an ice cream party and said to one child that he did not think he would see him the following semester.

If your child or adolescent is showing some of these behaviors or is asking more direct questions, you or a chosen member of the medical team can ask your child what he understands is happening with his illness and what his hopes and his fears about it are. How he answers those questions will determine how the conversation should continue. What he says may make it obvious how he wishes treatment to proceed (and can be shared with others), or he may make it obvious that he does not want to discuss it at the moment. His statements can always be used as the basis for further conversations.

If he seems ready to talk more about the situation, but you would find it painful to question him further, delegate the task to medical or psychosocial staff. Sometimes it is easier for a child or adolescent to talk about his wishes, concerns, or worries to an outsider whom he is less concerned about upsetting than he would be if he was talking with you. There are two booklets have been specially designed to help young people think about their wishes in this situation. One is titled "Voicing My Choices," and it is designed to help adolescents and young adults to think about what they want to communicate if their condition worsens.[10] It is a powerful document that gives your adolescent the opportunity to voice her preferences and her wishes in this sad situation. It is divided into several sections:

+ How I would like to be comforted.
+ How I would like to be supported.
+ Who I would like to make my medical decisions.
+ The types of life support treatment I would or would not want.
+ What I would like my family and friends to know about me.
+ My spiritual thoughts and wishes.
+ How I wish to be remembered.

The second booklet is titled "My Wishes," and it is intended for younger children to consider with their family or their caregivers how they want to be looked after and what they want their family and friends to know if they get sicker.[11] The content of both booklets is written simply and clearly and statements can be checked or crossed out. There is extra space for young people to write their own preferences and comments—about pain management, about who they would like with them, about where they would like to be if they die, about their favorite things, about their wishes for their family, and about their spiritual preferences among many things.

These booklets bring home the reality of what is happening and are likely to be painful to read. Some parents and children may not want to read them. The benefit for your reading them—whether or not you choose to go over them with your child—is that they may suggest to you questions to ask him. You can ask them in a hypothetical way (see the section below for examples of such questions). You can start by saying to your child that if he gets sicker, you want to be sure his wishes for his care are followed. If that feels too difficult, you can ask medical or psychosocial staff to begin the conversation. If your adolescent has been told he is likely to die, you or a chosen clinician can ask him whether he would like to look at the booklet "Voicing My Choices" and think about what he would want. You can tell him he can talk it over with you or one of his medical team or can write down his preferences and wishes. You can truthfully say that even if it is very hard to think about, other adolescents and parents have found having this information written down is beneficial.

MAKING SPEAKING TO YOUR CHILD MORE BEARABLE

How Language Can Help

Some parents find it very hard to use the words "death" or "dying" and prefer to talk with their child about the treatment not working, saying that the doctors will be giving them medicine to keep them comfortable as a way to indicate that their child cannot be cured. For example, Michael was initially unwilling to talk with the doctors or with his adolescent son, Adam, about his son's approaching death even though Adam was asking many questions about his condition. Michael finally asked the doctors, "Is he getting ready to leave us?" When the doctors said that yes, Adam was close to death, Michael agreed that the doctors could speak to Adam using Michael's words.

Some parents prefer to use metaphors to describe death, particularly with younger children. I have heard a parent describe death as a journey at the end of which his young child will find familiar people who love him or as a trip down a tunnel toward a bright, warm light.

Using an Earlier Conversation About Death as a Starting Point

If a child has indicated in an earlier conversation whether he would like to be told if he was going to die, that information can be the way to begin the conversation if that sad outcome becomes likely. So try to be open to such conversations should your child bring up the subject at any point during his treatment.

PAUL

Several years ago a remarkable eight-year-old boy, Paul, relapsed. He was going to need a stem cell transplant. Around the same time, we had to tell him that a good friend of his from the hospital had died. Paul told us how sad he was and then decided he wanted to write a letter to his friend's parents to tell them how sorry he was. He did this in my office. He asked if he was going to die also. I said everyone hoped not. I told him that what he had was very serious, but he was going to get lots of treatment for it, and everyone hoped that he would get better. He said he did not want to know if he was going to die. I asked why, and he said because it would be "so scary." I pointed out that we had been very honest with him so far about his health and we did not want him to be worrying about how he was doing when he did not need to. If we could not tell him bad news, how could he know when we were telling him the truth? Paul listened thoughtfully and then said after everything he had gone through, perhaps he would want to know. Death remained very much on his mind. The first thing he wanted to know after seeing a film about two children having a bone marrow transplant was if they had died. Luckily the answer was no. Despite his poor prognosis and the risky bone marrow transplant, happily, Paul has done well and we never needed to talk with him about another relapse. However, if his stem cell transplant had failed and he had been likely to die, I would have reminded him of our earlier conversation and would have asked him whether he did still want to know how he was doing. Based on his answer, I would have been more or less forthcoming about the situation he was facing.

Making the Conversation Hypothetical

Many parents find it easier to talk at first hypothetically.

- ◆ "If you were to get much sicker, what would you want? What would you be most worried about?"
- ◆ "If you did get much sicker, would you like to be at home or in the hospital?"
- ◆ "If you did get very sick, who would you like to visit you?"
- ◆ "If this treatment does not work, what would be most important for us to know about what you would want?"
- ◆ "If this treatment does not work, what you would want your friends to know or do? What would you like us to know or do?"
- ◆ "If you were in pain, would you like to be given medicine that allowed you to be comfortable even if it meant you were sleeping a lot of the time?"
- ◆ "If you were not to get better, would there be some special ways you would like to be remembered? Would there be special things you wanted your friends or your brothers and sisters to have? Would there be special wishes you had for your family?"

These earlier conversations may also be useful springboards for later conversations:

- ◆ "Do you remember when we talked in the hospital you said _____? Is that still what you want?"
- ◆ "Do you remember when I asked you about _____, you said_____? Is that still the way you feel?"

Speaking to Younger Children and School-Age Children

A young child has a limited sense of time and may become extremely anxious, confused, or angry if he is told too far in advance that he is likely to die. Too much honesty too soon can be difficult for a young child to handle.

Other young children who are given unwelcome bad news may transform it as the following story shows—reassuring to parents who worry that accurate information will remove a child's hope for cure.

ELIZABETH

Elizabeth, a nine-year-old girl, was receiving palliative treatment to relieve some painful symptoms. She repeatedly asked a doctor she knew well if she was going to die. He finally told her that she was. She began screaming and I was called. She ordered me to leave. I agreed, but told her I would come back later. When I returned, her mother was there (and had been told what had happened). Elizabeth told her mother in my presence that something sad had happened that morning. Her doctor had told her she was going to die. But she had been praying to God all day and he had told her he was not going to let her die. The next day when I visited I brought her a little book that contained "letters to God" that other children had written. She then wrote her own letter to God to add to the collection. And her faith that God would not let her die remained a comfort to her as she became sicker.

A school-age child may know more than you suspect and asking him what he is thinking may allow you to find out. You can then address what he wants and needs to know.

JUSTIN

A ten-year-old boy, Justin, who had never discussed his poor prognosis had remained relentlessly optimistic through a hard treatment and two stem cell transplants. One day I visited with him while his mother was talking with the doctors. I asked him what he thought they were talking about. He replied, "That I've relapsed, that there are no more treatments for me, and that they are giving up on me." I told him that I wished I could disagree with him about what they were talking about, but I couldn't—but I could tell him they would be trying as hard as they could to come up with the best plan for him that they could under the circumstances. He allowed me to share with his mother and his medical team what he had told me, and they were able to tell him the plan for his care (though not his cure) would be and asked him for his feedback.

. . . .

WHAT TO SAY AND HOW AND WHEN TO SAY IT

You may have already noticed times and places where your child has spontaneously brought up important questions—about values, spiritual beliefs or moral dilemmas. Hopefully, you will have been open to these conversations and shared some of your own views. Perhaps these talks occurred when you were coming home from school or from treatment. Perhaps it was in the bath. Perhaps it was when you were walking your dog together. These are good places and times for important conversations. You are together, you are unlikely to be interrupted (turn off your cell phone!), and your child may be feeling relaxed. If now you are in the sad situation of knowing bad news and wondering how much your child needs or wants to know, you can deliberately choose a similar setting and begin a conversation. If your child is in the hospital, choose a relatively quiet time of day when the doctors are not on their rounds. You can place a PLEASE DO NOT DISTURB sign on your child's hospital room door. If your child has a roommate, find a spare conference room and put the same sign up. With a child of any age, it is a good idea to check what he thinks is going on before you tell him bad news. You may be surprised at what he is already thinking, and at least you will know how much distance there is between what you tell him and what he already thinks.

Below are suggestions about how to give the bad news to a younger child that he has had a terminal relapse:

- ◆ Ask him, "How do you think you are doing medically?" in order to understand whether he has some idea about what is happening.
- ◆ If he fears he has relapsed, "I'm afraid you are right—the cancer has come back again."
- ◆ If he thinks the treatment was going well, "You are right the treatment was going well for a while, but unfortunately the cancer has come back again."
- ◆ If the treatment now is to manage symptoms and delay the disease: "The doctors are giving you medicine to help your headaches and to see that you are comfortable. . . ."

If your child asks, "Am I going to die?" ask him what he thinks, and based on his answer, either build on what he has said or tell him that things, sadly, are now moving in a directions that is different from what everyone wanted.

Consider the specific answers given below. Some emphasize hope but encourage the child to bring up questions. Others are more factual and informative. Depending on your child and how sick he is, you may find different answers more appropriate at different times. If your child is younger and very anxious, she may need hope for a cure for as long as possible. If she is a little older and likes being in control, she may benefit from getting the likely facts sooner and from being asked about her wishes and preferences as she gets sicker.

- "We hope not, but we cannot be sure. We will let you know how you are doing. Ask us again if you are worried, and we will tell you what is happening."
- "The doctors are worried because you have relapsed, but new medicines are being discovered all the time and maybe that will happen with you. Ask us whenever you want to know how you are doing"
- "Right now you are very sick, but sometimes people get better and even the doctors do not know why. We don't know if that will happen with you, but we hope so with all our hearts."
- "Right now the doctors don't have any more medicine that will cure you. They do have medicines that can slow it down. They also have medicines that can make you as comfortable as possible and help you do what you want to do."
- "You are not dying right now, but it could happen at some point. If you did get that sick, what would you worry about? Would you want to know? What would you want us to know?"
- "Yes, you will die, but not for a little while, and until then we will be together and we will try to do the things you want. If you like, we will tell you when it is close and you can ask us any time if you are worried."
- "Yes, you are close to dying and it is all right to let go when you need to. We love you very much and you will be in our hearts forever."

Heartbreaking as the idea of these conversations may be, many parents have said that having such conversations (and it is important not to think of it as a single conversation but as multiple conversations) can provide relief and can leave more space for other meaningful activities or conversations.

DISCUSSING WHAT HAPPENS AFTER DEATH

Even young children sometimes ask, "What happens when I die?" Young children are imaginative and suggestible. If you describe to your child your picture of heaven or an afterlife, that may become your child's vision—supplemented by his imagination. Or if you ask, you may discover that he has already his own particular vision of what happens after someone dies. One six-year-old child was sure there would be lots of ice cream in heaven. If you have a less sure vision, you can always say "some people think . . ." and ask him what he thinks.

Younger children may see death (or have death described to them) as a journey at the end of which they will meet someone who knows and loves them—like a grandparent who has died—and this can be a comforting image.

If you do not believe in a God and do not follow a particular spiritual or religious practice, you may still find words that will give your child some comfort. If his fear is not to be with you when he dies, telling him he will continue to be in your heart may allay his fears somewhat. And whether you believe in a God or whether you do not, you can surely truthfully say to your child that he will live forever in your heart.

Remember that your child may already have some ideas (or hopes) that you may want to listen to before you tell him anything.

Here are a few examples of responses you might give—depending on your religious tradition or personal beliefs—to your child's question "What happens after you die?"

- ◆ You can ask your child "What do you think happens when you die?" And then build on what he says.

- ◆ Depending on your own beliefs you can be clear: "You will go to heaven, which is the wonderful place people go when they die," or "You will live on in other people's memories," or "You will be born again as another being. It could be as an animal or as another person."

- ◆ Or you can be more vague: "No one knows exactly" or "Some people believe . . ."

- ◆ Or you can say something more general, such as "We are all part of nature and return to nature when we die. Our bodies become part of the earth and help other things grow. Our spirits live on in the hearts of people who love us." Or "We are all part of the cycle of life."

+ If you talk of heaven, you can ask your child: "What do you think heaven is like?"

+ If your child asks you, "What do you think heaven is like?" you can help him develop some comforting images along the lines of "Where God and his angels live," or "Where you will see other people who love you, like Grandma." Here are more suggestions: "Who and what would you like to be there? Let's think who is there waiting for you who will be so happy to see you." "We will come there too in a little while."

MAURICE

A four-year-old boy, Maurice, who was dying, was told by his parents he was going to walk along a tunnel and at the end of the tunnel he would see a beautiful light and his much-loved grandmother (who had just died the year before) would be waiting there for him. This appeared to be very comforting to Maurice, who had been quite agitated previously, and he died a few hours later with both parents holding his hands.

PAULINE

A ten-year-old girl, Pauline, had a stem marrow transplant that was not successful. After her doctors told her (with the consent of her parents) that she did not have long to live, her parents asked if she had a particular wish. She said she would like her dog to come to the hospital so that she could say good-bye to him. So, contrary to every hospital rule, the dog was smuggled into the hospital in a suitcase and spent the night with Pauline. Pauline also telephoned close family members and friends to say good-bye and also said good-bye to the hospital staff who had worked with her. She died peacefully in the hospital with her family at her bedside.

ADOLESCENTS

Adolescents approach their own deaths in very different ways. Some adolescents close to death may decide where they want to be or what medications they want to take. They may plan particular goals, including who gets possessions they value. They may call friends and family to say good-bye and may even plan their funerals and consider what kind of memorial they want. Some adolescents will talk with their friends, rather than parents, doctors, or therapists, about their approaching death. Some adolescents will delay any discussion or acknowledgment of the likelihood of death until the last possible moment. Others will not acknowledge it at all.

Adolescents, whose religious beliefs and values are likely to be more in flux than a younger child's, may develop their own spiritual beliefs as the illness progresses. These may influence their attitude toward death, what kind of funeral they want, and how they want to be remembered.

Balance what you say to your adolescent against his attitude and apparent concerns. It may well be that he understands more than he is letting on and simply does not want to talk about it. In this case, let him know you are available to talk if he wants. Or if you feel you cannot do this, encourage the doctor to probe gently whether your adolescent has any questions that he is not asking.

The doctor may want to inform your child about his medical condition, and you will need to decide how to respond. Once again, doctors are unlikely to agree to lie to your child. Based on your child's age and level of maturity, the questions he is asking, and your wishes, the doctor is likely to be more or less explicit in his answers. He too will want to preserve your child's hope for as long as possible. One wonderful doctor at Dana-Farber used to say to parents that only a miracle could save their child's life. He continued that, very rarely, he had seen a miracle happen, but usually, sadly, the miracle did not happen, and he feared the family should base their expectations on the more likely scenario. It is also true that doctors have different styles. Some are more blunt than others; some emphasize the facts, others the hopes; some have more difficulty delivering bad news than others; some show more emotion than others. But speaking generally, the older and more mature your child, the more reluctant a doctor will likely be not to answer his questions directly. If a younger child asks if he will die, and the doctor knows your wish is that he not be told, he may evade the question and suggest the child can ask again if he is worried or talk directly with you. The doctor will likely continue to discuss with you the benefits of open communication.

If your adolescent asks you or the doctors directly, "Am I going to die?" ask him first about what he is thinking. You can then adjust what you say accordingly. If the doctors have told you there is no curative treatment available, see what you think about these answers—again trying to be truthful but giving your adolescent continuing choices.

- ♦ "The doctors are worried. Right now they don't have medicine that can cure your cancer, but they can see that you are comfortable and can do some things that you want to do."
- ♦ "If the doctors can't stop the cancer from growing, you are likely to die—not right now, but at some point . . ."
- ♦ "If that does happen, what is important for us to know about what you would want?"
- ♦ "Is there anything particular you are worried about?"
- ♦ "Do you have questions for the doctor about how it might happen?"
- ♦ "Would you like us to tell you if the doctors think it is close?"

The following stories show how differently adolescents handle their approaching deaths.

Julie's Advance Planning

I was once sitting with a fourteen-year-old, Julie, who had shown little recognition of the seriousness of her condition despite two relapses and a stem cell transplant when I got a call from her doctor to tell me she had relapsed again and no more curative treatment remained. My face must have showed my feelings because Julie said, "That was Dr. _____, wasn't it, and he said I've relapsed," and she burst into tears. I asked her if she had suspected it, and she told me she had been talking with her boyfriend the previous night and had told him she thought she had relapsed. We were then able to go on and talk about the choices she still had and, sadly, the choices she no longer had. Julie was able to plan specific goals for herself, including:

- ♦ To be in her brother's wedding.
- ♦ To be at home as much as she could be.

- To be as comfortable as possible.
- To see her friends and her boyfriend as much as possible.
- To come and see us sometimes.

Julie was then able to tell her doctor and her parents what we had come up with—and her end-of-life care was designed to see she met as many of those goals as possible. She visited the clinic with her mother two days before she died. She harassed her doctor whom she loved dearly for keeping her waiting. I gave her a card to take home with her which I read to her to tell her how much she had meant to me. She told us how she was comforted by praying with her mother for herself and for others worse off than she was, how her schoolmates were dedicating the end-of-year concert to her, how she held a smooth stone and stroked it to calm herself. Her doctor and I went with her to the parking lot where we hugged her and said good-bye. Julie died peacefully in her sleep two nights later at home. Her mother—a woman of immense strength and faith—said, "I did not know death could be beautiful."

Jenn's Last-Minute Acknowledgment

Jenn, a lovely, courageous, and vibrant adolescent aged fourteen, had relapsed after a difficult and complicated treatment. Till that point Jenn had attended every medical meeting with her parents and had been a primary decision maker in matters relating to her treatment. She and her parents were told by her medical team that she had relapsed and there was no curative treatment. Jenn was enraged and extremely upset. She ordered her oncologist to explore more treatment options. She stated she was "not ready to die" and was not going to die. She subsequently refused to talk with her oncologist about her Do Not Resuscitate (DNR) status or her declining health. Jenn's parents seemed uncomfortable having discussions with the medical team without Jenn present. The medical team wanted to honor Jenn's wishes and admired her spirit, but they thought it was in her best interest that some decisions be thought about in advance of a medical crisis—particularly since the family lived a long way from the clinic. Her parents did discuss options for end-of-life treatment and DNR status. They knew Jenn wanted to be at home, not in the hospital, and opted for caring for her at home. They had to get some medical support locally.

In her parents' words:

> It felt awful. It was not what we were used to. It felt we were sneaking behind her back. But we had to. Despite Jenn's objections, we

had to call the local hospice, as the local visiting nurse association was not comfortable working with an adolescent who was that sick. Jenn told the first hospice nurse who came, "If you come here, I don't want any of that cloak-and-dagger routine." But the nurse thought we were all in denial (which we were not) and felt she needed to step in and talk with Jenn—told her she was being self-ish and making things difficult! When we found out, we fired her. She just did not understand what Jenn needed. The next nurse who came was wonderful. She supported all of us and knew how to talk with Jenn. She helped us feel safe. Jenn did tell us after one of her radiation treatments that she had known in her heart from the beginning that she would not make it. But the rest of the time she (and we) wanted to keep it as positive as possible.

I was allowed to visit Jenn on her birthday provided I agreed not to discuss her condition with her! I instead gave her a birthday card that listed some of her many accomplishments—noting that most people would not accomplish in their lives as much as she had already accom-plished. The night before Jenn died, the family acknowledged to one another and with Jenn that she was dying, how sad they were, how much they loved her, and how she would continue to be part of their lives. They called their priest and Jenn was able to tell him about the funeral she wanted.

In her mother's words, "The priest came and gave her the last rites . . . Jenn had good friends in school who were in a band. She told the priest she did not want a 'fuddy-duddy funeral' and she wanted her friends to play her favorite music at it. He agreed and they played."

Mark's Minimum Acknowledgment

An eighteen-year-old young man, Mark, was adamant that he would live despite the odds. He had a terrible prognosis. He made it through his first stem cell transplant and managed to get to his high school graduation. He was determined to go to college. He was accepted and began attending. He relapsed and persuaded his doctors to consider a second transplant, which was highly unusual at that time. His father remarked to me at this point that he appeared stuck in denial. How-ever, around this time Mark said to me: "I don't think my doctor real-izes I understand what my prognosis is—that I have one chance in a thousand of surviving, but I am choosing to focus on that one chance." He got through his second transplant and read up on courses he wanted to take the next semester. He was eagerly planning to return to college when he relapsed again and was admitted to the hospital in critical condition. When I visited him, he asked the other people in the room to leave. I assumed he wanted to speak about his imminent death. Instead he told me he was having trouble with his attitude and his ability to continue to think positively. I told him that everyone needed to give themselves a break sometimes. He died a few hours later.

Brian's Selective Acknowledgment

Brian was sixteen years old, the youngest of four children who lived with his parents and siblings. He had relapsed and had a poor prognosis. He was a fine student and athlete, much loved at home and popular in school. He was a resourceful, thoughtful, and caring young man who was having considerable pain from his treatment and his disease progression. He was referred to me to see if hypnosis would be helpful. It turned out he was already using a form of self-hypnosis that was extremely helpful in managing his pain, and he needed little additional help from me. I spent more time with his parents, who were suffering terribly because of his deteriorating and terminal condition. Neither felt they could discuss it with Brian because they said it would be too painful for everyone. They also thought that he was unaware of how seriously ill he was. One day he became very ill at home and told his sister who was there that he knew he was dying and he would like her to call the priest and get in touch with his parents at work. He also told her he had been talking about dying with his friends. They spent the rest of the day talking with each other about many things, including how things would be in the family after he died. His parents came home, and they and the priest were all there when he died. His mother asked his sister three months later whether Brian had known he was dying and if they had talked together about it. She was very relieved to hear that he had had someone to talk to.

....

THE IMPORTANCE OF HOPE

Holding on to hope may be as important to your child as it is to you. You may not want to share bad news because you fear it will take away hope. One parent described hope almost as a religious belief. But let's remember there is a difference between hope and understanding. A wonderful adolescent I knew who had just learned he had an incurable condition, said to me: "I guess I will have to hope for one thing and prepare for another." How can you help your child to hold onto hope of some kind? Can you help your child notice that she may have several hopes at the same time (as you perhaps do also) that may even be contradictory? For example, a child can hope she is cured, may hope she can stay at home whatever happens, and may hope she can go to her graduation. As your child gets sicker, it may be that some of her hopes are more realizable than others. Your hopes may shift, too. Perhaps you can encourage your child to transfer her hope from one goal, namely being cured, to other shorter-term goals that would give her satisfaction and pleasure in the short run, such as being at home or achieving a particular goal, like going to her graduation.

In the same way, do not be surprised if your child is sometimes able to discuss his likely death and sometimes not—if he appears to be going back and forth between recognizing his medical condition and planning for the future. Just as life would be unbearable if you focused solely on your child's illness and likely death, a brief excursion into the subject of death may be all your child can tolerate or need before returning to the experience of his or her day-to-day life. Hope may have a hand when fluctuations like the following occur:

- A teenager plans her funeral one week, and the following week, chooses the courses she wants to take next semester.

- A twelve-year-old child talks in quick succession about his likely death, his worry about how his parents will manage, and the progress of his local baseball team.

- A terminally ill seven-year-old boy describes in a play session how sad a baby dinosaur is because his mother has died, but notes that he will be all right because he will remember his mother and have his father with him. He then ends the intense play session by saying, "That's enough of that. Now let's play a game."

SAYING GOOD-BYE WITHOUT SAYING GOOD-BYE

Some families find meaningful ways to say good-bye—to demonstrate the power of their love—without ever explicitly saying the words.

- An adolescent who rarely spoke of her imminent death bought her boyfriend a cologne called Eternity.

♦ An eleven-year-old boy asked to have a party for his classmates.

♦ A ten-year-old boy used his Make-A-Wish money to buy presents for his family and his friends two days before he died.

For some parents, the quality of your child's life—adequate pain management, being at home, or achieving a particular goal—may be the most important way to express love as your child approaches death. Reminiscing about treasured family moments, recognizing your child's achievements, making a photograph book together, or expressing love verbally or nonverbally may be valuable substitutes for explicitly verbally acknowledging with your child his imminent death. You may do these things consciously or unconsciously. And after your child's death, you may be very glad you did them.

In this chapter I have described ways to begin conversations with your child about his condition and his prognosis. You can listen to what she is thinking and take that or an earlier conversation you had together as a starting point. You can give your child openings to talk but not force a conversation. Remember the importance of hope, but also remember that hopes can shift to match a sad reality. Children and adolescents have different styles, beliefs, and attitudes that will influence how they want to face or not face directly their upcoming death. And even if your child can talk sometimes about her likely death, she may be able to have such conversations only in small doses before her focus returns to her current life. If your child is able to speak to others but not you about his likely death, that may reflect his love and wish to protect you from pain, so don't feel bad about it. If you are able to have these conversations, as I said earlier, they may comfort you later, but if you do not, perhaps that is what allows you to be with your child in the way you want. You and your child will be the ones who negotiate the extent and nature of the conversations that feel right for you.

CHAPTER 23

. . . .

Grief and Bereavement

What you feared most has happened. Your child has died. If you were caring for her at home, you may have been looking after her around the clock and your home may be full of medical equipment and not feel like it is your own. Your family's routine has likely been focused exclusively on your sick child's care. If you were in the hospital, you probably got little sleep and felt immersed in an alien world of medical realities: medications; syringes; transfusion bags; oxygen masks; tubes; machines beeping; X-ray machines; life support monitors; the smell of alcohol wipes and antiseptic. If your child died in the ICU after some time on life support, you may have had many days in the hospital surrounded by these things. If she died suddenly, having been rushed to the hospital for an unexpected emergency, then shock will be added to your exhaustion. Whatever the circumstances surrounding your child's death, you will probably be completely physically exhausted and mentally drained. You have probably been running on overdrive looking after and supporting your child for some time. The rest of your life was on hold and you gave little thought to much else. Suddenly, the picture is reversed. The rest of the world is there, but your child is not. People are doing things or asking you to do things that bring home that terrible fact. Your child's body needs to be prepared to leave where it is. You have to let her body go with strangers to the funeral home or to the hospital morgue. A nurse at home or in the hospital will dispose of all your child's medications. If you are in the hospital, you will need to pack up your belongings and leave. Maybe the medical equipment company will come and take the equipment away from your home; that, astoundingly, can feel as if it is making your loss real. You are left with your grief and the new heartbreaking reality. No wonder you feel bereft.

People experience grief differently. No way is right or wrong. Your family and cultural values, your religious beliefs, your personality and your external circumstances will all influence how you mourn your child's death. Usually grief is a roller coaster, an extremely painful process that allows people to heal slowly and naturally, but sometimes grief becomes stuck or takes a path that makes it more difficult to recover, and we will talk about that as well in this chapter. People can experience their grief emotionally (what they feel), mentally (what they think), physically (how their body feels and reacts), or in different combinations at different times. Your way of experiencing grief, your personality, your values and your environment will all influence how you absorb your terrible loss and go on to become reinvolved in your life and the lives of those around you. Your grief process will be individual. You could have any one or many of the following reactions:

- You feel numb at first. Numbness may protect you temporarily from immediate and overwhelming pain.

- You feel empty, lost, and alone, particularly after your child's funeral. You may have been occupied with all the arrangements, and friends and family members have now returned home to their regular lives while you are left facing the reality of your life without your child's physical presence. You may feel the day has no structure and no purpose.

- You suffer waves of grief experienced physically and mentally. The waves of grief may begin immediately or later—and they will be of varying degrees of intensity. You may be someone who experiences intense sadness as part of your grief. You may feel waves of other emotions like anxiety, guilt, or anger. These waves, large or small, are often part of the grieving process. They usually gradually decrease in frequency and intensity over time.

- You do not experience waves of grief at all.

- You experience physical symptoms like headaches, stomach upsets, or difficulty sleeping. Or you may find you get sick more frequently than usual.

- You have recurring negative thoughts or nagging questions about your child's illness that give you little peace.

♦ You have recurring painful images of your child, often from his last days. It will take time for you to see whether you begin recovering more positive memories and images of your child, or whether these traumatic images need professional help to shift.

♦ You feel so exhausted that even the physical effort of getting out of bed seems too great.

♦ You feel you cannot go on and find the daily demands of life overwhelming.

♦ You experience grief in different ways at different times—sometimes emotionally, sometimes mentally, and sometimes physically. Some parents experience grief in every aspect of their being, while others experience it more in one mode than another—or block feelings out for long periods of time.

♦ You wonder if you are betraying your child if you have moments of feeling better.

♦ You and your spouse find it very difficult to comfort each other. You may each be suffering too much to have energy left to help the other. You may also experience grief differently.

♦ You may feel you have little emotional energy for or patience with your other children—and even want to get away from them at times.

♦ You find there are continuing unique external and internal triggers for your grief over time. These could be anniversaries, holidays, personal associations, or special memories connected with your child. The triggers may sometimes unexpectedly cause you bouts of intense grief. We build protections against what causes us pain, and when we are prepared, we can endure what we cannot endure when confronted by an unexpected reminder of what was.

Parents have described having some or many of these acute grief reactions soon after their child dies. As varied as the reactions to grief are, so too are the ways of enduring the pain, and gradually, sometimes very gradually and often in fits and starts, moving back into the light. Several bereaved parents as well as experienced grief counselors have written moving accounts of their own and others' experiences recovering from their child's death or from the death of other loved ones. The advice they give comes from the heart and from their own difficult journeys. The "For Parents Whose Child Has Died" section in the bibliography (p. 397) briefly describes some of these books and what each book focuses on. If you are feeling utterly isolated in your pain, some of these books may offer comfort and companionship along the way.

Here are a range of suggestions that other parents have found helped them cope in the time following their child's death. I hope very much that some of them will help you:

- Plan a funeral and/or memorial service that acknowledges who your child was. Several religious traditions have frameworks for these services, and usually you can honor your child's unique qualities in some way—through photographs, videos, scrapbooks or through what you, your other children, other family members, and class-mates write, draw, or say. Preparing these tributes may provide a focus and objective for those who are grieving. If you have no religious affiliations you may find a place, inside or outside—perhaps special to your family—where friends and family can gather to remember your child together. Perhaps you can find poems or writings that reflect your child's qualities and your sadness about her premature death.

- Allow yourself some positive moments each day, when you are able to laugh or hug someone. Share a positive memory about your child, without blaming yourself for having these moments. Consider these moments of reprieve and renewal that will help you recover physically and emotionally.

- Allow and experience the waves of grief as opposed to fighting or avoiding them. If you feel after a year or longer the waves have not decreased at all in either intensity or frequency, consider a consultation with a grief counselor.

- Recognize the rawness of your emotions (positive and negative) and tolerate the up-and-down mood swings.

- Allow yourself to do just the basics for a while—and congratulate yourself for doing them. Recognize getting out of bed each morning is an achievement. Take tasks one at a time, a day at a time.

♦ Allow associations with your child to enter your mind in whatever form they take and be open to sensing his presence.

♦ Keep busy. Do whatever tasks you feel up to—even if it is just a few each day—at first that occupy your mind and body.

♦ Divide your focus between your loss and the challenges of the new world without the physical presence of your child.

♦ Find what helps your particular style of grieving.

  ▸ If you feel strong emotions, can you let yourself safely experience them? Does talking about what you feel help? If so, are there people you can talk with? If you share your emotions comfortably and feel better having done so, you may benefit from joining a group with other bereaved parents. The group may help you feel less isolated, may allow you to share your intense feelings and to help others. But beware of joining a group too soon after your loss—say for at least six months afterward. Many parents said they felt too vulnerable early on and hearing other people's stories made them feel worse, not better.

  ▸ If you have consistent negative thoughts, what helps them shift? Does speaking about them help? What happens if you imagine the feelings that might be connected to the thoughts? Can you experience the feeling—be it sadness or anger—that likely goes along with the thought, and does that help the thought shift? Does finding other projects to occupy your mind, either connected or unconnected to your child's memory, give relief? If the thoughts have become repetitive ruminations that do not shift your perspective, allow no resolution, and are preoccupying you more and more, consider consulting with a grief counselor. These ruminations may prevent any movement in your grief.

  ▸ If you feel physically restless and become agitated, try a physical task—either one that is connected with your child, like keeping up his grave site, or one that is unrelated to him, like jogging, swimming, or exercising.

  ▸ If you have somatic/physical symptoms like high blood pressure or tension headaches or are getting sick more frequently than usual, consult your primary care physician. You may need blood pressure medication. You may benefit from exercising and/or using relaxation strategies to release or lower tension. Consider trying yoga. Physical activity is really important.

▶ If you cannot sleep, consider consulting with your doctor to get sleeping medication to use for a while. Lack of sleep makes healing more difficult. If you start exercising, you may get to sleep more easily.

◆ Recognize your style of grieving may be different from your partner's or your other children's, and that what helps one of you may not help the others. If some of you feel better sharing your emotions but others do not, a bereavement group may be good for some of you but not others.

◆ Recognize you are each doing your best to handle your mutual loss and don't take personally the differences in style or criticize one another for the differences.

◆ Ignore those who tell you your task is to let go of grief or "get over it."

◆ See your task as finding a way to accommodate your grief, which may in some form be part of you always—perhaps finding meaningful ways to continue feeling connections with your child in a manner that makes sense to you. (See the examples that follow.)

◆ Recognize you are likely not to be taking good care of yourself, so force yourself to have regular medical checkups. You are more vulnerable to major health problems when you are deeply grieving.

◆ Recognize grief is a process with ups and downs and that recovery may not be returning to where you were but finding where you are now and how to live with that.

◆ Recognize the only grief to avoid is "stuck" grief—where you always feel devastated and overwhelmed, or continue to have the same recurring negative thoughts, questions, or images in your head or avoid anything that reminds you of your child.

CONTINUING CONNECTIONS

More than three quarters of forty-eight bereaved parents contacted by two social workers in our department reported feeling a strong spiritual connection with their child at various points after his or her death.[1] The spiritual connection could take the form of a sensed presence or touch, a special object in the world like a bird, a star, or a meteor, a sign or special message from their child, dreams about their child, or an image of their child with family members who had died. Most of these parents had found these spontaneously occurring spiritual connections comforting. The parents also reported deliberate activities that maintained daily connections with their child that included praying, visiting their child's grave, talking with their child, or listening to music their child enjoyed.

CONTINUING CONNECTIONS

Here are examples of ways that parents have found to maintain continuing connections with their child, often combining this with helping others:

- The parents of a fourteen-year-old boy established a scholarship in his name that would be given each year to a member of the ninth-grade class in his high school who shared some of his qualities. The students wrote an essay about a project they wanted to do and the winners were chosen by his parents and others on the selection committee.

- The parents of a three-year-old boy raised money from an annual golf tournament which they donated to the department doing research on his disease.

- The parents of a seven-year-old boy made a remembrance area in the playground of his school with a plaque including his name and the dates he had lived.

- The parents of a fourteen-year-old girl took some of her classmates out for a celebration dinner the summer that she would have graduated from high school.

- The parents of a ten-year-old boy cooked Thanksgiving dinner for five years and brought it into the oncology floor for the families who were in the hospital. They also raised money through various ingenious fund-raising events which they gave to the resource specialist in our program to make available for families with financial emergencies because of their child's illness. (This family had received financial help themselves).

- The mother of a four-year-old boy went to nursing school and became a critical-care nurse.

- Several parents honored their child by joining the advisory board of our Pediatric Advanced Care Team (PACT) set up to improve palliative care for our families or by becoming active in Jimmy Fund Clinic activities.

- Some parents honored their child by organizing a team in the Boston Marathon Jimmy Fund Walk in their child's memory.

- The parents of a seventeen-year-old boy supported the founding of a Clinic for Survivors of Childhood Cancer.

· ·

COMPLICATED GRIEF REACTIONS

Some parents may find it harder than others to heal after their child's death. Perhaps you already had a painful loss or traumatic experiences in your own childhood. Perhaps you have had problems with depression and anxiety or other psychiatric conditions before your child got ill. Perhaps you were heartbroken and depressed before your child's death, or perhaps you denied to yourself that it was going to happen. Perhaps you have little outside support and limited resources. Perhaps you have experienced additional stressors after your child's death. Any of these factors may make you more vulnerable and less able to recover from your grief—and several of these factors may make it cumulatively more difficult. So be aware if you have some of these added stressors and be particularly gentle with yourself. There are signs you can look out for to judge whether your grief is progressing along a painful but gradual path to recovery or whether you are hitting serious roadblocks along the way. You may want to schedule a consultation with a grief counselor if you experience:

+ Extreme differences between how you are grieving and feeling and how your partner or other family members are feeling and grieving.

+ Intrusive memories, images, and flashbacks that keep recurring with no diminished frequency or intensity over time.

+ Feeling numb or flooded with emotions over many months.

+ Negative and repetitive thoughts (ruminations) that intrude and preoccupy you, do not change, even get worse over many months.

+ Inability to feel pleasure, laugh, have pleasant memories, enjoy special moments, or focus on your daily tasks over many months.

+ Extreme feelings of guilt.

+ Increasing symptoms of depression (increased feelings of hopelessness, helplessness, depressed mood, changes in eating and sleeping patterns, decreased energy and motivation affecting general functioning) or of anxiety (increased jitteriness, nervousness, difficulty concentrating, affecting general functioning).

+ Avoiding thoughts, memories, conversations, and people connected with your child.

+ Using drugs or alcohol to avoid the painful feelings.

+ Having many new physical complaints (headaches, stomach problems, palpitations, high blood pressure, etc.).

SONYA AND SAM

I worked with Sonya and Sam, parents of an eight-year-old girl, May, an only child. Sonya was emotionally available, loving and devoted throughout the extended terminal phase of May's illness. She took a leave of absence from her work to be with May. Despite repeated attempts by the medical staff, she avoided discussions of the seriousness of May's condition and always maintained that May would pull through. In fact, she became angry with Sam if he showed any pessimism regarding May's chance for survival. In other ways, the couple seemed to have a strong relationship. After May's death I talked with them by telephone, since, unfortunately, they lived far from the clinic. Sonya told me how she had not believed May was going to die. Her emotional pain was terrible, and she described May's death as losing part of herself.

Several months after May's death, she returned to work, began going out with people after work, and spent less and less time at home with Sam. She said it was too painful and that they were both so sad they could not comfort each other. I referred them to couples counseling locally and to a grief counselor, but they rarely went. Finally, they separated. I continued to be in telephone contact with Sam for several years. He came to understand Sonya's behavior as her way of avoiding her intense and unresolved sadness at May's death, which was triggered by his presence and any association with him and their past surroundings. He also came to understand that Sonya's denial of the likelihood of May's death may have been what helped her be with May till the moment she died. Although Sam was deeply unhappy about what had happened, he understood and forgave Sonya and was able to move on with his life.

Although in this instance May's death and Sonya's complicated grief reaction did put too much strain on Sonya and Sam's relationship, in general and contrary to popular belief, the data does not support the proposition that there is a higher risk of divorce among bereaved parents.[2] On the contrary, despite initial stress on the relationship, for many couples there is often a closer connection and growth that forms over time associated with having gone through this heartbreaking experience together.

In Janet's case, her traumatic personal history combined with the tragic death of her daughter triggered a major depression and a complicated grief reaction.

JANET

Janet was the mother of eighteen-year-old, Jody. Janet had had a history of physical and sexual abuse in childhood and early adulthood. Jody had died under difficult circumstances in the hospital from a complication of treatment as well as her illness. Her death was traumatic to witness. Although Janet had other children, she was closest to Jody. Janet experienced Jody's death as overwhelming, affecting every aspect of her life. She experienced intrusive memories and flashbacks. She also felt drawn to return to the medical setting and to talk with medical staff connected with Jody, although these visits re-traumatized her. She was angry at her husband for grieving differently. She focused on relationships that were connected to Jody and had difficulty with relationships that were not. She had many somatic symptoms and missed much time at work.

Her family and friends understood her emotional distress and supported her, but her distress increased over time. One year after Jody's death she was hospitalized for suicidal thoughts and self-destructive behavior. She was diagnosed with Major Depression and PTSD. She began taking an antidepressant. She continued meeting with a counselor. Therapy focused on her loss and how to reconnect with the world; on tolerating different styles of grieving from her own; on helping her shift back and forth more easily between her thoughts and feelings about Jody and the demands of her current life; on reframing the meaning of the loss; and on helping her understand how guilt, low self-esteem, and reluctance to accept treatment that might ease the traumatic memories were barriers to her recovery. She needed help to understand that recovery was not a betrayal of Jody and to discover what else in her current life gave it meaning, including positive ways to honor Jody's memory. She very gradually felt better and was able to reconnect with those around her.

If you recognize some or several of the signs of complicated grief, please look for an experienced therapist who works with people who are developing complicated grief reactions. These symptoms are responsive to therapy and other forms of treatment, including psychodynamic therapy, cognitive behavior strategies, meditation practice, and sometimes medications.[3] Several resources listed in the sections on End of Life and Bereavement in Appendices A (p. 332) and B (p. 359) and books described in the section "For Parents Whose Child Has Died" in the bibliography (p. 397) are designed to help those with complicated grief.[4] Many of the issues addressed in Jody's therapy may be shared by others experiencing complicated grief. The sooner you address what is contributing to your grief being stuck, the sooner you may begin to feel better. If your complicated grief reaction continues, it can lead to other negative consequences that perhaps could have been avoided if you had accepted help sooner.

HELPING YOUR OTHER CHILDREN GRIEVE

What can you do to help your other children walk their grief path and emerge more resilient and stronger than before when you are feeling so devastated yourself? Indeed, your other children will be suffering a double loss. Their brother or sister has died and you and your partner are grieving, which will likely and understandably make it very difficult for you to comfort them. Luckily, children are often remarkably resilient and can surprise us with their powers of recovery with just a little support from the adults around them.

Just as Explain, Involve, and Understand were the three key words to help your other children when your child was sick, they remain the three key words to help your other children after your child has died. The words are close to what adolescent bereaved siblings recommended as helpful for health providers to know about their bereavement.[5]

Can you explain that when grown-ups or children have lost someone they love, they have many different feelings? Explain your own reactions whatever they may be—that as well as feeling sad, you also feel angry, irritable, tired, and unwilling to do very much. Explain how much you love them even though you now feel very sad. Expressing and showing sadness in front of your other children gives them permission to express sadness. However, unrestrained crying in their presence may be scary, particularly to young children, so if necessary, find a private space where you can cry freely. Otherwise, you run the risk that your other children may feel that comforting you takes precedence over their own feelings. Explain also that over time you hope you will all gradually feel better and you will together figure out ways to help that happen.

Explain your answers to the direct questions the siblings may have. "Is it all right to play with his toys?" "Is it all right to go into his room?" For example, you might say, "For now I want to leave things the way they are, but I'll think about it again in a few weeks" (and remember to do so). Remember what you feel and think directly after your child's death may not be what you feel and think in several months, so it is probably wise to delay making any major decisions for a while. If you are able later to share at least some of your child's possessions with your other children, the toy may develop a special meaning for them, as Seamus's story shows later in the chapter (p. 325). And if you do, try not to show that you are upset if they do not treat the possessions as carefully as you would like. If something is breakable and precious to you, you can always explain you are saving it and will give it to your other children when they are older.

They may ask, "What do I say when someone asks me how many brothers or sisters do I have?" You may want to explain how you have decided to answer the question "How many children do you have?" You can explain many parents and brothers and sisters find this a hard question. For some parents it feels untruthful and a betrayal of the child who died not to include him in the number they give. Other parents prefer not to get into the discussion that could occur if they have to explain their answer. Some will vary their answers with the context in which they are asked. You can explain to your other children there is no right or wrong answer, and you can ask them what answer they would be most comfortable giving.

Your other children may have unstated questions: "Is it all right to talk about him?" "Is it all right to talk about feelings about his death?" and will take their lead from what you do and say. What you do and say will dictate how open or closed conversations are likely to be as well as how their brother or sister continues to be remembered and talked about (or not talked about) in the family. For example, when his birthday approaches, you could explain that you are likely to feel very sad. You could also tell them what you plan to do and see if they have ideas about what to do. It may be a chance to talk about memories of earlier birthdays. If you are able to have these more open conversations, your children are less likely to feel they are at fault for something they have done or said and will speak more freely. And as time goes on, it may even become more natural than painful to include references to your child who died in regular family conversations.

Involve your other children. We already talked about how your other children can be involved in their brother's or sister's illness and end-of-life care. They can also be involved in the wake and funeral. Young children can draw a picture or give a toy that will be put in your child's coffin. Older children can select other things that will go with him—a letter, a poem, a baseball that reflect who he was. They can also be asked if they would like particular jobs to do at the wake or funeral, like handing water around to people who come or standing by a photograph poster board if there is one and talking about the family photographs on it. It may be easier for them if they have a particular task to do. Some children may want to write something that they or an adult can read at the funeral. Younger children can be given choices whether and how they want to come to the wake and funeral. It is a good idea to have one adult close to a younger child who can take the child out if the child wants or needs to leave. If the casket will be open, you or someone else needs to tell the child how your child's body will look and what clothes he will be wearing. Involve friends and family to do special things with your other children that may both relieve you and also allow them some special time with and get support from people who are feeling less sad and overwhelmed than you are. It does seem that social support from others close to your children can help at this difficult time.[6] Involve siblings if you plan events to honor your child. They can walk part of a marathon or help raise money for the team. They can help plan and work at a fund raising event.

Understand if your other children act out, are more aggressive, show off, are disobedient, get worse grades, want to be with friends, don't want to be with friends, don't want to leave the house, don't want to stay in the house, have tantrums, have nightmares or a hard time sleeping initially. Children express grief in many different ways, and telling them about how sad you are feeling and that you understand how upset everyone else in the family is too may give them permission to look at their own feelings more directly. Understand if they have health concerns and visit the nurse's office frequently in school. Their symptoms may mimic some of their brother's or sister's symptoms or be unrelated. Understand if you have strong reactions to their health complaints. Call their pediatrician with any questions. He will understand why you become easily worried. Understand if your children want to spend more time out of the house with friends. For now, your house may feel like a sad place.

Understand that at some level your other children may wonder if you love them as much as you loved your child who died. They may even feel guilty that they survived and their brother or sister did not. If they do not remember their sibling, either because they were too young or were born after their sibling died, they and their older brothers or sisters may be quite sensitive to feeling compared to him or her (whether or not that was your intention) or they may compare themselves to their sibling. This can lead a child to feel inferior to and unable to compete with their brother or sister who died, particularly if you have emphasized only his positive qualities. Sometimes admiration for an older unknown sibling can also have very positive effects, as Seamus's story that follows demonstrates. If you have only one remaining child, it will be hard for that child not to feel an extra burden of responsibility. It will also be quite difficult for you not to focus very hard on how that child is doing. All your other children may need and benefit from direct and indirect reassurance from you that you love them equally and are glad they are with you and for the way they are—which is not the same way their brother or sister was. And that is okay.

COMPLICATED SIBLING GRIEF

When should you worry about your other children and what should you do if you are worried? Some factors that may make your children more vulnerable to their sibling's death are similar to what may increase a parent's vulnerability—an earlier loss, prior problems with anxiety, depression or other psychiatric conditions, denial or overwhelming sadness before their sibling's death, or stressful circumstances afterward. There may be a few factors unique to being a sibling that can make the loss harder for some brothers and sisters: namely a particularly close relationship with the sibling who died; being the stem cell donor for their sibling; or being the only other child in the family. If any of your other children have some of these vulnerabilities, you may need to be especially watchful.

What are the signs that your other child or children may need help? Notice if their sadness, anger, aggressive behavior, worries, anxieties, or other symptoms are becoming more frequent or intense or last longer over time instead of the other way around, or if new worrying behaviors occur, like using alcohol or drugs, or if their grades fall dramatically. Even if you notice upsetting behavior several years later, it may still be related to your child's death. Emotions and thoughts can be unconsciously or consciously triggered many years later. And the effect of a loss may rear its head again under different stressful circumstances and at different developmental stages later on.

What are the interventions that can help? Your understanding and patience is vital, but sometimes outside help may be valuable if your child is showing obvious signs of distress. If he is not and is reluctant to do anything, do not force him to. He may be healing in his own way. But if you are concerned, depending on your child's attitude and preferences, several options are open to you. You could take your child to an experienced grief counselor who works with children. You could enroll your child in a group for bereaved brothers and sisters if one exists locally. This may be most useful within the first few years after his sibling's death.[7] Often these groups meet for six to twelve times with some follow-up meetings. Such a group can allow your child to feel less alone and can provide a place where he or she can share feelings and experiences with the small group of children who have lost a close family member. He can learn how other children have coped and share his own story. If your child is reluctant to join anything on his own, you could consider looking into a weekend camp for bereaved families; you can accurately tell him that this is something that could be helpful for the whole family. Usually such a camp has separate groups and activities for parents and siblings, so he will have a chance to talk with other brothers and sisters whose sibling has died.

· ·

EFFECTS ON SIBLINGS' DEVELOPMENT

In her wonderful book *Shadows in the Sun*, Betty Davies points out that as siblings grow older, their brother's or sister's death will take on different meanings and they will think and feel different things at different times. For many siblings, it can influence their relationships, their values, their priorities, their sense of themselves, their choice of professions, and even their choice of partners in positive or in negative ways. For some siblings, for example, it can make it hard to develop close relationships later, as in Gregory's situation, particularly if the loss suffered was not addressed in childhood.

Gregory was nine when his eleven-year-old sister died. They were very close. Gregory lived with different relatives during his upbringing—some who treated him well and some who did not. He did not receive therapy despite obvious symptoms of depression and anxiety. As a young adult now, he notices he backs away from relationships as soon as they become serious and before the person leaves him. He has chosen to start therapy to address this issue.

Other siblings may have an increased concern for others and a wish to make a positive difference in the world. Many siblings in supportive environments grow in positive ways after their brother or sister's death.

Matthew was only four years old when his older brother, Nick, died. He participated for years in fund-raising events and activities his parents did to honor his brother. He is now a loving and caring young man who remembers his brother fondly and goes out of his way to be kind and considerate to others.

Mary was fourteen years old when her ten-year-old brother died. She had been actively involved in caring for him at home and spoke at his funeral. She participated for years in the Jimmy Fund Walk to raise money for the Jimmy Fund Clinic and wants to go to medical school to learn to be a doctor to "help sick kids."

Katie was eight years old when her three-year-old brother died. When he was at home her parents encouraged her to help in small ways in his care, and she sometimes visited him in the hospital. After his death, his mother became very active with other bereaved parents. Over time Katie also became involved with other bereaved brothers and sisters. She participated in bereaved sibling panels and spoke publically about her experience as a bereaved sibling. She has become a motivated and public-spirited young woman who will make a positive difference in the world.

The death of a sibling may significantly impact brothers and sisters even if they are born after their sibling dies, as Seamus's story poignantly shows.

Seamus was born three years after his three-year-old brother, Patrick, had died after a long and difficult fight against cancer. His parents continued to include the spirit of Patrick in the family in various ways. They talked about him and told stories about him. Each year they held a fund-raising event to raise money to fund the research Patrick's doctor continued to do. They kept up contact with some of the people who had looked after Patrick. Patrick's mother led groups for bereaved parents. And they allowed Patrick's toys—even his most precious one, Barney—to be used by and shared with Seamus.

Seamus, now eighteen years old, wrote a moving essay about the role in his life that Barney and the brother he never knew had played in his life.

Seamus begins: "The Barney doll's journey began inside Boston Children's Hospital, years before I was born. It originally belonged to Patrick, my older brother."

Seamus tells us that Barney, the dinosaur stuffed animal, had accompanied Patrick everywhere throughout his long hospital stays,

difficult treatments, and painful medical procedures. Barney had been
a very special comfort to Patrick as he fought for his life. Seamus continues:

> As Patrick passed from our world to another, Barney was left
> behind. Four years later, though, the small dinosaur found a
> new best friend. For the first six years of my childhood, Barney
> and I were inseparable. Whether it was day care, the doctor's
> office, or even a family vacation, I carried Barney with me wher-
> ever I went.
>
> As I grew older and became less attached to my Barney toy,
> the story behind it became a strong influence in my personality.
> While Barney is known for teaching kids the values of respect,
> compassion, and honesty, Patrick's story was my own child-
> hood mentor. As each year passed by, I seemed to become more
> motivated to make a difference not only in my life, but the lives
> of others. Everything I did, it seemed, I did for Patrick. All of
> the games that he couldn't play, problems he couldn't solve, and
> adventures he couldn't go on, I did with him in mind.
>
> One opportunity that Patrick brought to me that Barney
> couldn't was the game of golf. Since his death, my family has
> run a charitable golf tournament in Patrick's honor. Although
> he never had the chance to play it, he is the reason that the pas-
> sion for golf is embodied within me. The virtues that I have
> gained through playing, such as patience and poise, are indi-
> rectly related to Patrick.
>
> In the children's show, Barney is a figment of the kids'
> imaginations. He was only there in spirit, and not form. Even
> though his presence was lacking, the big purple dinosaur was
> still able to instill values into the hearts of his friends. While
> Patrick may not be here in body, he has handed me some of the
> most persistent virtues in my life. Although he isn't here to see
> it, Patrick has been the biggest influence in my life.

His mother wrote,

> When I read this essay I was overwhelmed. I honestly felt such
> a sense of relief and awe. It gave me the gift of knowing that
> through our pain we were able to give our children, both Katie
> and Seamus, the opportunity to build their character through
> Patrick's legacy and helped them to heal, that somehow we did
> things "right" keeping Patrick's spirit alive in our family.

THE FUTURE

As your life continues, you will find your particular path through your grief and the pain of your loss. If you need help sometimes, reach for it. If you have other children, as they get older, they too will include their brother or sister who died into the fabric of their lives. At some point in time, perhaps your family may take the opportunity to think again about your child's death and what it has meant for each of you. You may reassess what happened and consider the positive and negative ways your child's death has affected all your lives. You may want to sit down together or with a family therapist and put into words what some of those changes have been and what the experience has meant for different family members. You may clear up misunderstandings, understand different perspectives, and feel closer as a result.

There is no greater testimony to the resilience of the human spirit than the capacity to surmount a terrible loss and use it as an impetus to change and to make a positive difference in the world.[8] Many bereaved parents, interviewed years later, reported that though they wished with all their hearts that their child had not died, they felt they had become stronger, more resilient, compassionate, and empathetic to others because of who they had become and what they had done as a result of their loss.[9]

Acknowledgments

I would like to thank current and past colleagues at Dana-Farber Cancer Institute (DFCI) and Children's Hospital Boston, many of whom reviewed and improved parts of this book: in particular, Andrea Patenaude, who hired me at DFCI and has been a teacher, mentor, friend, and ruthless editor for more years than I can say; my colleagues in the Psychosocial Unit—Kathy Hewett (my office mate and co-teacher), Aurora Sanfeliz, Amy Grose, Judith August, Brian Delaney, Cori Liptak, Deborah Berk, Jorge Fernandes, Sarah Tarquini, Sarah Brandt, and Molly Mariano; its past leaders, Pat Dwyer and Pam Hogen, Nancy Frumer Styron and its current leader, Nina Muriel; Lisa Northman and Mary Beth Morris in the School Liaison program, who help so many children with treatment-induced learning problems; and Joe Chabot, whose kind heart and skill enables him to find resources where none previously existed. You all provide support and clinical excellence however stressful the circumstances. I applaud the efforts of Kira Bona to document the need of some of our families for extra support and I thank her for her input. I thank my colleagues in the David B. Perini Jr. Quality of Life Clinic for childhood cancer survivors for their help with the book and for their friendship; Christopher Recklitis, Sharon Bober, Rupa Gambhir, Lisa Kenney, Lynda Vrooman, Jill Brace O'Neill, and Eileen Duffey-Lind. I salute my colleagues in the pediatric advanced care team whose starting goal was to improve the end-of-life care for our patients: Joanne Wolfe, Michael Cuomo, and Janet Duncan. I recognize other doctors and nurse practitioners with whom I worked closely over the years, sometimes in heartbreaking situations: Holcombe Grier, Andy Androkides, Melissa Melone, Amy Billett, Leslie Lehman, Jennie Mack, Sarah Alexander, Sung-Yun Pai, Chuck Berde,

Scott Armstrong, and Lisa Diller, to name a few. I applaud the terrific Jimmy Fund Clinic nurses like Annie Beauchemin, Robin Griffey, and Trisha Robinson, ably assisted by Phyllis Booker and Philomena Grannell-Coburn and the inpatient nurses like Kathy Houlihan and Lisa Morrisey whose skills and compassion were so important to the families they cared for. I feel very lucky to have worked with such a remarkable group of people over so many years whose dedication to the children and families under their care was exemplary.

I am grateful to Rachael Coakley, who kindly reviewed and improved my chapters on helping children and their parents manage pain and anxiety, and to Lori Wiener at the National Institutes of Health, who is so generous in sharing her knowledge and her resources.

A very special thanks goes to the participants in the writing seminar at Cambridge Hospital led by Nancy Chodorow. They suffered through different iterations of the book, gave thoughtful, careful, and useful feedback and meant I had to meet deadlines for review. This book would never have been completed without them.

I am very grateful to my research assistant, Kaitlin Herbert, who helped me face the endnotes and assemble a formidable list of resources with humor and efficiency while viewing technology as a friend rather than a foe.

I would like to thank my editor, Becky Cole, who improved the book immeasurably, making it clearer, more direct, and a little more authoritative than is my natural bent! I also appreciate that Becky managed to keep reading even when she found the material extremely upsetting. And I appreciate the tactful guidance of Sara Carder, who had the misfortune to take on the book when I considered it done! I am grateful to Rebecca Strobe and Heather Brennan, who showed patience and efficiency in helping me get the manuscript into publishable form.

I thank my husband, Stephen, who has consistently supported and encouraged me to write this book, my children, Chloe, Nell, and Michael, who because of my workplace had to suffer my extreme worries about their health while they were growing up, and my grandchildren, Clara, Ansel, Eli, Samuel, and Angela, whose charms may have contributed to the length of time this book has taken to write. As I look at them, I am reminded daily of the blessings of good health.

And of course my biggest thanks go to the many wonderful families with whom I had the privilege to work over many years, whose courage and endurance were never-ending sources of inspiration. An unexpected joy in writing this book was in renewing contact with many of them, receiving their enthusiastic support, and in some instances including their advice and experiences in the book that they generously agreed to share with other parents who might benefit. This book is a tribute to them and to their children, as well as hopefully providing suggestions and ideas based on many years of experience and observation about what can help parents whose child develops a major health challenge.

APPENDIX A

. . . .

Resources from Foundations, Organizations, or Government Agencies

All foundation information accessed via foundation websites between September 2016 and March 2017.

. . . .

ON TREATMENT AND SURVIVORSHIP

Alex's Lemonade Stand Foundation

http://www.alexslemonade.org/

Description: A childhood cancer foundation dedicated to researching potential cures for childhood cancer and offering financial and emotional support to families

Resources Provided:

- ◆ Travel for Care Program (travel reimbursements):
  - ▷ Eligibility: children (under 21) actively diagnosed with pediatric cancer whose family's income does not exceed $75,000 and who are moving into or out of a specific set of hospitals

> ▶ Process to Apply: online application completed by a social worker or other medical representative

- ◆ SuperSibs! Program (sibling support):
  - ▶ Eligibility: children (between 4 and 18) who have a sibling who has (or had) cancer
  - ▶ Process to Apply: online referral by a parent or hospital representative

American Cancer Society

http://www.cancer.org/

Description: Organization aimed to provide information and support to cancer patients while also funding research and advocating for cancer patients

Resources Provided:

- ◆ Road to Recovery (car rides):
  - ▶ Eligibility: individuals currently receiving cancer treatment who are ambulatory
  - ▶ Process to Apply: check website for local Road to Recovery program
- ◆ Hope Lodge (housing):
  - ▶ Eligibility: vary by location
  - ▶ Process to Apply: check website for local Hope Lodge site

American Childhood Cancer Organization (ACCO)

http://www.acco.org/

Description: Organization aimed to provide information and support to families dealing with pediatric cancer (previously named Candlelighters Childhood Cancer Foundation)

Resources Provided:

- ◆ Candlelighters Groups (regional meetings and support services):
  - ▶ Eligibility: vary by location
  - ▶ Process to Apply: see website for closest regional group

- ◆ Comfort Kit and books on treatment and late effects of childhood cancer:
  - ▶ Eligibility: child or teenager recently diagnosed with cancer
  - ▶ Process to Apply: join ACCO to receive free kit and books

Andrew McDonough B+ Foundation

http://bepositive.org/
Description: Childhood cancer foundation aimed to raising awareness about pediatric cancer while funding research and providing financial assistance to families

Resources Provided:

- ◆ B+ Foundation Family Assistance Program (variety of expenses):
  - ▶ Eligibility: children (under 21) diagnosed with pediatric cancer
  - ▶ Process to Apply: paper application completed by family and social worker

Be the Match Foundation

https://bethematch.org/
Description: Foundation that manages a bone marrow registry and provides support and information to individuals in need of a transplant

Resources Provided:

- ◆ Transplant Support Assistance Funds (travel reimbursements and co-pays):
  - ▶ Eligibility: received a bone marrow or cord blood transplant within the last 12 months through the Be the Match registry
  - ▶ Process to Apply: application completed by transplant center personnel

Bone Marrow Foundation

http://bonemarrow.org/
Description: Foundation created to provide financial assistance to patients and families affected by bone marrow or stem cell transplants

Resources Provided:

- Lifeline Fund (variety of expenses):
  - Eligibility: patients who will or have recently received a bone marrow, stem cell, or cord blood transplant at a certified transplant center
  - Process to Apply: paper application completed by parent and social worker or nurse coordinator
- Scholarship Grant:
  - Eligibility: student enrolled part-time or full-time at a public school, university, trade school, or homebound education program who has previously undergone a transplant and demonstrates financial need
  - Process to Apply: paper application completed by student and letters of recommendation from educator or health care professional

Bryan's Dream Foundation

http://bryansdream.org/

Description: Foundation aimed at providing information and support for children diagnosed with brain tumors and other childhood cancers

Resources Provided:

- Family Financial Assistance (variety of expenses up to $1,000):
  - Eligibility: children diagnosed with a brain tumor who receive care at eligible hospitals (see website)
  - Process to Apply: paper application completed by oncologist or social worker

Camp Mak-A-Dream

http://www.campdream.org/

Description: Organization designed to provide children with pediatric cancer, and their siblings, with memorable camp experiences. Camp is in Montana.

Resources Provided:

- Kids Camp (one-week camp):

> ▶ Eligibility: children (6 to 14) previously diagnosed with or currently receiving treatment for cancer
> ▶ Process to Apply: online application completed by parent

- ◆ Sibs Camp (one-week camp):
  - ▶ Eligibility: children (6 to 17) who either have a parent or sibling currently diagnosed with cancer or had a parent or sibling pass away from cancer
  - ▶ Process to Apply: online application completed by parent

- ◆ Teen Camp (one-week camp):
  - ▶ Eligibility: children (15 to 18) previously diagnosed with or currently receiving treatment for cancer
  - ▶ Process to Apply: online application completed by parent

CancerCare

http://cancercare.org/
Description: Organization aimed to provide support and information to cancer patients and siblings

Resources Provided:

- ◆ Financial Assistance (transportation, home care, child care):
  - ▶ Eligibility: children (under 18) actively receiving cancer treatment who demonstrate financial need
  - ▶ Process to Apply: call 1-800-813-HOPE (4673) to speak with a CancerCare social worker about eligibility

- ◆ Co-Payment Assistance Foundation (co-pays):
  - ▶ Eligibility: must pass detailed financial, medical, and insurance eligibility criteria (see website)
  - ▶ Process to Apply: call 1-866-55-COPAY (2-6729) or online application completed by patient or parent

Cancer Survivors' Fund

http://www.cancersurvivorsfund.org/
Description: Organization dedicated to supporting children and young adults diagnosed with cancer

Resources Provided:

- ◆ Scholarship Programs (college scholarship):
  - ▶ Eligibility: young adult who is a cancer survivor or currently diagnosed with cancer accepted into an undergraduate institution
  - ▶ Process to Apply: online application completed by student

- ◆ Prosthetic Limb Assistance Program (prosthetics):
  - ▶ Eligibility: children or young adults who have survived cancer or who are currently diagnosed with cancer in need of a prosthetic limb
  - ▶ Process to Apply: online application completed by patient, parent and physician

Childhood Leukemia Foundation

https://www.clf4kids.org/

Description: Foundation aimed at providing hope for children diagnosed with all forms of cancer

Resources Provided:

- ◆ Hugs-U-Wear (wigs):
  - ▶ Eligibility: children who have a leukemia diagnosis and experienced hair loss
  - ▶ Process to Apply: online form completed by a social worker or child life specialist

- ◆ Wish Basket Program (wish baskets):
  - ▶ Eligibility: children who have a leukemia diagnosis
  - ▶ Process to Apply: online form completed by a social worker or child life specialist

- ◆ Hope Binder (phone app or binder to keep medical information):
  - ▶ Eligibility: families with children diagnosed with cancer
  - ▶ Process to Apply: online form completed by a social worker or download the phone app

Children's Cancer Association

http://joyrx.org/

Description: Organization aiming to provide joy and positive experiences to families dealing with pediatric cancer

Resources Provided:

- Alexandra Ellis Caring Cabin (retreat):
  - Eligibility: children (5 to 19) receiving active treatment for cancer, a related blood disease, or a terminal illness, in the Pacific Northwest region (Oregon and SW Washington)
  - Process to Apply: e-mail CCA through website

- Chemo Pal Mentoring Program (one-on-one mentorship):
  - Eligibility: children receiving active treatment for cancer in the Pacific Northwest region (Oregon and SW Washington)
  - Process to Apply: e-mail CCA through website

Children's Cancer Recovery Foundation

http://childrenscancerrecovery.org/

Description: Foundation created to improve the overall well-being of children diagnosed with childhood cancer

Resources Provided:

- Helping Hands Fund (household expenses up to $300):
  - Eligibility: children (under 18) actively receiving cancer treatment
  - Process to Apply: application completed by a parent and social worker

- Camp Scholarships Fund (camp scholarship up to $400):
  - Eligibility: children (under 18) previously diagnosed with cancer who are in remission
  - Process to Apply: application completed by a parent and social worker

Children's Health Insurance Program (CHIP)

**https://www.healthcare.gov/medicaid-chip/childrens-health
-insurance-program/**

Description: Government program providing low-cost health care coverage to children in families that do not qualify for Medicaid

Resources Provided:

- ♦ CHIP (health insurance):
  - ❯ Eligibility: differs by state
  - ❯ Process to Apply: call 1-800-318-2596 or fill out an online application at https://www.healthcare.gov/get-coverage/

Children's Organ Transplant Association (COTA)

http://cota.org/
Description: Charity organization that helps families fund-raise for transplant-related expenses through an online platform and community events

Cory's Crusaders

http://coryscrusaders.org/
Description: Charitable organization aimed at providing financial support to families caring for a child with a brain tumor

Resources Provided:

- ♦ Financial Assistance (variety of expenses):
  - ❯ Eligibility: child (under 18) currently receiving treatment for a brain tumor
  - ❯ Process to Apply: online application completed by parent and physician

Dream Street Foundation

https://dreamstreetfoundation.org/
Description: Foundation providing camp experiences to children and young adults with cancer and chronic or life-threatening illnesses

Resources Provided:

- ♦ Kids Camp (one-week camp):
  - ❯ Eligibility: children (4 to 14) with cancer, a life-threatening illness, or a chronic illness

- Process to Apply: online application completed by parent and doctor

- Young Adult Camp (one-week camp):
  - Eligibility: young adults (18 to 24) with cancer, a life-threatening illness, or a chronic illness
  - Process to Apply: online application completed by young adult and doctor

Eagle Mount Bozeman

https://eaglemount.org/

Description: Organization offering summer camps and outdoor programming for children and young adults with a variety of disabilities and illnesses

Resources Provided:

- Big Sky Kids (weeklong camp for child and parent):
  - Eligibility: children (5 to 11; 11 to 18) who are currently receiving cancer treatment or who recently completed treatment
  - Process to Apply: online application completed by parent
- Young Adult Retreat (weeklong camp):
  - Eligibility: young adults (16 to 23) previously diagnosed with cancer who are currently in remission
  - Process to Apply: online application completed by young adult

Family Reach Foundation

http://familyreach.org/

Description: Foundation created to help financially support families of children diagnosed with childhood cancer

Resources Provided:

- Family Reach Grants (variety of expenses):
  - Eligibility: children (under 17) or young adults (18 to 30) who have been diagnosed with cancer and are within one year of receiving treatment at an eligible hospital (see website)

- Process to Apply: social worker must contact organization to receive further information

First Descents

http://firstdescents.org/

Description: Organization that organizes multiday retreats that involve active outdoor activities (rock climbing, surfing, etc.) for young adult cancer patient and survivors

Resources Provided:

- First Descents Retreats (multiday programs):
  - Eligibility: young adult (18 to 39) cancer patients or cancer survivors
  - Process to Apply: online application

GoFundMe

https://www.gofundme.com

Description: Website dedicated to helping individuals raise money via an online platform for a variety of purposes, including expenses associated with medical issues

Help Hope Live

https://helphopelive.org/

Description: Website dedicated to helping individuals receiving a transplant, living with a catastrophic illness, or dealing with a catastrophic injury raise money via an online platform for covering uninsured medical expenses

The Hole in the Wall Gang Camp

http://www.holeinthewallgang.org/

Description: Organization that provides memorable camp experiences to seriously ill children and their families

Resources Provided:

- Summer Camp (one-week camp):
  - Eligibility: children (7 to 15) diagnosed with a serious illness
  - Process to Apply: online application completed by parent

+ Summer Camp for Siblings (one-week camp):
    ▶ Eligibility: children (7 to 15) with a sibling who is diagnosed with a serious illness
    ▶ Process to Apply: online application completed by parent
+ Hero's Journey (one-week retreat):
    ▶ Eligibility: teens (16 to 18) diagnosed with a serious illness
    ▶ Process to Apply: online application completed by parent and teen
+ Hero's Journey for Siblings (one-week retreat):
    ▶ Eligibility: teens (16 to 18) with a sibling who is diagnosed with a serious illness
    ▶ Process to Apply: online application completed by parent and teen
+ CampOut (home visit program):
    ▶ Eligibility: children (under 17) who have previously attended the Hole in the Wall Gang Camp
    ▶ Process to Apply: request a visit online
+ Family Weekend Programs (family weekend retreats):
    ▶ Eligibility: children (5 to 15) affected by a serious illness
    ▶ Process to Apply: online application completed by parent

Imerman Angels

https://imermanangels.org/
Description: Organization aimed to provide cancer patients, survivors, and caregivers with one-on-one support from a similarly matched individual

Resources Provided:

+ Mentor Angels (one-on-one support):
    ▶ Eligibility: cancer patients, cancer survivors, or caregivers of any age
    ▶ Process to Apply: online application completed by patient or parent

Immune Deficiency Foundation

http://primaryimmune.org/
Description: Organization aimed at improving the quality of life for individuals with primary immune deficiency disorders

Resources Provided:

- ◆ IDF Teen Escape (weekend trip):
  - ◗ Eligibility: teens (12 to 18) who have been diagnosed with a primary immunodeficiency disease (PI)
  - ◗ Process to Apply: online registration completed by teen or parent
- ◆ IDF Get Connected Groups (in-person support groups):
  - ◗ Eligibility: individuals and families affected by PI
  - ◗ Process to Apply: see website for local group meetings
- ◆ IDF Retreats (biannual event):
  - ◗ Eligibility: individuals and families affected by PI
  - ◗ Process to Apply: online registration completed by parent

The InterNational Council for Infertility Information Dissemination (INCIID)

http://www.inciid.org/

Description: Organization aimed at providing information and support to individuals and families exploring family-building options due to infertility

Resources Provided:

- ◆ IVF Scholarship (fertility aid):
  - ◗ Eligibility: members of the INCIID community with medical infertility
  - ◗ Process to Apply: online application completed by patient and medical professional

Jeffrey Modell Foundation

http://www.info4pi.org/

Description: Nonprofit dedicated to increasing awareness and treatment options for primary immunodeficiency disorders while supporting families

Resources Provided:

- ◆ Roots & Wings (travel reimbursements and other expenses):

> ▶ Eligibility: children who have been identified at birth with SCID or other T-cell lymphopenias who are receiving treatment at an eligible hospital (see website)
> ▶ Process to Apply: online application completed by parent and doctor

Joe Andruzzi Foundation

http://joeandruzzifoundation.org/
Description: Foundation created by retired NFL player to financially support pediatric and adult cancer patients and caregivers

Resources Provided:

- ◆ Financial Assistance (living expenses):
  - ▶ Eligibility: individual actively diagnosed with cancer receiving treatment in New England, New York, or New Jersey
  - ▶ Process to Apply: online application completed by a social worker or other hospital professional

Leukemia & Lymphoma Society (LLS)

http://www.lls.org/
Description: Organization aimed at funding research for blood cancers and providing information and access to treatment for blood cancer patients

Resources Provided:

- ◆ Co-Pay Assistance Program (co-pays):
  - ▶ Eligibility: individuals with financial need with a confirmed blood cancer diagnosis
  - ▶ Process to Apply: online applications completed by patient, parent, or doctor
- ◆ Chronic Myeloid Leukemia (CML) Test Costs (up to $1,000):
  - ▶ Eligibility: individuals with financial need with a chronic myeloid leukemia (CML) diagnosis who have received a BCR-ABL PCR test
  - ▶ Process to Apply: online application completed by patient or parent

- Pay-It-Forward Patient Travel Assistance Program (travel expenses):
  - Eligibility: individuals with financial need with a confirmed blood cancer diagnosis
  - Process to Apply: online application completed by patient, parent, or doctor
- First Connection Program (peer-to-peer support via phone or in person):
  - Eligibility: recently diagnosed patients and family members
  - Process to Apply: online application completed by patient or parent
- Family Support Groups (local monthly meeting):

  - Eligibility: any individual affected by blood cancer
  - Process to Apply: check website for local LLS chapter

Locks of Love

http://www.locksoflove.org/
Description: Organization dedicated to providing hairpieces to financially needy children who have suffered from medical hair loss

Resources Provided:

- Hairpieces:
  - Eligibility: children (under 21) who have suffered medical hair loss
  - Process to Apply: online application completed by parent and medical professional

Look Good Feel Better for Teens

http://lookgoodfeelbetter.org/programs/teens
Description: Organization dedicated to improving teen girls' self-image and appearance throughout their cancer treatment

Resources Provided:

- Look Good Feel Better Workshops:
  - Eligibility: differs by location
  - Process to Apply: see website for workshops in your area

Lucy's Love Bus

http://lucyslovebus.org/
Description: Organization aimed at providing access to integrative therapies for children diagnosed with pediatric cancer

Resources Provided:

- Lucy's Children Integrative Therapies (therapy expenses):
  - Eligibility: children (under 21) in the New England area who are currently diagnosed with childhood cancer or are still experiencing lasting effects from cancer treatment
  - Process to Apply: online application completed by parent

Matthew Larson Foundation for Pediatric Brain Tumors

http://ironmatt.org/
Description: foundation aimed at supporting brain tumor research and providing support to families currently dealing with a child with a pediatric brain tumor

Resources Provided:

- Family Assistance (variety of expenses):
  - Eligibility: children (under 21) with a brain tumor (malignant or benign) who receive treatment at a specific set of hospitals
  - Process to Apply: online application completed by a social worker

Medicaid

https://www.medicaid.gov/
Description: Government program that provides health insurance coverage to children, low-income families, the elderly, and medically needy and/or disabled individuals

Resources Provided:

- Medicaid (health insurance):
  - Eligibility: see eligibility requirements on website (differ by state)
  - Process to Apply: apply online at https://www.medicaid.gov/apply-for-coverage/apply-for-coverage.html

National Cancer Survivors Day Foundation

http://www.ncsd.org/

Description: Nonprofit organization dedicated to providing inspiration and support to individuals diagnosed with cancer

Resources Provided:

- National Cancer Survivors Day (one-day event):
  - Eligibility: any person wishing to celebrate cancer survivors
  - Process to Apply: check to see if there is a NCSD event in your area

National Center for Learning Disabilities

www.ncld.org/

Description: Organization dedicated to improving the quality of life for children diagnosed with a learning or attention issue

Resources Provided:

- Allegra Ford Thomas Scholarship ($2,500 award):
  - Eligibility: graduating high school senior with financial needs who has a documented LD and/or ADHD who plans to attend a two-year community college or vocational program
  - Process to Apply: online application completed by student

- Anne Ford Scholarship ($10,000 award):
  - Eligibility: graduating high school senior with financial needs who has a documented LD and/or ADHD who plans to attend a four-year college
  - Process to Apply: online application completed by student

National Children's Cancer Society (NCCS)

https://thenccs.org/#

Description: Organization that provides support and information to families of children with pediatric cancer and pediatric cancer survivors

Resources Provided:

- Transportation Assistance Fund (travel expenses):
  - Eligibility: child (under 18) diagnosed with cancer whose family displays financial need (for travel expenses)
  - Process to Apply: online application completed by parent

- Emergency Assistance Fund (variety of expenses up to $200):
  - Eligibility: child receiving inpatient cancer treatment for a consecutive thirty days or who has spent at least thirty days away from home over the course of three months
  - Process to Apply: online application completed by parent
- Prescription Drug Card (prescription discounts):
  - Eligibility: not applicable (most beneficial to those who are underinsured or uninsured)
  - Process to Apply: print card online (http://thenccs.agelity.com/)
- Beyond the Cure Ambassador Scholarship (college scholarship up to $3,500):
  - Eligibility: survivors of childhood cancer
  - Process to Apply: online application completed by student

National Patient Travel Center

http://www.patienttravel.org/
Description: Foundation created to ensure pediatric and adult patients with financial need are not denied access to treatment due to an inability to travel to a given hospital

Resources Provided:

- Travel Accommodations (commercial airline, private flight, ground transportation):
  - Eligibility: patients displaying financial and medical need to receive diagnosis and/or treatment at a distant location
  - Process to Apply: online application completed by parent

Next Step Foundation

http://www.nextstepnet.org/
Description: Massachusetts-based organization aimed at providing emotional support to young adults with life-threatening illnesses through retreats and workshops

Resources Provided:

- Next Step Campference (annual event):

> Eligibility: young adults (16 to 24) who have a variety of life-threatening illnesses (sickle cell anemia, cancer, HIV, rare genetic disease)
> Process to Apply: online application completed by patient

Okizu

http://okizu.org/

Description: Organization created to support families of children with pediatric cancer through different types of family programs

Resources Provided:

◆ Oncology Camp:
> Eligibility: children (6 to 17) who currently have or previously had pediatric cancer
> Process to Apply: online application completed by parent

◆ SIBS Camp:
> Eligibility: children (6 to 17) who have a sibling who currently has or previously had pediatric cancer (passed away or in remission)
> Process to Apply: online application completed by parent

◆ Family Camp:
> Eligibility: all members of the immediate family of a child who currently has or previously had pediatric cancer
> Process to Apply: online application completed by parent

◆ Teens-N-Twenties Camp:
> Eligibility: young adults (18 to 25) who currently have cancer or previously had cancer or who have a sibling who currently has or previously had cancer
> Process to Apply: online application completed by young adult

Patient Advocate Foundation

http://www.patientadvocate.org/

Description: Foundation dedicated to protecting patients by serving as a liaison in order to ensure access to care, maintenance of employment, and financial stability

Resources Provided:

- ◆ Co-Pay Relief (co-pay and prescription assistance):
  - ▸ Eligibility: individuals with financial need and insurance who have a confirmed medical diagnosis (see list of eligible diagnoses)
  - ▸ Process to Apply: online application completed by patient (https://www.copays.org/)

- ◆ Scholarships for Survivors ($3,000 per year):
  - ▸ Eligibility: young adults (under 25) who have been diagnosed with or treated for cancer or a chronic, or a life-threatening disease within the last five years who are pursuing a college education
  - ▸ Process to Apply: online application completed by student and medical professional

Patient Airlift Services

http://www.palservices.org/

Description: Nonprofit organization that provides free flights to pediatric and adult patients with financial need who are seeking treatment, diagnosis, or follow-up for a medical condition

Resources Provided:

- ◆ Private Flights:
  - ▸ Eligibility: patients with significant financial need who live in the northeastern US who have the mobility to enter a plane
  - ▸ Process to Apply: online application completed by parent

Patient Services, Inc.

http://www.patientservicesinc.org/

Description: Nonprofit that helps chronically ill patients afford expensive medical costs

Resources Provided:

- ◆ A.C.C.E.S.S Programs (legal representation):
  - ▸ Eligibility: individuals with rare chronic disorders (see website for eligible groups)
  - ▸ Process to Apply: call 1-888-700-7010

- Copayment Assistance:
  - Eligibility: individuals with rare chronic disorders (see website for eligible groups)
  - Process to Apply: online application completed by parent and medical professional

Pediatric Brain Tumor Foundation

http://www.curethekids.org/

Description: Foundation that funds pediatric brain tumor research and provides assistance and information to families with a child diagnosed with a pediatric brain tumor

Resources Provided:

- The Butterfly Fund (emergency assistance):
  - Eligibility: children diagnosed with a pediatric brain tumor who are receiving treatment at an eligible hospital (see website)
  - Process to Apply: application completed by social worker
- College Scholarship Fund (college scholarships of $500):
  - Eligibility: high school graduates or college students diagnosed (before age 19) with a pediatric brain tumor or spinal cord tumor who plan to attend or currently attend an academic institution
  - Process to Apply: application completed by student

River Discovery

http://riverdiscovery.org/

Description: Organization dedicated to providing child and young adult cancer survivors with river adventures

Resources Provided:

- Youth Survivors 1-Day Adventure (family retreat):
  - Eligibility: children (6 and older) who are pediatric cancer survivors
  - Process to Apply: application completed by parents

- ◆ Salmon River Adventure (weeklong retreat):
  - ▶ Eligibility: teens and adults (13 and older) who have survived cancer
  - ▶ Process to Apply: application completed by participant

Ronald McDonald House Charities of Southern California

http://rmhcsc.org/

Description: A branch of the Ronald McDonald House Corporation that also runs medically supervised camps

Resources Provided:

- ◆ Camp Ronald McDonald for Good Times Family Camp (weekend camp):
  - ▶ Eligibility: children (infants to 9) who have or have had pediatric cancer (siblings and parents may also attend)
  - ▶ Process to Apply: online application completed by parent

- ◆ Camp Ronald McDonald for Good Times Sleep-Away Camp (summer camp):
  - ▶ Eligibility: children (9 through high school graduation) who have had or currently have pediatric cancer (siblings older than 9 may also attend)
  - ▶ Process to Apply: online application completed by parent

Ronald McDonald House Corporation

http://www.rmhc.org/

Description: Foundation that provides housing for families with a child who is seeking medical treatment for a serious illness

Resources Provided:

- ◆ Ronald McDonald House (in specific cities):
  - ▶ Eligibility: differs by location (see website)
  - ▶ Process to Apply: through the hospital where your child will be seeking treatment

The Samfund

http://www.thesamfund.org/

Description: Foundation that provides financial support to young adults diagnosed with cancer

Resources Provided:

- ◆ Samfund Grant (financial support):
  - ▶ Eligibility: young adults (21 to 39) who have completed cancer treatment or are currently in remission
  - ▶ Process to Apply: online application completed by survivor

The Sibling Support Project

https://www.siblingsupport.org/

Description: Organization dedicated to supporting siblings of individuals with special health, developmental and mental health concerns

Resources Provide:

- ◆ SibShops (in-person support group):
  - ▶ Eligibility: differs by location but usually siblings (8 to 13) of children with developmental concerns
  - ▶ Process to Apply: see website for SibShops in your area

Stupid Cancer

http://www.stupidcancer.org

Description: organization created to empower and connect young adult cancer patients and survivors

Resources Provided:

- ◆ OMG! Cancer Summit for Young Adults (annual event):
  - ▶ Eligibility: young adult (21 to 39) cancer patients, survivors, caregivers, or advocates
  - ▶ Process to Apply: register online to attend

Supplemental Security Income (SSI)

https://www.ssa.gov/ssi/

Description: Government program that provides financial assistance to disabled children whose families demonstrate financial need

Resources Provided:

- ◆ Financial Assistance (variety of expenses):
  - ▶ Eligibility: children (under 18) displaying financial need who have a medical condition that results in severe functional

limitations for at least twelve consecutive months or who have been given a terminal diagnosis
  ▶ Process to Apply: application completed by parent and medical personnel

Take a Swing at Cancer

http://www.takeaswing.org/
Description: Nonprofit organization dedicated to helping families deal with the financial burden of cancer

Resources Provided:

♦ Financial Assistance (variety of expenses):
  ▶ Eligibility: children (under 21) in the New England area who are actively receiving treatment for pediatric cancer
  ▶ Process to Apply: application completed by parent

True North Treks

http://www.truenorthtreks.org/
Description: Organization dedicated to providing teen and young-adult cancer survivors with canoeing and backpacking experiences along with other young cancer survivors

Resources Provided:

♦ True North Treks (weeklong retreats):
  ▶ Eligibility: young adults (18 to 39) who have survived cancer
  ▶ Process to Apply: application completed by participant

The Ulman Cancer Fund

http://ulmanfund.org/
Description: Foundation created to support young adults and their families during and after cancer diagnosis

Resources Provided:

♦ Patient Navigation (patient and family support):

▶ Eligibility: young adults (15 to 39) currently or previously diagnosed with cancer

▶ Process to Apply: call 1-410-964-0202 to receive services

♦ Scholarships ($2,500/yr):

▶ Eligibility: college student who was a young adult (15 to 39) during their own cancer treatment or the treatment of a parent or sibling

▶ Process to Apply: online application completed by student

Wiskott-Aldrich Foundation

http://www.wiskott.org/

Description: Foundation aiming to provide support and information to families touched by Wiskott-Aldrich syndrome

Resources Provided:

♦ For Pete's Sake Family Support Program (variety of expenses):

▶ Eligibility: children displaying financial need diagnosed with a rare disease

▶ Process to Apply: online application completed by parent

Women, Infants, and Children (WIC)

http://www.fns.usda.gov/wic/women-infants-and-children-wic

Description: Government program designed to support women, children, and infants' health and nutrition development

Resources Provided:

♦ Food Vouchers:

▶ Eligibility: children (under age 5) who are deemed to be at "nutritional risk"

▶ Process to Apply: set up an appointment at a local WIC office to determine eligibility

END-OF-LIFE AND BEREAVEMENT

American Childhood Cancer Organization (ACCO)

http://www.acco.org/

Description: Organization aimed to provide information and support to families dealing with pediatric cancer

Resources Provided:

+ Founding Hope Fund (personalized memorial funds):
  ▶ Eligibility: individuals who want to honor a child who has died from cancer by founding their own fund through ACCO
  ▶ Process to Apply: fill out information form online

Bereaved Parents of the USA

http://bereavedparentsusa.org/

Description: Organization dedicated to emotionally supporting bereaved families facing the death of a child

Resources Provided:

+ BP/USA National Gathering (annual event):
  ▶ Eligibility: family members, including siblings, of a child who has died
  ▶ Process to Apply: register online

Clayton Dabney Foundation for Kids

http://www.claytondabney.org/

Description: Organization dedicated to providing emotional and financial support to families facing the last stages of their child's terminal illness

Resources Provided:

+ Financial Assistance (up to $2,000):
  ▶ Eligibility: financially needy children (up to 21) facing the final stages of terminal pediatric cancer

> Process to Apply: online application completed by parent and medical professional

The Compassionate Friends

http://www.compassionatefriends.org/

Description: Organization created to providing emotional support to bereaved families

Resources Provided:

♦ TCF National Conference (annual event):
  > Eligibility: family members (grandparent, parent, sibling) of a child who has passed away
  > Process to Apply: call 1-877-969-0010 for information on attending

The InterNational Council for Infertility Information Dissemination (INCIID)

http://www.inciid.org/

Description: In addition to providing infertility resources (see page 343), the website also includes a shared section of the website (Memorial Gardens) to post a tribute for a child who has died.

MISS Foundation

http://missfoundation.org/

Description: Organization dedicated to providing counseling, advocacy, and education to bereaved families dealing with the loss of a child

Resources Provided:

♦ Selah Retreat (weekend retreat):
  > Eligibility: bereaved individuals suffering the loss of a loved one
  > Process to Apply: register online for an event

Okizu

http://okizu.org/

Description: Organization created to support families of children with pediatric cancer through different types of family programs

Resources Provided:

- Bereaved Family Camp (one-week camp):
  - Eligibility: immediate family members of a child who has passed away from cancer
  - Process to Apply: online application completed by parent
- Bereaved Teen Camp (one-week camp):
  - Eligibility: teens (13 or older) who have a sibling who has died from cancer
  - Process to Apply: online application completed by parent

. . . .

Online Support and Information Websites

All website information accessed via foundation websites between September 2016 and March 2017.

. . . .

ON TREATMENT AND SURVIVORSHIP

Alex's Lemonade Stand Foundation

http://www.alexslemonade.org/

Description: A childhood cancer foundation dedicated to researching potential cures for childhood cancer and offering financial and emotional support to families, including siblings.

Also Offers:

- Parent-to-Parent Network (online one-on-one support)
- Childhood Cancer Treatment Journal
- My Childhood Cancer Database (online survey)
- List of Camps for Siblings (by state)

American Cancer Society

http://www.cancer.org/

Description: Organization funding cancer research and providing information to cancer patients on cancer diagnoses, treatment options, financial aid, educational challenges, and current cancer research.

Also Offers:

- Cancer Survivors Network (online community support): https://csn.cancer.org/

American Childhood Cancer Organization (ACCO)

http://www.acco.org/

Description: Organization to support families dealing with pediatric cancer. Website provides extensive information on a variety of topics including pediatric cancer diagnoses, treatment options, lists of oncology treatment centers and comprehensive late effects clinics, current research, sibling issues, educational issues and advocacy. It provides referrals for patient navigation services, foundations, and camps as well as US Candlelighter affiliates. Call 1-855-858-2226.

Also Offers:

- Online peer-to-peer support
- Blog
- iCANcer (phone app)
- "Light Up the Holidays with Hope, National Childhood Cancer Awareness Tree," Childhood Cancer Awareness Event in Washington, DC, every December

American Psychological Oncology Society (APOS)

http://apos-society.org/

Description: Society created for psychosocial oncology professionals to share information and research in order to improve the lives of families affected by cancer.

Also Offers:

- Helpline (emotional support for parents): call 1-866-276-7443

American Society of Clinical Hypnosis (ASCH)

https://www.asch.net/

Description: Society created for health care and mental health care professionals who use clinical hypnosis. It provides information on hypnosis and finding doctors who are trained in hypnosis.

Association for Applied Psychophysiology & Biofeedback (AAPB)

http://www.aapb.org/

Description: Organization dedicated to providing information on applied psychophysiology and biofeedback to improve health and the quality of life for patients. It provides information on finding doctors who use biofeedback.

Association of Cancer Online Resources (ACOR)

http://www.acor.org/

Description: Website providing more than 100 online community support groups for cancer and related disorders that allow caregivers and patients to share useful information with one another.

Association of Pediatric Hematology Oncology Education Specialists (APHOES)

http://www.aphoes.wildapricot.org/

Description: Website managed by a group of medical and psychology professionals dedicated to addressing the educational needs of pediatric hematology and oncology patients. It provides information to educators and medical professionals on educational challenges faced by patients.

Be the Match Foundation

https://bethematch.org/

Description: Foundation that manages a bone marrow registry and provides support and information to individuals in need of a transplant; the website provides information on blood cancer diagnoses, transplant procedures, and identifying a donor.

Also Offers:

- ◆ Parent's Companion Program (parent support)
- ◆ Personal Stories

Blood & Marrow Transplant Information Network

http://www.bmtinfonet.org/

Description: Organization aimed to provide emotional support and information on transplant procedures and transplant center options to patients.

Also Offers:

+ Caring Connections Program (online community support for patients and families)

Canadian Cancer Society

http://www.cancer.ca/

Description: Canadian organization dedicated to improving the quality of life of cancer patients. The website provides detailed information on cancer diagnoses, treatment options, and prevention.

Also Offers:

+ Online Support (http://cancerconnection.ca/)
+ Informational Specialist Supports. Call 1-888-939-3333

CancerCare

http://cancercare.org/

Description: Organization aimed to provide support and information to cancer patients on diagnoses, current research, and helping children (patients and siblings) cope with cancer.

Also Offers:

+ Counseling services (phone or in person)
+ Support groups (online, via phone, in person)
+ Connect Education Workshops (webinars)

Cancer.Net

http://www.cancer.net/

Description: Website created by the American Society of Clinical Oncology to provide accessible information to cancer patients. It provides detailed information on a variety of topics including cancer diagnoses, navigating cancer care, coping with cancer, current research and advocacy.

Also Offers:

♦ List of camps for children and families

CancerSourceKids

http://www.cancersourcekids.com/

Description: Website created for children to learn more about cancer through easy-to-understand language and games. It also provides information for parents of children with pediatric cancer.

Also Offers:

♦ CancerVive Teacher's Guide

Cancer Support Community

http://www.cancersupportcommunity.org/

Description: Organization dedicated to providing support and information to individuals affected by cancer. It provides information on cancer diagnoses, living with cancer, current cancer research and advocacy.

Also Offers:

♦ Cancer Support Helpline: Call 1-888-793-9355
♦ Live Web Chats
♦ The Living Room (online community support)
♦ Group Loop (teen online support group)
♦ Frankly Speaking About Cancer (radio show): https://www.voiceamerica.com/show/965

Canteen

https://www.canteen.org.au/

Description: Australian organization aimed at supporting teens and young adults (12 to 25) who have been diagnosed with cancer by providing emotional support and accessible information on diagnoses, treatment options, and living with cancer.

Also Offers:

- ◆ CanTeen Community (teen online support group)
- ◆ CanTeen Counseling Services. Call: 1-800-835-932

Caregiver Action Network

http://caregiveraction.org/

Description: Organization dedicated to improve the quality of life of family caregivers. The website provides detailed information on a variety of topics related to caregiving including managing medicine, attending doctor's appointments, and managing emotional stress.

Also Offers:

- ◆ Family Caregiver Forum (online peer forum)

Caring Bridge

https://www.caringbridge.org

Description: Nonprofit dedicated to making individuals' health journeys easier and increasing compassion for individuals struggling with a medical diagnosis.

Also Offers:

- ◆ Caring Bridge (personal website)

Children's Brain Tumor Foundation

http://www.cbtf.org/

Description: Organization dedicated to supporting and providing information on brain tumor diagnoses, treatment options, and follow-up care to families who have a child with a brain or spinal cord tumor.

Also Offers:

- ◆ Social Worker Support (online or by phone)
- ◆ Jenna's Corner Online Community (online support)
- ◆ Family to Family Network (peer support)

Children's Cancer Association

http://joyrx.org/

Description: Organization provides an extremely through online resource list for families facing all phases of the treatment process including disease-specific resources, aid and assistance, family resources, child/teen resources, and support for end of life.

Children's Cause for Cancer Advocacy

http://www.childrenscause.org/

Description: National advocacy organization dedicated to improving access to healthier treatment options and to enhancing families' abilities to cope with pediatric cancer diagnoses. It provides information to families on how to become advocates for pediatric cancer research.

Children's Oncology Group

https://childrensoncologygroup.org/

Description: COG is the largest pediatric research group in the world, made up of more than two hundred hospitals. It funds pediatric cancer research and provides extensive information on many topics related to pediatric cancer including diagnoses, treatment options and clinical trials.

Also Offers:

+ Survivorship Guidelines (http://www.survivorshipguidelines .org/)
+ COG Family Handbook
+ A Treatment Summary Template for Survivors
+ Risk-Based Clinical Practice Guidelines
+ Health Links (http://www.survivorshipguidelines.org /pdf/COG_LTFU_Guidelines_AppendixII_v4.pdf)
+ Reducing Risk of Second Cancers

Chronic Granulomatous Disease Association

http://www.cgdassociation.org/

Description: Nonprofit dedicated to helping individuals with chronic granulomatous disease (CGD) by providing information on diagnosis, treatment options, and current clinical trials.

CureSearch

http://curesearch.org/

Description: Nonprofit dedicated to improving cures for childhood cancer by funding innovative research. It also provides information for parents on pediatric cancer including diagnoses, current research, coping with cancer, and understanding the cancer treatment process.

Also Offers:

+ Legacy or Champion Funds (personal funds)
+ Personal Stories
+ Blog

Fanconi Anemia Research Fund

http://fanconi.org/

Description: Organization designated to researching Fanconi anemia and providing information to families about Fanconi anemia diagnosis, current Fanconi anemia research, treatment options, and testing centers.

Also Offers:

+ Online support groups
+ Annual publication (FA Courier & FA Family Newsletter)

FinAid

http://www.finaid.org/scholarships/

Description: Organization dedicated to providing information about financial aid and scholarship to students. It specifically provides a detailed list of scholarship for cancer survivors (http://www.fastweb .com/college-scholarships/articles/cancer-scholarships).

Hope Portal

http://searchhope.chla.org/

Description: online resource created by Children's Hospital of Los Angeles to make searching for cancer information easier for parents, patients, siblings, and health care professionals. It provides detailed resource lists for specific populations.

IDF SCID Initiative

http://primaryimmune.org/
Description: Branch of the IDF website that focuses on supporting families affected by severe combined immune deficiency (SCID).

Also Offers:

+ IDF SCID Newborn Screening Campaign
+ IDF SCID Newborn Screening Toolkit
+ National and Regional Programming
+ Online Support Group

Immune Deficiency Foundation (IDF)

http://primaryimmune.org/
Description: Organization aimed at improving the quality of life for individuals with primary immune deficiency disorders (PI). It provides information on PI disorders, treatment options, PI testing centers, and living with a PI disorder.

Also Offers:

+ Peer Support Program
+ IDF Friends (online support community for adult family members)
+ IDF Common Ground (online support community for teens)
+ Primary Immune Tribune and IDF Advocate (monthly newsletters)
+ IDF Reel Stories (personal stories)

Inner Kids

http://www.susankaisergreenland.com/inner-kids-1/
Description: Website dedicated to providing information on teaching children about mindfulness. It has songs, games, and downloadable resources for children's use.

The InterNational Council for Infertility Information Dissemination (INCIID)

http://www.inciid.org/

Description: Organization aimed at providing information and support to individuals and families exploring family-building options due to infertility.

Also Offers:

- Community Forums (online support)
- Newsletter

Jeffrey Modell Foundation

http://www.info4pi.org/

Description: Nonprofit dedicated to increasing awareness and treatment options for primary immunodeficiency disorders. It also provides information on primary immunodeficiency (PI) disorder diagnosis, PI screening, PI disorder symptoms, and current PI research.

Also Offers:

- Public service announcement videos
- Vicki's Voice (blog)

LD Online

http://www.ldonline.org/

Description: Website dedicated to providing information to parents of children with learning disabilities or ADHD. It provides information on LD or ADHD diagnoses, school-based support options, and tips to supporting a child with LD or ADHD.

Also Offers:

- Kids' Voices (personal stories and artwork)
- LD OnLine Newsletter (monthly)
- Discussion boards (online support)

Leukemia and Lymphoma Society (LLS)

http://www.lls.org/
Description: Organization aimed at funding research and improving access to treatment for blood cancers. It also provides information on blood cancer diagnoses, treatment options, follow-up care, current clinical trials, and advocacy.

Also Offers:

♦ Information Specialists Support (call 1-800-955-4572 or chat live online)

♦ LLS Community (online community support)

♦ Education videos and webcasts

Living with CGD

http://www.livingwithcgd.org/
Description: Website created by the Immune Deficiency Foundation to support and provide information to families on CGD diagnosis and treatment options.

LiveStrong Foundation

https://www.livestrong.org/
Description: Organization that aims to support and provide information to individuals diagnosed with cancer. It provides information on treatment and survivorship through the LiveStrong Guidebook and Planner and brochures. It also provides information on current cancer research in the LiveStrong Research Library.

Also Offers:

♦ LiveStrong Care Plan (follow-up care online program)

♦ LiveStrong Rally (phone app for people interested in following an individual's cancer journey)

♦ LiveStrong at School (tools for educators)

Look Good Feel Better for Teens

http://lookgoodfeelbetter.org/programs/teens
Description: Organization dedicated to improving teenage girls' self-image and appearance throughout their cancer treatment. It provides beauty tips and instructional videos.

Macmillan Cancer Support

http://www.macmillan.org.uk/
Description: Organization based in the UK that provides extremely detailed information about various types of pediatric cancer. It also provides information on the treatment process, treatment options, and the emotional effects of pediatric cancer on the family.

My LifeLine

http://www.mylifeline.org/
Description: Organization that helps cancer patients and caregivers create personalized websites to share information on their cancer journey.

National Bone Marrow Transplant Link (NBMT Link)

http://www.nbmtlink.org/
Description: Organization aimed at providing emotional support and information to bone marrow and stem cell transplant recipients and their families from diagnosis to survivorship.

Also Offers:

- ◆ Peer Support On-Call Program (1-800-546-5268)
- ◆ Books and publications

National Brain Tumor Society

http://braintumor.org/
Description: Organization created to fund research to find a cure and better treatment options for individuals with a brain tumor. It provides information on brain tumor research, diagnoses, treatment options, and advocacy.

National Cancer Institute (NCI)

https://www.cancer.gov/types/childhood-cancers
Description: Government agency run by the NIH that is responsible for cancer research and training. The website provides information on pediatric cancer including diagnoses, treatment options, treatment centers, coping with cancer, and survivorship.

National Center for Complementary and Integrative Health (NCCIH)

https://nccih.nih.gov
Description: Government agency associated with the NIH that researches complementary and integrative health approaches for many types of diseases. The website provides information on current complementary and integrative health approaches and discusses products, practices, and research.

National Center for Learning Disabilities

www.ncld.org/
Description: Organization dedicated to improving quality of life for children diagnosed with learning or attention difficulties. It also provides information on current learning disabilities research and advocacy.

Also Offers:

- ◆ Friends of Quinn (website for young adults with LD)
- ◆ Understood (parent website)

National Children's Cancer Society (NCCS)

https://thenccs.org/#
Description: Organization that provides support and information to families of children with pediatric cancer and pediatric cancer survivors. NCCS provides information on many topics including survivorship (Beyond the Cure), long-term follow-up care, emotional issues, caregiver role, fertility issues, and health insurance.

Also Offers:

- ◆ Late Effects After Treatment Tool (customized assessment): http://leatt.thenccs.org/

♦ Long-Term Follow-Up Clinics (listed by state): https://thenccs.org/long-term-clinics

National Coalition for Cancer Survivorship

http://www.canceradvocacy.org/

Description: Organization that advocates for cancer patients and survivors in order to provide greater quality of care and quality of life. It also provides information on public policy initiatives and cancer advocacy including health insurance and employment rights.

Office of Cancer Complementary and Alternative Medicine (OCCAM)

https://cam.cancer.gov/

Description: Government agency dedicated to improving the quality of care for all cancer patients by conducting research on complementary and alternative medicine (CAM) and sharing this information with patients.

Parent's Guide to Cord Blood Foundation

https://parentsguidecordblood.org

Description: Foundation dedicated to educating parents about the potential medical uses for cord blood as well as cord blood storage options. The website includes a detailed table of private cord blood banks which includes their location, fees, and current number of released cord blood units.

Path International

http://www.pathintl.org/

Description: Nonprofit dedicated to improving lives of children with special needs by providing access to horse-related activities and therapies. The website provides a list of Path centers in different areas of the country.

Patient Advocate Foundation

http://www.patientadvocate.org/

Description: Foundation dedicated to protecting patients by serving as a liaison in order to ensure access to care, maintenance of employment, and financial stability.

Also Offers:

- ◆ Webinars
- ◆ My Resource Search (phone app providing health care, financial, and insurance help)
- ◆ Coverage Access Guide (insurance guide)

Patient Services, Inc.

http://www.patientservicesinc.org/

Description: Nonprofit that helps chronically ill patients afford expensive medical expenses. It also provides information on varying medical diagnoses, insurance issues, and legal support.

Pediatric Brain Tumor Foundation

http://www.curethekids.org/

Description: Foundation that funds pediatric brain tumor research and provides assistance to families with a child diagnosed with a pediatric brain tumor. It also provides information on current pediatric brain tumor research, pediatric brain tumor diagnoses, pediatric brain tumor treatment options, and fund-raising opportunities.

Also Offers:

- ◆ Family Support Learning Series (video interviews with brain tumor experts)
- ◆ Starfolio (booklet for newly diagnosed patients and families)

Ped-Onc Resource Center

http://www.ped-onc.org/

Description: Website dedicated to support and provide information to families with children with cancer about treatment, survivorship, and advocacy.

Also Offers:

- ◆ Support groups (www.acor.org/)
- ◆ Resource lists for children and teens dealing with cancer

- List of scholarship opportunities (http://ped-onc.org/scholarships/)
- List of camps by state (http://ped-onc.org/cfissues/camps.html)

SCID Angels for Life

http://www.scidangelsforlife.com/

Description: Organization that funds SCID research and provides information to families affected by SCID on diagnosis, newborn screening, and current clinical trials.

The Sibling Support Project

https://www.siblingsupport.org/

Description: Organization dedicated to supporting siblings of individuals with special health, developmental. and mental health concerns.

Also Offers:

- Online support groups (by age)
- Books for siblings

Sickle Cell Information Center

https://scholarblogs.emory.edu/scinfo/

Description: Website designated to providing information and support to patients with sickle cell anemia regarding diagnosis and current research efforts.

Also Offers:

- Individual stories
- Newsletter (monthly)

Society for Cognitive Rehabilitation

http://www.societyforcognitiverehab.org/

Description: Organization created to increase the use of cognitive rehabilitation therapy. The website provides information on cognitive rehabilitation therapy practices and how to find a CRT therapist.

StupidCancer

http://stupidcancer.org/

Description: Organization created to empower and connect young adult cancer patients and survivors. It also provides extensive information on topics relevant to young adult cancer patients and survivors including finances, fertility, employment, and emotional support.

Also Offers:

- ◆ Online community forums
- ◆ Regional meetings
- ◆ Podcast ("The Stupid Cancer Show") and blog
- ◆ Events (CancerCon, Cancer Summit, Cancer Road Trip)

T.H.E. BRAIN TRUST

http://www.braintrust.org/

Description: Nonprofit dedicated to providing emotional support to cancer patients and their families through online support groups including groups for parents of children with brain tumor and related conditions.

The Samfund

http://www.thesamfund.org/

Description: Foundation that provides financial support to young adults diagnosed with cancer. It also provides extensive information on topics important to young adult cancer patients and survivors including fertility, finances, caregiver support, and advocacy.

Also Offers:

- ◆ Webinars

13Thirty Cancer Connect

http://13thirty.org/

Description: Organization dedicated to providing emotional support and information to adolescents and young adults affected by cancer. It provides information on cancer diagnoses, undergoing treatment, coping emotionally, and interacting with others.

Vital Options International

http://www.vitaloptions.org/
Description: Nonprofit focused on increasing cancer conversations between researchers, survivors, medical professionals, and advocates.

Also Offers:

+ The Group Room (videos)
+ Advocacy in Action (interviews on key cancer issues)
+ Vital Conversations (interviews on cancer research and cancer care)
+ Living With Cancer (interviews on cancer diagnosis, treatment, and survivorship)

Wiskott-Aldrich Foundation

http://www.wiskott.org/
Description: Foundation aiming to provide support and information to families touched by Wiskott-Aldrich syndrome (WAS). It provides information on WAS diagnosis, treatment options, and current clinical trials.

Also Offers:

+ Discussion Forum (online support)

World Cancer Research Fund International

http://www.wcrf.org/
Description: Organization dedicated to funding cancer prevention research related to nutrition, physical activity, and diet on cancer and cancer survival. It provides information on current scientific research, prevention recommendations, and policy initiatives.

Youth Cancer Services

http://www.youthcancer.com.au/
Description: Service provider network supported by CanTeen and the Australian government aimed at providing age-appropriate treatment and emotional support for teens and young adults (15 to 25) diagnosed with cancer.

....

END-OF-LIFE AND BEREAVEMENT

American Childhood Cancer Organization (ACCO)

http://www.acco.org/

Description: Organization aimed to providing support and information on bereavement to families dealing with pediatric cancer.

BabySteps Children's Fund

http://babysteps.com/

Description: Nonprofit dedicated to supporting families facing the death of a child. It provides information on facing grief, as well as resource lists for bereaved families, including support for siblings and grandparents.

Also Offers:

- ♦ Bereavement Sharing Rooms (forums for children, adults, and professional caregivers)
- ♦ Remembrance Rooms (personalized memorials)

Bereaved Parents of the USA

http://bereavedparentsusa.org/

Description: Organization dedicated to emotionally supporting bereaved families facing the death of a child. It provides informational brochures in English and Spanish around common bereavement topics.

Also Offers:

- ♦ Regional support group meetings
- ♦ *A Journey Together* (online quarterly newsletter)

CancerCare

http://cancercare.org/

Description: Organization aimed to provide support and information to cancer patients on diagnoses, current research, and helping children (patients and siblings) cope with cancer. It also provides information for bereaved families.

Also Offers:

- Counseling services (phone or in person)
- Support groups (online, via phone, in person)
- Connect Education Workshops (webinars)

Centering Corporation & *Grief Digest* Magazine

https://centering.org/
Description: Organization created to provide support and information for bereaved families.

Children's Hospice International

http://www.chionline.org/
Description: Organization dedicated to improving access to hospice and palliative care to terminally ill children. It provides information on hospice care for children and includes personal stories from families.

The Compassionate Friends

http://www.compassionatefriends.org/
Description: Organization created to providing emotional support to bereaved families.

Also Offers:

- Online community forums
- Regional meetings
- *We Need Not Walk Alone* (biannual magazine)
- *Open to Hope* (weekly radio show)

CureSearch

http://curesearch.org/
Description: Nonprofit dedicated to improving cures for childhood cancer by funding innovative research. It also provides information on end-of-life care and grief for families.

The Dougy Center

http://www.dougy.org/

Description: Organization dedicated to emotionally supporting bereaved individuals.

Also Offers:

- Regional support groups (Dougy Center–trained) for children, young adults, and adults
- Podcast ("Dear Dougy Podcast")
- Books & DVDs (bereavement materials)

GriefNet

http://www.griefnet.org/

Description: Website designed to provide online support and information to bereaved individuals.

Also Offers:

- Online support group
- KIDSAID (online support group for children)

Grief Recovery Method

https://www.griefrecoverymethod.com

Description: Branch of the Grief Recovery Institute dedicated to emotionally supporting bereaved individuals.

Also Offers:

- Books on Bereavement
- Workshops (two-day, in person)
- Grief Support Groups (regional, in person)

GriefSong

https://www.griefsong.com

Description: Collection of songs created by Paul Alexander to help families cope with the death of a loved one through music.

MISS Foundation

http://missfoundation.org/
Description: Organization dedicated to providing counseling, advocacy, and education to bereaved families dealing with the death of a child. It provides information on grief topics including funerals, therapy services, coping methods, and supporting children during the grief process.

Also Offers:

- Compassionate Bereavement Care Providers (searchable tool to find regional counselors)
- HOPE Mentor (one-on-one peer support)
- Regional support groups (monthly)
- Online Discussion Forums (support groups)

Rainbows for All Children

https://rainbows.org/
Description: Organization dedicated to providing support for children as they navigate the grief process. It provides educators and families with curriculum and materials to purchase for children in the bereavement process.

Notes

CHAPTER 1

1   Wendy Pelletier and Kira Bona, "Assessment of Financial Burden as a Standard of Care in Pediatric Oncology." *Pediatric Blood & Cancer* 62, no. s5 (2015): S620.

2   Eleni Petridou, Theodoros N. Sergentanis, Christina Perlepe, Paraskevi Papathoma, Gerasimos Tsilimidos, Evangelina Kontogeorgi, Maria Kourti et al., "Socioeconomic Disparities in Survival from Childhood Leukemia in the United States and Globally: A Meta-analysis." *Annals of Oncology* 26, no. 3 (2015): 596.

CHAPTER 2

1   Children's Oncology Group (COG), http://www.childrensoncologygroup.org.

CHAPTER 4

1   Lori Wiener, Haven Battles, Cynthia Mamalian, and Sima Zadeh, "Shop-Talk: A Pilot Study of the Feasibility and Utility of a Therapeutic Board Game for Youth Living with Cancer." *Supportive Care in Cancer* 19, no. 7 (2011): 1050. Therapists who are interested in obtaining a copy of the game should contact Dr. Lori Wiener at weinerl@mail.nih.gov.

2   AA = Aplastic Anemia.

CHAPTER 5

1   Bregje A. Houtzager, Martha A. Grootenhuis, Huib N. Caron, and Bob F. Last, "Quality of Life and Psychological Adaptation in Siblings of Pediatric Cancer Patients, 2 Years After Diagnosis." *Psycho-Oncology* 13, no.8 (2004): 506.

2 Robin F. Kramer, "Living With Childhood Cancer: Impact on the Healthy Sibling." *Oncology Nursing Forum* 11, no. 1 (1984), 44–51.

3 "Internalizing" symptoms refer to behaviors that indicate withdrawal, depression, or anxiety; "externalizing" symptoms refer to behaviors like acting out, aggression, or violence.

4 Ignace P.R. Vermaes, Anna M.J. van Susante, and Hedwig J.A. van Bakel, "Psychological Functioning of Siblings in Families of Children with Chronic Health Conditions: A Meta-Analysis." *Journal of Pediatric Psychology* 37, no. 2 (2011): 172.

5 Bregje A. Houtzager, Frans J. Oort, Josette EHM Hoekstra-Weebers, Huib N. Caron, Martha A. Grootenhuis, and Bob F. Last, "Coping and Family Functioning Predict Longitudinal Psychological Adaptation of Siblings of Childhood Cancer Patients." *Journal of Pediatric Psychology* 29, no. 8 (2004): 600.

6 www.alexslemonade.org/campaign/supersibs.

7 "Sibling Voices," YouTube video, 13:26, posted by "DanaFarberCHBSibsProgram," August 2011, https://www.youtube.com/watch?v=c4mqXYm0yfc.

8 Designed by Dr. Joshua Wootton, who was a psychologist at DFCI.

9 https://www.cc.nih.gov/ccc/patient_education/pepubs/siblings_workbook.pdf.

10 Visit Alex's Lemonade Stand Foundation to learn more about SuperSibs!: https://www.alexslemonade.org/campaign/supersibs-sibling-support -childhood-cancer-familiesslemonade.org/supersibs.

CHAPTER 7

1 Rachael Coakley, *When Your Child Hurts: Effective Strategies to Increase Comfort, Reduce Stress, and Break the Cycle of Chronic Pain* (New Haven, CT: Yale University Press, 2016).

2 Eric T. Boie, Gregory P. Moore, Chad Brummett, and David R. Nelson, "Do Parents Want to be Present During Invasive Procedures Performed on Their Children in the Emergency Department? A Survey of 400 Parents." *Annals of Emergency Medicine* 34, no. 1 (1999): 72.

3 Scott W. Powers, "Empirically Supported Treatments in Pediatric Psychology: Procedure-Related Pain." *Journal of Pediatric Psychology* 24, no. 2 (1999): 136.

4 Paul B. Jacobsen, Sharon L. Manne, Kenneth Gorfinkle, Ora Schorr, Bruce Rapkin, and William H. Redd, "Analysis of Child and Parent Behavior During Painful Medical Procedures." *Health Psychology* 9, no. 5 (1990): 572.

CHAPTER 8

1 Lisa Roberts, *Breathe, Chill: A Handy Book of Games and Techniques Introducing Breathing, Meditation and Relaxation to Kids and Teens* (CreateSpace Independent Publishing Platform, 2014). You can look through the book and pick out scripts and ideas that appeal to you.

2 Coakley, *When Your Child Hurts*, 151.

3 Some useful websites: www.anxietybc.com/adults/how-to-do-progressive -muscle-relaxation, www.the-guided-meditation-site.com/progressive -muscle-relaxation-script-html, www.the-guided-meditation-site.com /rapid-relaxation-script.html.

4 The Comfort Ability: https://www.thecomfortability.com/.

5 Scripts for younger children are available at: http://hprc-online.org /family-relationships/families/managing-emotions/progressive -muscle-relaxation-for-younger-children-pdf. Additional scripts are designed for slightly older children: https://www.anxietybc.com/parenting/how -do-progressive-muscle-relaxation.

6 Coakley, *When Your Child Hurts*, 151.

7 See: http://www.the-guided-meditation-site.com/passive-relaxation-script .html.

8 Coakley, *When Your Child Hurts*, 151–53.

CHAPTER 9

1 Duck-rabbit (*Kaninchen und Ente*), illustration from *Fliegende Blatter,* vol. 97, no. 2465, October 23, 1982.

CHAPTER 10

1 Mary Jane Ott, "Imagine the Possibilities! Guided Imagery with Toddlers and Pre-schoolers." *Pediatric Nursing* 22, no. 1 (1996): 34–35.

2 *No Fears, No Tears,* directed by Leora Kuttner (Boston: Fanlight Productions, 1986), DVD. One of the many techniques shown in this excellent video is a parent taking his hospitalized daughter on an imaginary journey to Candy Land.

3 Daniel P. Kohen and Karen Olness, *Hypnosis and Hypnotherapy with Children* (New York: Guilford Press, 1996): 204–8.

4 Gary R. Elkins and Bryan D. Carter, "Use of a Science Fiction–Based Imagery Technique in Child Hypnosis." *American Journal of Clinical Hypnosis* 23, no. 4 (1981), 274–77.

5 Nancy Klein, *Healing Images for Children: Teaching Relaxation and Guided Imagery to Children Facing Cancer and Other Serious Illnesses* (Watertown, WI: Inner Coaching, 2001), 135–41.

6   CHOC Children's Hospital has free guided-imagery exercises for pain management, anxiety, general relaxation, progressive muscle relaxation, and sleep done by psychologists available online: http://www.choc.org/programs-services/integrative-health/guided-imagery/.

7   Several organizations offer training in hypnosis and will have lists of certified professionals. Their websites describe the history, use, and possible purposes of hypnosis with children.
National Pediatric Hypnosis Training Institute: www.nphti.net
Society of Developmental and Behavioral Pediatrics: www.sdbp.org
International Society of Hypnosis: www.ishhypnosis.org
American Society of Clinical Hypnosis: www.asch.net
The Milton H. Erickson Foundation: www.erickson-foundation.org

8   Daniel P. Kohen and Pamela Kaiser. "Clinical Hypnosis with Children and Adolescents—What? Why? How?: Origins, Applications, and Efficacy." *Children* 1, no. 2 (2014): 74–98.

9   Kohen and Olness, *Hypnosis*, 99–319.

10   Josephine R. Hilgard and Samuel LeBaron, *Hypnotherapy of Pain in Children with Cancer* (Los Altos, CA: Kaufmann, 1984).

CHAPTER 11

1   *No Fears, No Tears: 13 Years Later*, directed by Leora Kuttner (2000; Vancouver, BC: Crown House Publishing, 2010), DVD. This remarkable video includes interviews with the children who starred in the earlier video, *No Fears, No Tears*, and shows how they used the techniques they learned in different, mainly positive ways in the intervening thirteen years.

CHAPTER 12

1   Barbara A. Cromer and Kenneth J. Tarnowski, "Noncompliance in Adolescents: A Review." *Journal of Developmental & Behavioral Pediatrics* 10, no. 4 (1989): 208–9.

2   *Medicine and Your Child: A Guide for Parents on Adherence and Administration* (National Cancer Institute, 2011). This booklet can be downloaded for free at https://ccr.cancer.gov/Pediatric-Oncology-Branch/psychosocial/education.

3   This is very difficult for a parent to know, but in some instances may be shown by a blood test or other tests like a urine sample.

CHAPTER 13

1   Karen K. Ballen, Juliet N. Barker, Susan K. Stewart, Michael F. Greene, and Thomas A. Lane, "Collection and Preservation of Cord Blood for

Personal Use." *Biology of Blood and Marrow Transplantation* 14, no. 3 (2008): 358.

2 See p. 35.

3 See p. 34.

4 Additional possible late effects on organs, fertility, growth, and mobility, and other health complications, are discussed in chapter 17 in the Survivorship section.

5 Victoria W. Willard, Wing Leung, Qinlei Huang, Hui Zhang, and Sean Phipps, "Cognitive Outcome After Pediatric Stem-Cell Transplantation: Impact of Age and Total-Body Irradiation." *Journal of Clinical Oncology* 32, no. 35 (2014): 3984–85.

6 Susan K. Parsons, Sean Phipps, Lillian Sung, K. Scott Baker, Michael A. Pulsipher, and Kirsten K. Ness, "NCI, NHLBI/PBMTC First International Conference on Late Effects after Pediatric Hematopoietic Cell Transplantation: Health-Related Quality of Life, Functional, and Neurocognitive Outcomes." *Biology of Blood and Marrow Transplantation* 18, no. 2 (2012): 164.

7 See the appendixes. For example, the Blood & Marrow Transplant Information Network: http://www.bmtinfonet.org/.

8 See the "For Patients and Families" section on https://bethematch.org/.

CHAPTER 14

1 Sue P. Heiney and Sheldon Lamphier, *The Gift: For Children Who Are Bone Marrow Donors* (Columbia, SC: Palmetto Health South Carolina Cancer Center, 2004).

CHAPTER 15

1 Susan K. Stewart, *Autologous Stem Cell Transplants: A Handbook for Patients* (Highland Park, IL: Blood and Marrow Transplant Information Network, 1999), 72.

2 See pages 170–171.

CHAPTER 16

1 See Appendix A, Resources from Foundations, Organizations, or Government Agencies—On Treatment and Survivorship—and Appendix B, Online Support and Information Websites—On Treatment and Survivorship.

2 Anne Kazak et al., "Posttraumatic Stress Symptoms During Treatment in Parents of Children with Cancer." *Journal of Clinical Oncology* 23, no. 30 (2005): 7405.

CHAPTER 17

1   Siobhan M. Phillips et al., "Survivors of Childhood Cancer in the United States: Prevalence and Burden of Morbidity." *Cancer Epidemiology, Biomarkers & Prevention* 24, no. 4 (2015): 656.

2   The multi-institutional Childhood Cancer Survivor Study (CCSS), supported by the National Cancer Institute (NCI), is the largest of these survivor groups. It includes more than 20,000 five-year survivors treated for various cancers between 1970 and 1986 and some of their siblings as a comparison group . A group of approximately 15,000 survivors treated between 1987 and 1999 and some siblings have been recruited for further study. Many of the studies about childhood cancer survivorship comes from follow-up with subsets of the first group.

3   Children's Oncology Group (COG), http://www.childrensoncologygroup .org; Scottish Intercollegiate Guidelines Network (SIGN), http://www .sign.ac.uk/; United Kingdom Childhood Cancer Study (UKCCS), http:// www.ukccs.org/.

4   David G. Tubergen et al., "Prevention of CNS Disease in Intermediate-Risk Acute Lymphoblastic Leukemia: Comparison of Cranial Radiation and Intrathecal Methotrexate and the Importance of Systemic Therapy: A Children's Cancer Group Report." *Journal of Clinical Oncology* 11, no. 3 (1993): 524.

5   Jacqueline Casillas et al., "Identifying Predictors of Longitudinal Decline in the Level of Medical Care Received by Adult Survivors of Childhood Cancer: A Report from the Childhood Cancer Survivor Study." *Health Services Research* 50, no. 4 (2015): 1036.

6   The National Children's Cancer Society provides existing follow-up clinics listed by state: https://www.thenccs.org/long-term-clinics.

7   Your clinic's recommendations for your child's medical follow-up will likely be based on the most current information available as indicated in the Children's Oncology Group (COG) Guidelines. You can also check the COG website, which has materials that have been prepared specially for parents of childhood cancer survivors. The materials are called Health Links. They cover various topics, and you can download any material that could be relevant to your child's care (http://www.survivorshipguidelines .org/).

8   Ibid.

9   Janette McDougall and Miranda Tsonis, "Quality of Life in Survivors of Childhood Cancer: A Systematic Review of the Literature (2001–2008)." *Supportive Care in Cancer* 17, no. 10 (2009): 1243.

10   Judith A. Punyko et al., "Physical Impairment and Social Adaptation in Adult Survivors of Childhood and Adolescent Rhabdomyosarcoma: A Report from the Childhood Cancer Survivors Study." *Psycho-Oncology* 16, no. 1 (2007): 28.

11 Theresa B. Haddy, Revonda B. Mosher, and Gregory H. Reaman, "Late Effects in Long-term Survivors After Treatment for Childhood Acute Leukemia." *Clinical Pediatrics* 48, no. 6 (2009): 606.

12 Marilyn A. Crawshaw and Patricia Sloper, "'Swimming Against the Tide'—The Influence of Fertility Matters on the Transition to Adulthood or Survivorship Following Adolescent Cancer." *European Journal of Cancer Care* 19, no. 5 (2010): 616–17.

13 Brad J. Zebrack, Sallie Foley, Daniela Wittmann, and Marcia Leonard. "Sexual Functioning in Young Adult Survivors of Childhood Cancer." *Psycho-Oncology* 19, no. 8 (2010): 817–19.

14 Sean Phipps, "Psychosocial Issues for Transplant Patients and Donors," in *Pediatric Psycho-Oncology: A Quick Reference on the Psychosocial Dimensions of Cancer Symptom Management,* eds. Lori S. Wiener et al. (New York: Oxford University Press, 2015), 152–53.

15 Nancy Keene, ed., *Educating the Child with Cancer: A Guide for Parents and Teachers* (Kensington, MD: Candlelighters Childhood Cancer Foundation, 2003), 83–90, 215–22.

16 Keene, *Educating the Child,* 101–8.

17 The Association of Pediatric Hematology Oncology Educational Specialists (Stony Brook, NY: Searles Graphics; 2011); http://www.aphoes.org/.

18 See Appendix A. Special Education Advocacy, http://www.specialeducation advocacy.org/.

19 Council of Parent Attorneys and Advocates; www.copaa.org/?page =guidelinesadv.

20 Robert W. Butler et al., "A Multicenter Randomized Clinical Trial of a Cognitive Remediation Program for Childhood Survivors of a Pediatric Malignancy." *Journal of Consulting and Clinical Psychology* 76, no. 3: 376.

21 Widely used computer-based cognitive remediation programs include www.lumosity.org, www.cogmed.com, and www.braintrain.com.

22 Brian P. Daly and Ronald T. Brown, "Cognitive Sequelae of Cancer Treatment," in *Pediatric Psycho-Oncology: A Quick Reference on the Psychosocial Dimensions of Cancer Symptom Management,* eds. Lori S. Wiener et al. (New York: Oxford University Press, 2015), 170, 172–73.

23 Heather M. Conklin et al., "Long-Term Efficacy of Methylphenidates in Enhancing Attention Regulation, Social Skills, and Academic Abilities of Childhood Cancer Survivors." *Journal of Clinical Oncology* 28, no. 29 (2010): 4468.

24 Daly and Brown, "Cognitive Sequelae," 173.

25 Robert B. Noll et al., "Social, Emotional, and Behavioral Functioning of Children with Cancer." *Pediatrics* 103, no. 1 (1999): 73–74.

26 Kathryn Vannatta et al., "A Controlled Study of Peer Relationships of Children Surviving Brain Tumors: Teacher, Peer, and Self-Ratings." *Journal of Pediatric Psychology* 23, no. 5 (1998): 284.

27 Lisa A. Schwartz, Julia Rowland, and Aziza Shad, "Pediatric Cancer Survivors: Moving Beyond Cure," in *Pediatric Psycho-Oncology: A Quick*

Reference on the Psychosocial Dimensions of Cancer Symptom Management, eds. Lori S. Wiener et al. (New York: Oxford University Press, 2015), 362.

28   It remains to be seen how this will be affected by any new health care legislation.

....

CHAPTER 18

1   Lonnie K. Zeltzer et al., "Psychosocial Outcomes and Health-related Quality of Life in Adult Childhood Cancer Survivors: A Report from the Childhood Cancer Survivor Study." *Cancer Epidemiology Biomarkers & Prevention* 17, no. 2 (2008): 444.

2   *No Fears, No Tears: 13 Years Later,* directed by Leora Kuttner (2000; Vancouver, BC: Crown House Publishing, 2010), DVD.

3   Kazak et al., "Posttraumatic Stress Symptoms," 7405.

4   Bregje A. Houtzager, Frans J. Oort, Josette EHM Hoekstra-Weebers, Huib N. Caron, Martha A. Grootenhuis, and Bob F. Last, "Coping and Family Functioning Predict Longitudinal Psychological Adaptation of Siblings of Childhood Cancer Patients." *Journal of Pediatric Psychology* 29, no. 8 (2004): 600–2.

....

CHAPTER 19

1   Karen Emmons et al., "Predictors of Smoking Initiation and Cessation Among Childhood Cancer Survivors: A Report from the Childhood Cancer Survivor Study." *Journal of Clinical Oncology* 20, no. 6 (2002): 1610.

2   Anne E. Lown et al., "Alcohol Consumption Patterns and Risk Factors Among Childhood Cancer Survivors Compared to Siblings and General Population Peers." *Addiction* 103, no. 7 (2008): 1144.

....

CHAPTER 20

1   Graham J. Reid, M. Jane Irvine, Brian W. McCrindle, Renee Sananes, Paul G. Ritvo, Samuel C. Siu, and Gary D. Webb, "Prevalence and Correlates of Successful Transfer from Pediatric to Adult Health Care Among a Cohort of Young Adults with Complex Congenital Heart Defects." *Pediatrics* 113, no. 3 (2004): e200.

2   Paul C. Nathan, Mark L. Greenberg, Kirsten K. Ness, Melissa M. Hudson, Ann C. Mertens, Martin C. Mahoney, James G. Gurney et al., "Medical Care in Long-Term Survivors of Childhood Cancer: A Report from the Childhood Cancer Survivor Study." *Journal of Clinical Oncology* 26, no. 27 (2008): 4406.

3   Craig Sable, Elyse Foster, Karen Uzark, Katherine Bjornsen, Mary M. Canobbio, Heidi M. Connolly, Thomas P. Graham et al., "Best Practices in Managing Transition to Adulthood for Adolescents with Congenital Heart Disease: The Transition Process and Medical and Psychosocial Issues." *Circulation* 123, no. 123 (2011): 1477.

4   Long-Term Follow-Up Guidelines (COG Guidelines) at the Children's Oncology Group website: http://www.survivorshipguidelines.org.

5   Eugene Suh, Christopher K. Daugherty, Kristen Wroblewski, Hannah Lee, Mackenzie L. Kigin, Kenneth A. Rasinski, Jennifer S. Ford et al., "General Internists' Preferences and Knowledge About the Care of Adult Survivors of Childhood Cancer: A Cross-Sectional Survey." *Annals of Internal Medicine* 160, no. 1 (2014): 16.

6   Susan M. Fernandes, Joanne O'Sullivan-Oliveira, Michael J. Landzberg, Paul Khairy, Patrice Melvin, Gregory S. Sawicki, Sonja Ziniel et al., "Transition and Transfer of Adolescents and Young Adults with Pediatric Onset Chronic Disease: The Patient and Parent Perspective." *Journal of Pediatric Rehabilitation Medicine* 7, no. 1 (2014): 50. Children's conditions included in the study are cancer, Type 1 diabetes, congenital heart disease, juvenile rheumatoid arthritis, hematologic disease, inflammatory bowel disease, cystic fibrosis, solid organ transplant, genetic disorders, and renal disease requiring dialysis.

7   Natasha N. Frederick, Sharon L. Bober, Lexie Berwick, Mary Tower, and Lisa B. Kenney, "Preparing Childhood Cancer Survivors for Transition to Adult Care: The Young Adult Perspective." *Pediatric Blood & Cancer* 64, no. 10 (2017): e26549.

8   Tziona Lugasi, Marie Achille, and Moire Stevenson, "Patients' Perspective on Factors That Facilitate Transition from Child-Centered to Adult-Centered Health Care: A Theory Integrated Metasummary of Quantitative and Qualitative Studies." *Journal of Adolescent Health* 48, no. 5 (2011): 438.

9   Nina S. Kadan-Lottick, Leslie L. Robison, James G. Gurney, Joseph P. Neglia, Yutaka Yasui, Robert Hayashi, Melissa Hudson, Mark Greenberg, and Ann C. Mertens, "Childhood Cancer Survivors' Knowledge About Their Past Diagnosis and Treatment: Childhood Cancer Survivor Study." *JAMA* 287, no. 14 (2002): 1839.

10 Fernandes et al., "Transition and Transfer," 46.

11 Richard S. Lazarus, "The Costs and Benefits of Denial," in *Fifty Years of the Research and Theory of R. S. Lazarus: An Analysis of Historical and Perennial Issues* (Mahwah, NJ: Lawrence Erlbaum Associates, 1997), 247.

12 Lugasi et al., "Patients' Perspective," 437–39.

CHAPTER 21

1   Joanne Wolfe, Neil Klar, Holcombe E. Grier, Janet Duncan, Susanne Salem-Schatz, Ezekiel J. Emanuel, and Jane C. Weeks, "Understanding

of Prognosis Among Parents of Children Who Died of Cancer: Impact on Treatment Goals and Integration of Palliative Care." *JAMA* 284, no. 19 (2000): 2473.

2   Jeffrey P. Burns, Jeffrey Edwards, Judith Johnson, Ned H. Cassem, and Robert D. Truog, "Do-not-resuscitate Order After 25 Years." *Critical Care Medicine* 31, no. 5 (2003): 1545.

3   Mary E. Lauer, Raymond K. Mulhern, Jelena B. Bohne, and Bruce M. Camitta, "Children's Perceptions of Their Sibling's Death at Home or Hospital: The Precursors of Differential Adjustment." *Cancer Nursing* 8, no. 1 (1985): 26–27.

4   Jennifer Giovanola, "Sibling Involvement at the End of Life." *Journal of Pediatric Oncology Nursing* 22, no. 4 (2005): 224–25.

....

CHAPTER 22

1   There have been striking shifts over time in how doctors in the Western world have talked with parents and their children about prognosis. In the Victorian era, child mortality was widespread and there was little effort to protect children from the knowledge of their imminent death— indeed, repentance, prayer, and absolution might require explicit acknowledgment. In the first half of the twentieth century, with the gradual improvement in medical skill and subsequent decline in child mortality in the Western world, along with greater emphasis on protecting the child, children were rarely told of their terminal prognosis. Then the hospice movement began and a famous study conducted by Vernik and Marion (1965) in a leukemia ward showed that many young children did know they were dying and felt alone and scared. Since then, a gradual trend for more open communication is evident worldwide—but still many cultures and ethnic groups including within the United States, have different beliefs, values, and practices that may affect what doctors believe should be disclosed and what families want disclosed to adults, let alone to children.

2   Giuseppe Masera, John J. Spinetta, Momcilo Jankovic, Arthur R. Ablin, Giulio J. D'Angio, Jeanette Van Dongen-Melman, Tim Eden et al., "Guidelines for Assistance to Terminally Ill Children with Cancer: A Report of the SIOP Working Committee on Psychosocial Issues in Pediatric Oncology." *Medical and Pediatric Oncology* 32, no. 1 (1999): 46.

3   Shana Jacobs, Jennie Perez, Yao Iris Cheng, Anne Sill, Jichuan Wang and Maureen E. Lyon, "Adolescent End of Life Preferences and Congruence with Their Parents' Preferences: Results of a Survey of Adolescents with Cancer." *Pediatric Blood & Cancer* 62, no. 4 (2015): 713.

4   Bryan A. Sisk, Myra Bluebond-Langner, Lori Wiener, Jennifer Mack, and Joanne Wolfe, "Prognostic Disclosures to Children: A Historical Perspective." *Pediatrics* 138, no. 3 (2016): 5.

5   Dan Schaefer and Christine Lyons, *How Do We Tell the Children?: A Step-by-Step Guide for Helping Children and Teens Cope When Someone Dies*, 4th ed. (New York: Newmarket Press, 2011), 11–25.

6   Ibid., 16–20.

7   Earl A. Grollman, "Explaining Death to Children." *Journal of School Health* 47, no. 6 (1977): 337–39.

8   Ulrika Kreicbergs, Unnur Valdimarsdóttir, Erik Onelöv, Jan-Inge Henter, and Gunnar Steineck, "Talking About Death with Children Who Have Severe Malignant Disease." *New England Journal of Medicine* 351, no. 12 (2004): 1184.

9   Ivana M.M van der Geest, Marry M. van den Heuvel-Eibrink, Liesbeth M. van Vliet, Saskia M.F. Pluijm, Isabelle C. Streng, Erna M.C. Michiels, Rob Pieters et al., "Talking About Death with Children with Incurable Cancer: Perspectives from Parents." *Journal of Pediatrics* 167, no. 6 (2015): 1325.

10 Lori Wiener, Sima Zadeh, Haven Battles, Kristin Baird, Elizabeth Ballard, and Janet Osherow, "Allowing Adolescents and Young Adults to Plan Their End-of-life Care." *Pediatrics* 130, no.5 (2012): 903. The book may be purchased from Aging with Dignity (https://agingwithdignity .org/).

11 "My Wishes" can be purchased from Aging with Dignity (https://agingwith dignity.org/).

....

CHAPTER 23

1   Mary Sormanti and Judith August, "Parental Bereavement: Spiritual Connections with Deceased Children." *American Journal of Orthopsychiatry* 67, no. 3 (1997): 460.

2   Reiko Schwab, "A Child's Death and Divorce: Dispelling the Myth." *Death Studies* 22, no. 5 (1998): 460, 462.

3   Henk Schut and Margaret S. Stroebe, "Interventions to Enhance Adaptation to Bereavement." *Journal of Palliative Medicine* 8, no. 1 supplement (2005): s-146.

4   For example, Therese A. Rando, *Treatment of Complicated Mourning* (Champaign, IL: Research Press, 1993).

5   Malin Lövgren, Tove Bylund-Grenklo, Li Jalmsell, Alexandra Eilegård Wallin, and Ulrika Kreicbergs, "Bereaved Siblings' Advice to Health Care Professionals Working with Children with Cancer and Their Families." *Journal of Pediatric Oncology Nursing* 33, no. 4 (2016): 302–4.

6   Mary-Elizabeth Bradley Eilertsen, Alexandra Eilegård, Gunnar Steineck, Tommy Nyberg and Ulrika Kreicbergs, "Impact of Social Support on Bereaved Siblings' Anxiety A Nationwide Follow-Up." *Journal of Pediatric Oncology Nursing* 30, no. 6 (2013): 306–8.

7   Joseph M. Currier, Jason M. Holland, and Robert A. Neimeyer. "The Effectiveness of Bereavement Interventions with Children: A Meta-analytic Review of Controlled Outcome Research." *Journal of Clinical Child and Adolescent Psychology* 36, no. 2 (2007): 257.

8   Jeanna A. Schaefer and Rudolf H. Moos, "The Context for Posttraumatic Growth" in *Posttraumatic Growth: Positive Changes in the Aftermath of Crisis,* ed. Richard G. Tedeschi, Crystal L. Park, and Lawrence G. Calhoun (Mahwah, NJ: Lawrence Erlbaum Associates, 1998): 105.

9   Linda P. Riley, Lynda L. LaMontagne, Joseph T. Hepworth, and Barbara A. Murphy, "Parental Grief Responses and Personal Growth Following the Death of a Child." *Death Studies* 31, no. 4 (2007): 277–99.

Bibliography for Parents

Note: All books are available from Amazon.com, new or used, unless otherwise noted.

FOR PARENTS WITH CHILDREN IN TREATMENT

Allen, Jeffrey S., and Roger J. Klein. *Ready, Set, Relax: A Research-Based Program of Relaxation, Learning and Self-esteem for Children*. Watertown, WI: Inner Coaching, 1996. This book provides scripts and exercises to help children relax and manage anxiety. This book could serve as a tool for both parents and clinicians to use with children experiencing stress of any kind.

Bluebond-Langner, Myra. *In the Shadow of Illness: Parents and Siblings of the Chronically Ill Child*. Princeton, NJ: Princeton University Press, 2000. An anthropologist considers the impact of having a child with cystic fibrosis on well siblings and their parents through the close observation of nine families. Available from Princeton University Press at http://press.princeton.edu/.

Bombeck, Erma. *I Want to Grow Hair, I Want to Grow Up, I Want to Go to Boise: Children Surviving Cancer*. New York: Harper & Row, 1989. Erma Bombeck's uplifting and funny book about children fighting and surviving cancer is based on conversations she had with children with cancer and feedback they gave her about what she should write. The humor and the spirit of these children as well as her own empathy and admiration for them is clear. Used copies are available from Amazon.

Bracken, Jeanne Munn. *Children with Cancer: A Comprehensive Reference Guide for Parents*. New York: Oxford University Press, 2010. Written in 1986, updated in 2010, the current edition provides information on different types of childhood cancer, the range of treatments available, and ways to cope with the challenges of treatment. It also includes a list of domestic and international clinics and organizations.

Brown, Ronald T., ed. *Comprehensive Handbook of Childhood Cancer and Sickle Cell Disease: A Biopsychosocial Approach*. New York: Oxford

University Press, 2006. This book is written for researchers and professionals in the fields of pediatric cancer and sickle cell disease. It stresses how research findings should be incorporated into clinical practice. However, parents may find particular chapters to be of interest depending on their child's specific medical situation.

Clark, Lynn. *SOS Help for Parents: A Practical Guide for Handling Common Everyday Behavior Problems*. Bowling Green, KY: SOS Programs & Parents Press, 2014. A very useful, clearly written book that provides commonsense suggestions such as time-out, "reflective listening," and "beating the timer" for managing children's challenging behaviors. This book may have helpful hints for parents who have found disciplining their sick child challenging.

Coakley, Rachael. *When Your Child Hurts: Effective Strategies to Increase Comfort, Reduce Stress, and Break the Cycle of Chronic Pain*. New Haven, CT: Yale University Press, 2016. This excellent book, written by a clinical pediatric psychologist, is for parents of children experiencing chronic pain. The book provides effective strategies and research-based practices for reversing the cycle of chronic pain and returning to more normal daily functioning.

Janes-Hodder, Honna, and Nancy Keene. *Childhood Cancer: A Parent's Guide to Solid Tumor Cancers*, 2nd ed. Sebastopol, CA: O'Reilly Media Inc., 2002. First printed in 1999, this updated edition describes the different types of solid tumor cancers and the treatments given for them. It covers emotional challenges and coping strategies for the child and the family as well as other useful topics including identifying available resources.

Hoffman, Ruth, and Sandra E. Smith, eds. *A Parent's Guide to Enhancing Quality of Life in Children with Cancer*. American Childhood Cancer Organization, 2014. Focusing on pediatric palliative care as a means to provide symptom relief and emotional support for any life-threatening illness, this book has chapters written by multidisciplinary experts intended to improve the quality of life for a child with cancer.

Keene, Nancy. *Childhood Leukemia: A Guide for Families, Friends & Caregivers*. Bellingham, WA: Childhood Cancer Guides, 2010. First printed in 1997, this fourth edition provides comprehensive information about childhood leukemia—including diagnosis and treatment, emotional challenges, school and external resources, some survivorship issues, and dealing with treatment failure.

Keene, Nancy. *Your Child in the Hospital: A Practical Guide for Parents*, 3rd ed. Bellingham, WA: Childhood Cancer Guides. First printed in 1997, the third edition (2015) offers useful and wise tips for any parent whose young child has to go to the hospital.

Klein, Nancy C. *Healing Images for Children: Teaching Relaxation and Guided Imagery to Children Facing Cancer and Other Serious Illnesses.* Watertown, WI: Inner Coaching, 2001. The book has guided imagery and relaxation scripts to help sick children and their parents manage typical stressful encounters they may have in the medical world. It includes a useful bibliography for children suffering from various childhood illnesses.

Roberts, Lisa. *Breathe, Chill: A Handy Book of Games and Techniques Introducing Breathing, Meditation and Relaxation to Kids and Teens.* Create Space Independent Publishing Platform, 2014. Written by a registered children's yoga teacher who works with sick children, this book provides simple exercises and activities for children to relax and meditate. This book can help children manage hospitalization, stress, anxiety, and pain.

Shiminski-Maher, Tania, Catherine Woodman, and Nancy Keene. *Childhood Brain & Spinal Cord Tumors: A Guide for Families, Friends & Caregivers,* 2nd ed. Bellingham, WA: Childhood Cancer Guides, 2014. First printed in 2001, this updated edition informs parents about brain and spinal cord tumors and the symptoms, treatments, and side effects that may accompany the diagnosis. It covers sources of support, family issues, and other important topics related to brain and spinal cord tumors.

Stewart, Susan K.. *Autologous Stem Cell Transplants: A Handbook for Patients.* Highland Park, IL: Blood and Marrow Transplant Information Network, 2000. This is a very useful short book written for patients and parents whose child requires an autologous stem cell transplant. Much of the book is addressed to parents and addresses topics such as infections, pain relief, nutrition, and caregiving after the transplant.

Webb, Nancy Boyd. *Play Therapy with Children and Adolescents in Crisis: Fourth Edition.* New York: Guilford Press, 2015. This book illustrates the positive uses of play therapy with children and adolescents in crisis. One section describes working with children going through different medical challenges and how play therapy can be invaluable.

Wiener, L., M. Pao, A. Kazak, et al., eds. *Pediatric Psycho-Oncology: A Quick Reference on the Psychosocial Dimensions of Cancer Symptom Management.* New York: Oxford University Press, 2015. This paperback is designed to be a basic reference for multidisciplinary caregivers on the psychosocial issues relevant to children who get cancer and their families. Authors are from a range of disciplines in the medical field. Parents could find the succinct summaries of current practice illuminating.

Woznick, Leigh A., and Carol D. Goodheart. *Living with Childhood Cancer: A Practical Guide to Help Families Cope.* Washington, DC: American Psychological Association, 2010. Written by the mother and grandmother of a child with cancer, this book provides parents and families with a thorough guide for what to expect and how to cope throughout their child's treatment. The book includes personal stories from more than one hundred families who were interviewed for the book, providing a personal touch. There is also an extensive resource list.

FOR PARENTS WITH CHILDREN WHO ARE SURVIVORS

Goldman, Stewart, and Christopher D. Turner, eds. *Late Effects of Treatment for Brain Tumors.* New York: Springer, 2009. This book describes the range of late effects that brain tumor survivors can experience. Each chapter details late effects by organ type and provides up-to-date information on the newest treatments and technologies designed to deal with these effects. While the book is primarily written for medical personnel, parents may also find particular chapters relevant to what their child is currently experiencing or could experience later.

Grinyer, Anne. *Life After Cancer in Adolescence and Young Adulthood: The Experience of Survivorship.* New York: Routledge, 2009. This book focuses not only on physical late effects for childhood cancer survivors but also on potential emotional, social, and psychological effects. By using case studies and interviews with pediatric cancer survivors, this book blends the personal experience of survivorship with the scientific literature in the field.

Keene, Nancy, Wendy Hobbie, and Kathy Ruccione. *Childhood Cancer Survivors: A Practical Guide to Your Future.* Los Angeles: Childhood Cancer Guides, 2012. This book speaks directly to childhood cancer survivors and their parents. It discusses the varied survivorship journey and the different needs of different survivors at different times. It describes how to navigate the system in regards to educational, insurance, and disability needs and offers comprehensive information on possible late effects and how to manage them. It modulates potentially distressing information with personal, often uplifting, stories from more than one hundred cancer survivors, woven into the text.

Mucci, Grace A., and Lilibeth R. Torno. *Handbook of Long Term Care of the Childhood Cancer Survivor* (Specialty Topics in Pediatric Neuropsychology series). New York: Springer, 2015. This book is a fund of information on all aspects of childhood cancer survivorship. It is written for caregivers and gives a clear rationale and framework for appropriate follow-up care of childhood cancer survivors. It could also be a valuable resource for parents wanting to research particular topics such as neuropsychological late effects and how to manage them.

Schwartz, Cindy, Wendy Hobbie, Louis Constine, and Kathleen Ruccione, eds. *Survivors of Childhood and Adolescent Cancer: A Multidisciplinary Approach*. New York: Springer, 2005. This book provides comprehensive information on the long-term consequences of cancer therapy on survivors' health and well-being. The book details how different organ systems could be affected and offers a detailed guide to appropriate follow-up assessment and care. Parents may want to check how their child's follow-up medical care matches with what is recommended.

Wallace, Hamish, and Daniel Green, eds. *Late Effects of Childhood Cancer*. London: Arnold Publications, 2004. This book provides a comprehensive review of the late effects that survivors of pediatric cancer can face. Fertility and treatment-related effects on typical development are some of the topics discussed that could be of particular interest to many parents and patients.

Woodruff, Teresa K. and Karrie A. Snyder, eds. *Oncofertility: Fertility Preservation for Cancer Survivors*. New York: Springer, 2007. This book examines fertility options for cancer patients. The book has a few specific chapters about fertility preservation in children and adolescent cancer patients that may be of interest to parents and adolescents.

FOR PARENTS WHOSE CHILD HAS DIED

Davies, Betty. *Shadows in the Sun: The Experiences of Sibling Bereavement in Childhood*. Philadelphia: Brunner/Mazel, 1999. A sensitive and beautifully written book that describes the powerful impact that a sibling's death has during childhood and across the lifespan.

Doka, Kenneth J. and Nancy Boyd Webb. *Helping Bereaved Children: A Handbook for Practitioners*. New York: Guilford Press, 2011. A well-written and thoughtful book describing how skilled clinicians can help children of all ages cope with loss through a variety of therapeutic interventions. One chapter is devoted exclusively to coping with the death of a sibling, and parents could find it helpful to read.

Grollman, Earl A., ed. *Bereaved Children and Teens: A Support Guide for Parents and Professionals*. Boston: Beacon Press, 1996. A book with chapters by people who have worked with bereaved children over many years. It covers different ways to help grieving children, including how to effectively communicate and how to incorporate different religious perspectives.

Grollman, Earl A. *Living When a Loved One Has Died*. Boston: Beacon Press, 1995. A wonderful book, written by a grief counselor who is also a rabbi, that shares nuggets of advice for anyone facing a loved one's death. It elaborates on the themes that "grief is universal and at the same time extremely personal," and that you will "heal in your own way."

Emswiler, Mary Ann, and James P. Emswiler. *Guiding Your Child Through Grief*. New York: Bantam Books, 2000. A very helpful book written by professionals who have considerable personal experience working with grieving children. The book discusses the many ways in which a child can express grief and provides advice on how parents can help their child and themselves over time. An appendix also provides useful tips for teachers and other professionals.

Finkbeiner, Ann K. *After the Death of a Child: Living with the Loss Through the Years*. New York: Simon & Schuster, 2012. A book written by a bereaved parent describing the various ways in which life changes after the loss of a child based on her conversations with many other bereaved parents. The book movingly and compassionately describes the different paths parents can take over time and the impact these decisions have on a parent's perspective about life.

Mehren, Elizabeth. *After the Darkest Hour the Sun Will Shine Again: A Parent's Guide to Coping with the Loss of a Child*. New York: Simon & Schuster, 1997. A bereaved mother offers an understanding perspective and inspiration by telling her own story and the stories of other bereaved parents both today and historically. She describes different paths that have brought some parents comfort over time.

Rosof, Barbara D. *The Worst Loss: How Families Heal from the Death of a Child*. New York: Henry Holt & Company, 1995. A sensitive account of how the death of a child shatters the presumptions on which we operate, and how we can slowly rebuild our lives.

Rothman, Juliet Cassuto. *The Bereaved Parents' Survival Guide*. New York: Continuum International Publishing Group, 1997. An insightful, compassionate, and practical book written by a bereaved parent who has worked in the area of grief counseling for many years. The book transmits the message that there is light at the end of a very dark tunnel. However, contrary to the findings of more recent studies, it overestimates the number of parents who divorce after the death of their child.

Schaefer, Dan. *How Do We Tell the Children?: A Step-by-Step Guide for Helping Children and Teens Cope When Someone Dies.* New York: Newmarket Press, 2010. An empathetic book that gives practical advice about what to say and do in order to help children of any age who have lost someone they love.

Schiff, Harriet Sarnoff. *The Bereaved Parent.* New York: Penguin Books, 1978. A moving and helpful book written by a bereaved mother that gives practical and reassuring advice to bereaved parents.

Silverman, Phyllis R. *Never Too Young to Know: Death in Children's Lives.* New York: Oxford University Press, 2000. A book that uses stories from children and bereaved families as well as grief research to explore how death affects children and how to help them cope over time.

Children's Book List

Note: All books are available from Amazon.com, new or used, unless noted otherwise.

TREATMENT AND SURVIVORSHIP

Preschool to Early Elementary

Some books suitable for preschool children are included in the "Books for Children with Chronic Illnesses and Conditions" (113 titles listed).
http://www.goodreads.com/list/show/8536.Books_for_Children _with_Chronic_Illness

A detailed list of books on a variety of illnesses and conditions including ADHD, AIDS, allergies, asthma, autism spectrum disorder, bipolar disorder, Crohn's disease, cystic fibrosis, diabetes, lupus, migraines, multiple sclerosis, and rheumatoid arthritis.

Bourgeis, Paulette. *Franklin Goes to the Hospital.* Tonawanda, NY: Kids Can Press, 2000.

Ages 3 to 6

After suffering a cracked shell, Franklin must go to the hospital for surgery and stay overnight. Even though Franklin is afraid, he tries to be brave. This book is a good resource for parents who need to prepare a young child for a stay in a hospital.

Calloway, Jill Trotta. *There's An Elephant in My Room . . . : A Child's Unforgettable Journey Through Cancer Proved Hope Was Stronger Than Fear.* Bloomington, IN: Author House, 2010.

Ages 4 to 8

A book written by the parent of a classmate of a young girl with cancer. This book suggest the importance of positive values, like hope and determination, gleaned from watching a young child with cancer get through her treatment.

Cocca-Leffler, Maryann. *Bravery Soup*. Morton Grove, IL: Albert Whitman & Company, 2002.

Ages 3 to 7

A picture book that tells the story of Carlin the raccoon as he faces his fears and gains courage in order to help his friend.

Cole, Joanna, and Bruce Degen. *The Magic School Bus: Inside the Human Body*. New York: Scholastic, 1990.

Ages 5 to 10

This picture book takes the child on a trip through the human body in a fun, engaging way. The book explains the purpose of cells and describes the various systems in the body (e.g. digestive, circulatory and nervous).

Cole, Joanna, and Bruce Degen. *The Magic School Bus: Inside Ralphie, A Book About Germs*. New York: Scholastic, 1995.

Ages 5 to 10

This picture book takes a child on an adventure through the body of a sick child. Children learn about how germs can make a person sick and how our body works to keep us healthy.

Deland, M. Maitland. *The Great Katie Kate Tackles Questions about Cancer*. Austin, TX: Greenleaf Book Group.

Ages 4 to 8

A picture book written by a radiation oncologist to help young children understand their cancer diagnosis. It suggests how to deal with feelings of anxiety and worry that often accompany a cancer diagnosis in a playful and engaging way.

Drescher, Joan. *A Journey in the Moon Balloon: When Images Speak Louder Than Words*. London: Jessica Kingsley Publishers, 2015.

Ages 6 to 11

An interactive picture book that offers children ways to use their imagination and creative skills to manage difficult feelings. The new expanded edition provides additional resources for parents, teachers, and health professionals to help children cope emotionally with challenges.

Filigenzi, Courtney. *My Cancer Days*. American Cancer Society, 2015.

Ages 6 to 9

A picture book that describes the emotions a child with cancer may have during treatment. The story is told from the perspective of a young girl with cancer who uses colors to show the different emotions she feels.

Fisher, Jenevieve. *I'm a Kid Living with Cancer*. Carnation, WA: Isaiah 11:6 Publishing Company, 2010.

Ages 4 to 9

A picture book written by a cancer survivor who is now a radiation oncology therapist, it describes cancer and its treatment honestly and compassionately to children. The book offers detailed explanations about medical procedures like X-rays, CT scans, and MRIs. Also available in Spanish.

Gaynor, Kate. *The Famous Hat*. Dublin, Ireland: Special Stories Publishing, 2008.

Ages 4 to 8

A fictional story that describes how a young boy diagnosed with leukemia copes with his hair loss and cancer treatment.

Gosselin, Kim. *Taking Diabetes to School*. New York: JayJo Books, 2002.

Ages 4 to 9

A picture book, written by the mother of a child with type 1 diabetes, describing diabetes in simple terms. This book is designed to use in a classroom and explains the symptoms, causes, and treatment of diabetes to young children.

Gosselin, Kim. *Taking Seizure Disorders to School: A Story about Epilepsy*. New York: JayJo Books, 2002.

Ages 5 to 8

A picture book that describes epilepsy in simple terms and interesting pictures. This book can be used in classrooms to increase children's understanding of seizures and to reduce their anxiety when witnessing a seizure.

Hample, Stewart and Eric Marshall. *Children's Letters to God*. New York: Workman Publishing, 1991.

Ages 6 to 9

An enchanting book that contains letters written by children to God.

Mays, Lydia Criss and Barbara Meyers. *The Long and Short of It: A Tale About Hair*. Atlanta: American Cancer Society, 2010.

Ages 6 to 9

An endearing story about two girls with different hair challenges; one girl would like to grow her hair longer, while the other has recently lost her hair from cancer treatment and would like to have her hair back.

Piper, Watty. *The Little Engine That Could*. New York: Philomel Books, 2005.

Ages 3 to 7

A classic children's book that suggests to young readers the positive outcomes of determination, optimism, and hard work.

Saltzman, David. *The Jester Has Lost His Jingle*.

Ages 6 to 9

Written by a young adult who died of Hodgkin's disease, this story tells the tale of a jester who lives in a city that has lost its ability to laugh. After he visits a girl in a hospital ward and makes her laugh, laughter is released back into the world. This story reminds children that joy and laughter are inside of them, even in the worst of circumstances.

Middle Elementary

"Books for Children with Chronic Illnesses and Conditions" (113 titles listed). Some suitable for middle school children.

http://www.goodreads.com/list/show/8536.Books_for_Children
_with_Chronic_Illness

A detailed list of books on a variety of illnesses and conditions
including ADHD, AIDS, allergies, asthma, autism spectrum
disorder, bipolar disorder, Crohn's disease, cystic fibrosis, diabetes,
lupus, migraines, multiple sclerosis and rheumatoid arthritis.

Beth, Barbara. *My Life by Me: A Kid's Forever Book*. Washington, DC:
Magination Press, 2012.

Ages 8 to 12

An interactive book designed by a psychologist to help children
process questions, thoughts, and feelings provoked by a life-
threatening illness. The book also offers space for children to
document important moments and memories of their life.

Available through the American Psychological Association: http://
www.apa.org/pubs/

Crowe, Karen. *Me and My Marrow: A Kid's Guide to Bone Marrow Transplants*. Deerfield, IL: Fujisawa Healthcare, 1999.

Ages 6 to 14

An excellent resource that provides detailed, age-appropriate
explanations of the transplant process to children who are
preparing for a transplant themselves. The book includes tips
and advice from children and teenagers who have survived a
transplant, providing a personal element to the text.

Available for free at www.bridges4kids.org

Heiney, Sue P., and Sheldon Lamphier. *The Gift: For Children Who are
Bone Marrow Donors*. Columbia, SC: Palmetto Health South Carolina
Cancer Center, 2004.

Ages 6 to 14

A great resource written for child bone marrow donors and their
parents. The first half of the book includes a touching fable that
serves as a metaphor for the sibling's role as a donor and offers
interactive activities to complete before and after the stem cell
harvest. The second half of the book is designed for adult caregivers to understand the donor process and suggests ways to support
the child throughout this process.

Jampolsky, Gerald, *There Is a Rainbow Behind Every Dark Cloud*. Millbrae, California: Celestial Arts, 1978.

> Ages 8 to 12
>
> An interactive book, written and illustrated by children 8 to 19 years of age facing life-threatening illnesses, that provides additional space for the reader to draw or write about his or her own illness. The book is separated into two sections: the first section illustrating the children's personal experiences and the second section illustrating "things that can help."
>
> Available at the Center for Attitudinal Healing: http://www.healingcenter.org/

Keene, Nancy. *Chemo, Craziness and Comfort: My Book about Childhood Cancer.* Washington, DC: Candlelighters Foundation, 2002.

> Ages 6 to 12
>
> The book tells children and families what to expect during the treatment process, including physical and emotional effects. It also provides space following each chapter for children to write questions or draw pictures.
>
> Available at American Childhood Cancer Organization (ACCO): http://store.acco.org/collections/acco-books-and-information-resources

Polacco, Patricia. *The Lemonade Club*. New York: Philomel Books, 2007.

> Ages 7 to 11
>
> A story about a fifth-grade class who come together to support their classmate Marilyn, who has recently been diagnosed with leukemia.

Adolescence

Goldman Koss, Amy, *Side Effects*. New York: Square Fish, 2010.

> Ages 12 and up
>
> A story told with humor and poignancy from the perspective of a fifteen-year-old girl who gets cancer, endures the difficult treatment, survives, and then thrives.

Huegel, Kelly. *Young People and Chronic Illness: True Stories, Help, and Hope*. Minneapolis, MN: Free Spirit Publishing, Inc., 1998.

Ages 10 and up

This book describes the lives of ten children who are living with a chronic illness (e.g., Crohn's disease, hemophilia, diabetes, epilepsy, asthma, cancer, inflammatory bowel disease, juvenile rheumatoid arthritis, congenital heart defect, and lupus). The first half of the book explains each disease and includes an interview with each child; the second part of the book focuses on how each child manages his or her illness and copes with the different diseases.

Krementz, Jill. *How It Feels to Fight for Your Life*. New York: Little, Brown & Company, 1989.

Ages 10 to 14

Inspiring stories of fourteen children who are living with chronic illnesses including cancer, cystic fibrosis, severe burns, and other difficult conditions. The children share the challenges, uncertainties and pain sometimes caused by these illnesses; however, their positive spirit shines throughout.

Marchiano, Melinda. *Grace: A Child's Intimate Journey Through Cancer and Recovery*. San Luis Obispo, CA: Happy Quail Press, 2010

Ages 12 and up

A moving memoir written by a fourteen-year-old cancer survivor documenting her treatment journey in a humorous and honest way.

Sandison, Sierra. *Sugar Linings: Finding the Bright Side of Type 1 Diabetes*. Create Space Independent Publishing Platform, 2015.

Ages 12 and up

A memoir written by a young woman who became Miss Idaho despite being (or because of being) diagnosed with type 1 diabetes as an adolescent. She describes what it feels like physically and socially to have diabetes. The book describes her journey to improve her self-esteem and accept her diagnosis, and conveys the hopeful message that challenges can present unique opportunities.

Trillin, Alice. *Dear Bruno*. New York: The New Press, 1996.

Ages 10 to 14

A book that shares a letter written to a twelve-year-old boy diagnosed with cancer from a young woman who had recently survived lung cancer. The letter is written in a reassuring, frank, and matter-of-fact tone.

Available at The New Press: http://thenewpress.com/books

Wainwright, Tabitha. *You and an Illness in Your Family.* New York: Taylor & Francis, 2001

Ages 10 to 14

The book focuses on helping teenagers cope with stresses caused by illness in the family.

For Siblings

American Cancer Society, *Because . . . Someone I Love Has Cancer.* 2002.

Ages 6 to 12

A therapeutic activity book with crayons attached intended to support and encourage a child during the cancer treatment of a close family member.

Beall-Sullivan, Christina. *Hi, My Name Is Jack.* Park City, Utah: Bopar Books, 2000.

Ages 8 to 12

A children's book focused on the feelings experienced by the healthy sibling of a very ill child.

Bentrim, William. *What About Me? Well Children with Sick Siblings.* CreateSpace Independent Publishing Platform, 2010.

Ages 4 to 8

A book written for well children of a very ill sibling that acknowledges the feelings and emotions, including guilt, abandonment, and anger, that children may feel throughout their sibling's treatment.

Dodd, Michael. *Oliver's Story: For Sibs of Kids with Cancer.* American Childhood Cancer Organization, 2004.

Ages 3 to 8

A book written by a clinical psychologist that suggests ways children can cope with various emotions they may feel when a sibling is diagnosed with a serious illness.

Also available in Spanish.

Available at American Childhood Cancer Organization (ACCO): http://store.acco.org/collections/acco-books-and-information -resources

Heegaard, Marge. *When Someone Has a Very Serious Illness: Children Can Learn to Cope with Loss and Change.* Minneapolis, MN: Woodland Press, 1992.

Ages 5 to 12

A book written by a clinical social worker and art therapist that encourages children to draw as one way to cope with feelings about having a sibling with a serious illness.

Kelly, Emmett. *My Sister Got Cancer: A Workbook for Siblings of Cancer Patients.* CreateSpace Independent Publishing Platform, 2016.

Ages 9 to 12

This first part of the book is written from the perspective of a young boy whose younger sister is diagnosed with cancer. The second part has common questions siblings have and the third part gives brothers and sisters space to record their own experiences

The book can be printed and downloaded for free from: http://www.porf.org/connect/emmetts-story-and -workbook/.

Sonnenblick, Jordan. *Drums, Girls, and Dangerous Pie.* New York: Scholastic, 2010.

Ages 12 to 16

A touching, heartbreaking, and funny novel written from the perspective of a teenage boy whose life gets upended when his brother is diagnosed with a life-threatening illness.

Wozny, Sharon. *Jamie's Journey: Cancer from the Voice of a Sibling*. Chandler, AZ: Little Five Star, 2016.

> Ages 8 to 12
>
> The first half of this book describes the experience of a teenage girl, Jamie, when her younger brother gets cancer. Jamie finds keeping a journal helps her. The second half of the book offers space for the reader, presumably a teenager with a sick sibling, to write about his experiences.

GRIEF AND BEREAVEMENT

Preschool to Early Elementary

Brown, Laurie Kransy. *When Dinosaurs Die: A Guide to Understanding Death*. Boston: Little, Brown Books for Young Readers, 1996.

> Ages 5 to 10
>
> A picture book using dinosaur figures that factually and honestly describes the different emotions, causes, and rituals associated with death. The story also suggests ways in which children can remember those who have died.

Buscaglia, Leo. *The Fall of Freddie the Leaf*. Thorofare, NJ: Slack Incorporated, 1982.

> Ages 4 to 8
>
> A picture book that explains life and death through the life of a leaf named Freddie. Through his wise friend, Daniel, another leaf on the tree, Freddie learns that everyone has a unique purpose in life and that death is a natural part of living.

Hanson, Warren. *The Next Place*. Minneapolis, MN: Waldman House Press, 1997.

> Ages 5 to 10
>
> An exquisitely illustrated book that expresses a spiritual belief in the beauty and peace of "The Next Place" without any particular religious affiliation.

Heegaard, Marge. *When Someone Very Special Dies: Children Can Learn to Cope with Grief.* Minneapolis, MN: Woodland Press, 1996.

> Ages 4 to 7
>
> A picture book written by a clinical social worker and art therapist designed to teach about death in an accessible way for young children. It encourages children to understand and express the emotions they are feeling after a death through drawings or writing.

Jeffers, Oliver. *The Heart and the Bottle.* New York: Philomel Books, 2010.

> Ages 4 to 8
>
> A story about a young girl facing the death of someone she loves; she puts her heart in a bottle to avoid feeling pain but gradually learns to face her grief.

Johnson, Marvin, and Joy Johnson. *Where's Jess?* Omaha, NE: Centering Corporation, 1992.

> Ages 3 to 6
>
> A simply illustrated picture book ideal for young children who have had a very young sibling die.
>
> Available at The Centering Corporation: https://centering.org/.

Karst, Patrice. *The Invisible String.* Camarilla, CA: DeVorss & Co. Publications, 2000.

> Ages 4 to 8
>
> A touching book for children who have lost someone they love. The book reminds children of the "invisible string" representing the love between two people that exists even after someone has died.

Mellonie, Bryan. *Lifetimes: The Beautiful Way to Explain Death to Children.* Toronto: Bantam Books, 1983.

> Ages 4 to 8
>
> A book that explains death as a natural part of living by describing the life cycles of plants, animals, and people, which all have "a beginning, an ending, and living in between."

Mundy, Michaelene. *Sad Isn't Bad: A Good-Grief Guidebook for Kids Dealing with Loss.* St. Meinrad, IN: Abbey Press, 2006.

Ages 4 to 8

A book written by a school counselor that provides reassuring, positive advice to help children who have suffered a loss.

Schulz, Charles. *Why, Charlie Brown, Why? A Story About What Happens When a Friend Is Very Ill.* New York: Little Simon, 2002.

Ages 4 to 8

A book intended for children who have had a close friend die. The book tells the story of Janice, a girl with leukemia, and describes the various reactions of friends, classmates, and family members to her death.

Stickney, Doris. *Water Bugs and Dragonflies: Explaining Death to Young Children.* Cleveland, OH: Pilgrim Press, 1997.

Ages 4 to 8

A touching picture book written by the wife of a Christian minister that describes the tale of a water bug who transforms into a dragonfly. Once the water bug leaves the water to become a dragonfly, it can no longer return to its friends under the surface but still is content in its new beautiful home.

Thomas, Pat. *I Miss You: A First Look at Death.* Hauppauge, NY: Barron's Educational Series, 2000.

Ages 4 to 8

A picture book written by a psychotherapist and counselor which helps children understand that grief and loss are natural reactions following the death of a friend or family member. Includes questions for parents, teachers, or caregivers to ask children as they go through the book.

Varley, Susan. *Badger's Parting Gifts.* New York: Mulberry Books, 1992.

Ages 4 to 8

A story that movingly tells through an assorted animal cast how remembering and sharing the parting gifts of a dear friend can transform grief into comfort.

Wilhelm, Hans. *I'll Always Love You.* New York: Crown Publishers, 1985.

Ages 4 to 8

A picture book that describes the close relationship between a boy and his dog, Elfie. They grow up together but one day Elfie dies; after his death, the boy feels very sad but treasures his love for his dog.

Middle Grades

Bahr, Mary. *If Nathan Were Here*. Grand Rapids, MI: Wm B. Eerdmans Publishing Company, 2000.

Ages 8 to 12

This book describes a young boy's grief over the death of his best friend. Through the help of supportive adults and creating a memory box at school, the young boy is able to start addressing his friend's death.

Coerr, Eleanor. *Sadako and the Thousand Paper Cranes*. New York: Puffin, 2004.

Ages 8 to 12

A true story based on the life of Sadako, a Japanese girl, who was diagnosed with leukemia. Following a Japanese legend, Sadako tried to fold one thousand paper cranes to make her well again, and after she died, her friends completed the task for her.

Munday, Michaelene. *What Happens When Someone Dies?: A Child's Guide to Death and Funerals*. St. Meinrad, IN: Abbey Press.

Ages 6 to 10

A picture book written by a school counselor that answers basic questions young children often have after someone close has died and prepares them to go to a funeral.

Rugg, Sharon, et al. *Memories Live Forever: A Memory Book for Grieving Children*. Marietta, GA: Rising Sun Center for Loss and Renewal.

Ages 5 to 12

An interactive book that offers exercises for children to complete in order to remember a loved one who has died.

Available through the Centering Corporation: https://centering
.org/ in English and Spanish.

Adolescents

Earl, Esther, Lori Earl, and Wayne Earl. *This Star Won't Go Out: The Life
and Words of Esther Grace Earl*. London: Penguin UK, 2014.

Ages 13 and up

The moving story in Esther Earl's own words and in the words of
her family and friends of her journey through life, including
cancer treatment and her early death at the age of sixteen. The
book eloquently shares the gifts she left behind for those who
knew her through her unquenchable spirit.

Fitzgerald, Helen. *The Grieving Teen: A Guide for Teenagers and Their
Friends*. New York: Simon & Schuster, 2001.

Ages 13 and up

Written by a bereavement counselor, this book focuses on the
special needs of adolescents struggling with loss and offers wise
suggestions about ways to cope.

Gootman, Marilyn. *When a Friend Dies: A Book for Teens About Grieving
& Healing*. Minneapolis, MN: Free Spirit Publishing, 2005.

Ages 12 to 17

A book for teenagers coping with the loss of a friend, providing
advice and answers to questions from teenagers in a respectful,
compassionate manner.

Grollman, Earl. *Straight Talk About Death for Teenagers: How to Cope with
Losing Someone You Love*. Boston: Beacon Press, 1993.

Ages 12 to 17

An understanding and compassionate book written by a grief
counselor that raises topics and questions commonly asked by
teenagers following a loved one's death. The teenager can read the
whole book or focus on sections most relevant to him or her.

O'Toole, Donna R. *Facing Change: Falling Apart and Coming Together
Again in the Teen Years*. Compassion Books, 1995.

Ages 13 and up

A short book written for teenagers by a bereavement counselor about the process of grief including how to endure it, how to know you are slowly emerging from it, and how you can eventually grow from the experience.

Scrivani, Mark. *When Death Walks In*. Omaha, NE: Centering Corporation, 2005.

Ages 13 and up

A booklet from the Centering Corporation designed to help teenagers with their grief. Different feelings that can occur after someone's death are described and advice is given about going back to school and reconnecting with friends following a death.

Available from The Centering Corporation: https://centering.org/

Sims, Alicia. *Am I Still a Sister?* Louisville, KY: Carraro's Art-Print and Publishing Company, 1998.

Ages 8 to 14

A moving book that shares letters over many years that a thirteen-year-old girl, Alicia, wrote to her younger brother who died when she was four years old.

Traisman, Enid Samuel. *Fire in My Heart, Ice in My Veins: A Journal for Teenagers Experiencing a Loss*. Centering Corporation, 2002. PO Box 4600, Omaha, NE 68104.

Ages 13 and up

A journal designed by a bereavement counselor for grieving teenagers that provides them with a place to express their thoughts and feelings following the death of a loved one and suggests ways to help them remember that person. Each page has a one- or two-sentence prompt that they can expand on or just think about.

Available at the Centering Corporation: https://centering.org/

Index